OFFICE GYNECOLOGY

OFFICE GYNECOLOGY

Robert H. Glass, M.D.

**Associate Professor in Residence,
Department of Obstetrics and Gynecology,
University of California, San Francisco**

THE WILLIAMS & WILKINS COMPANY / BALTIMORE

Library of Congress Cataloging in Publication Data
Main entry under title:

Office gynecology.

  Bibliography:
  Includes index.
  1. Gynecology. I. Glass, Robert H. [DNLM: 1. Office management. 2. Gynecologic diseases.
WP100 G54901
RG103 034   618.1   76-4849
ISBN 0-683-03549-5

Composed and printed at the
Waverly Press, Inc.
Mt. Royal and Guilford Aves.
Baltimore, Md. 21202, U.S.A.

Preface

Practitioners involved in the health care of women spend the largest portion of their working hours in an office or clinic. Despite this, the focus of most journal articles and textbooks in gynecology is on hospital practice. Up to date information on office practice must be obtained in a fragmented fashion from throw-away journals or medical newspapers. The aim of this book is to present, in one volume, current information on a variety of issues vital to the office practice of gynecology. No attempt is made to be encyclopedic, but rather there is a conscious effort to concentrate on common problems.

The authors are all clinicians who have special areas of expertise. They consistently have met the editor's goal to provide complete, concise, and practical information. Even the most experienced gynecologist will find material here that will be useful to him or her in clinical practice, and the book provides a standard against which all practitioners can measure their information and their response to women. The book should be helpful not only to the gynecologist but also to all others involved in the health care of women—family practitioners, internists, residents, interns, medical students, nurse practitioners, and nurse midwives.

I am indebted to the contributors who have given of their time, interest, and knowledge.

ROBERT H. GLASS, M.D.
San Francisco, California

Authors

JAMES L. BREEN, M.D.
Director, Department of
Obstetrics and Gynecology
Saint Barnabas Medical Center
Clinical Professor
Obstetrics and Gynecology
Jefferson Medical College

PAUL F. BRENNER, M.D.
Assistant Professor
Obstetrics and Gynecology
University of Southern California
   School of Medicine

DALE BROWN, JR., M.D.
Clinical Instructor
Obstetrics and Gynecology
Baylor College of Medicine

MICHAEL J. DALY, M.D.
Professor and Chairman
Obstetrics and Gynecology
Temple University
   Health Sciences Center

CARL GEMZELL, M.D.
Professor
Obstetrics and Gynecology
State University of New York,
   Downstate Medical Center

ROBERT H. GLASS, M.D.
Associate Professor in Residence
Obstetrics and Gynecology
University of California,
   San Francisco

MITCHELL S. GOLBUS, M.D.
Assistant Professor
Obstetrics and Gynecology
University of California,
   San Francisco

SADJA BREWSTER GOLDSMITH,
   M.D., M.P.H.
Medical Research Director
Planned Parenthood
San Francisco-Alameda

EARL GREENWALD, M.D.
Assistant Professor
Obstetrics and Gynecology
Temple University
   Health Sciences Center

ARTHUR L. HERBST, M.D.
Joseph Bolivar DeLee
   Professor and Chairman
Obstetrics and Gynecology
   University of Chicago

ROBERT B. JAFFE, M.D.
Professor and Chairman
Obstetrics and Gynecology
University of California,
   San Francisco

VALERIE JORGENSEN, M.D.
Assistant Professor
Obstetrics and Gynecology
University of Pennsylvania

NATHAN G. KASE, M.D.
Professor and Chairman
Obstetrics and Gynecology
Yale University
   School of Medicine

RAYMOND H. KAUFMAN, M.D.
Professor and Ernest William Bertner
   Chairman
Obstetrics and Gynecology
Baylor College of Medicine

WILLIAM R. KEYE, JR., M.D.
Postdoctoral Fellow,
Reproductive Endocrinology
Obstetrics and Gynecology
University of California,
   San Francisco

WILLIAM J. LEDGER, M.D.
Professor
Obstetrics and Gynecology
University of Southern California
   School of Medicine

JAY MANN, PH.D.
Associate Director
Human Sexuality Program
University of California,
   San Francisco

ALAN J. MARGOLIS, M.D.
Professor
Obstetrics and Gynecology
University of California,
   San Francisco

DANIEL R. MISHELL, JR., M.D.
Professor and Associate Chairman
Obstetrics and Gynecology
University of Southern California
   School of Medicine

JOHN MCL. MORRIS, M.D.
John Slade Ely Professor of
   Gynecology
Yale University
   School of Medicine

STANLEY J. ROBBOY, M.D.
Assistant Professor
Pathology
Harvard Medical School

ROBERT E. SCULLY, M.D.
Professor
Pathology
Harvard Medical School

ANN K. SPENCE, M.D.,
Clinical Lecturer
Family Medicine
University of Western Ontario

LEON SPEROFF, M.D.
Associate Professor
Obstetrics and Gynecology
Yale University
   School of Medicine

DUANE E. TOWNSEND, M.D.
Professor
Obstetrics and Gynecology
University of Southern California
   School of Medicine

Contents

1

PELVIC INFECTION AND VENEREAL DISEASE

WILLIAM J. LEDGER, M.D.

INTRODUCTION

Pelvic infection from sexually transmitted microorganisms represents the most important infectious disease problem facing the gynecologist in his office practice in the 1970's. This eminence is based partly on the large numbers of women involved. For example, although the reporting of *Neisseria gonorrhea* infections represents only a minority of such organism infections, and although these specific organism infections include only a portion of all sexually acquired pelvic infections, there were 874,161 reported cases of *N. gonorrhea* in the United States in 1974, indicating the epidemic proportions of this problem.[1] The fact that a minority of these cases, 350,863, were in women probably reflects under-reporting of asymptomatic women. The reported rate of gonorrhea increased each year from 1971 (624,371) to 1974 (874,161), an increase of 40%, with the greatest increase seen in the number of infected women (Table 1.1). In addition to the large numbers of women involved, pelvic infection is an important problem because there is good medical evidence that early detection and treatment of infections in females can achieve a clinical cure without the unacceptable residuals of infertility and pelvic pain. The seriousness of pelvic infection should not be downgraded. A recent study demonstrated tubal occlusion by laparoscopy in 12.8% of women after one clinical episode of salpingo-oophoritis.[2] With this serious outcome in mind, our goal as physicians should be appropriate employment of all diagnostic and therapeutic techniques so that the full female potential for reproduction and normal adult living can be assured. This is a major responsibility for the practicing physician.

PATHOPHYSIOLOGY OF SEXUALLY ACQUIRED PELVIC INFECTIONS

There is substantial evidence that the gram negative aerobe *N. gonorrhea* plays a significant role in the early manifestations of sexually acquired pelvic infections in women. In the pre-antibiotic era, Curtis performed a number of detailed microbiologic studies (including grinding up tubal material for culture) on pelvic tissue removed at operation.[3] His descriptions of the relationship between the microbiologic recovery of *N. gonorrhea* and clinical observations in the operating room were interesting. This organism was isolated from minced fallopian tubes removed at operation only when there was visual evidence of acute inflammation.

TABLE 1.1

Reported Cases of Gonorrhea

Fiscal year	Male	Female	Total	Percentage increase over previous year		
				Male	Female	Total
1971	448,731	175,640	624,371			
1972	494,652	223,749	718,401	10.2	27.4	15.1
1973	504,706	304,975	809,681	2.0	36.3	12.7
1974	523,298	350,863	874,161	3.7	15.0	8.0

In fact, in no cases were gonococci isolated from non-inflamed fallopian tubes in this pre-antibiotic era study. This circumscribed time interval of microbiologic recovery has been confirmed in modern studies based upon surface recovery of the gonococcus. Eschenbach and Holmes[4] and Chow et al.[5] recovered this organism from cervix and cul de sac aspirations in patients with clinical evidence of acute salpingitis. These investigators noted the gonococcus was recovered more frequently from the endocervix than from the peritoneal fluid. The common microbiologic isolation of this organism from the endocervix, minced fallopian tubes, and cul de sac aspirations in women with clinical evidence of acute salpingitis, and the absence of peritoneal or tubal recovery when there is no inflammation, strongly indicate the importance of this organism in acute salpingitis. An unfortunate additional observation is that although prior exposure to this potential pathogen elicits an immunologic response that can be measured in the serum, no absolute protection against future infection is established.

Obviously, not every pelvic infection is directly related to the gonococcus. A whole series of recent evaluations have confirmed the importance of other bacteria, particularly anaerobic microorganisms, in pelvic infections. Eschenbach and Holmes,[4] Chow et al.,[5] Thadepalli et al.,[6] Swenson et al.,[7] and our own anaerobic laboratory at the Los Angeles County-University of Southern California (LAC-USC) Medical Center[8] have frequently isolated anaerobic organisms from infection sites in women with sexually acquired pelvic infections. All these investigators have found anaerobic organisms in the majority of these serious soft tissue pelvic infections.

In fact, these investigations suggest that a number of classical beliefs about the mechanisms of bacterial soft tissue pelvic infections may not be correct. Emerging from these studies is a pattern of infection that will require re-orientation of gynecologic thinking about both the mechanisms and the treatment of pelvic infections. These new facts include the observations that anaerobes can be recovered from over 70% of soft tissue pelvic infections. These infections are a mixed microbiologic bag, i.e. more than one microorganism is frequently recovered. This is in contrast to the single-pathogen concept that applies so well to such infections as pyelonephritis. The antibacterial therapy of these mixed infections has not been established by prospective study. Some of the preliminary studies suggest that less than complete antibiotic coverage of the recovered organism may still yield a clinical cure.[9] Finally, we have been impressed at the LAC-USC Medical Center that operative drainage or removal of a pelvic abscess may be necessary for cure. What has been most significant to us has been the observation that the organisms recovered from the infected site have not been resistant in the laboratory to the antibiotics given to the patient prior to operation. Unlike observations by Gorbach that anaerobes were not recovered after 24 hours of clindamycin therapy, we have been able to recover anaerobes from previously undrained soft tissue infection sites despite prior clindamycin therapy.[8] If confirmed by other investigators, this will be a significant observation. In the past, physicians have generally equated therapeutic failure of response by the patient to the presence of resistant organisms at the site of infection. The physican's automatic response was to switch the patient to more powerful and potentially more toxic antibiotics. In view of these findings, our concern should be directed toward the discovery of a pelvic abscess with the appropriate operative intervention or the use of anticoagulants for the treatment of septic pelvic thrombophlebitis. This decision will be dealt with in detail in the section on therapeutics.

Besides the anaerobes, the other components in these mixed bacterial soft tissue pelvic infections are the aerobes. Recently, most of our attention has been directed toward the gram-negative aerobes, particularly *Escherichia coli*, which is one of the most common microorganisms recovered from these patients. In addition, there is new awareness of gram-positive cocci in such infections. Unlike the late 1950's when the predominant organism of concern was the coagulase-positive staphylo-coccus, more frequent pathogens recovered in the 1970's are the streptococci. The Group A beta-hemolytic streptococcus is not a frequent isolate, but can be associated with serious, life-threatening pelvic infections. A more frequent isolate on our service is the enterococcus. Although doubts have been expressed about the pathogenicity of this organism, it has been associated with serious infections in our patients.

The role of mycoplasma in pelvic infections has not been established as yet. Members of this group of organisms have been isolated in pure culture from a Bartholin's abscess[10] and, in combination with other organisms, from patients with a tubo-ovarian abscess. The clinical significance of these observations is not known.

No discussion would be complete without some comments on the influence of changes in social mores and medical practice upon the incidence of pelvic infection. There has been a worldwide revolution in sexual mores, reflected in an increasing rate of gonorrhea among an ever younger population. One factor influencing this more permissive sexual attitude has been the development of such methods of contraception as the oral contraceptives and the intrauterine device. These contraceptives are more effective than those previously available, and their employment is not related to the act of intercourse, as was the case with such mechanical methods as the condom, diaphragm, or jelly. Physicians have emphasized the lack of complete protection with mechanical methods. Fiumara quotes a description of a condom-like penile sheath of the 17th century as an "armor against enjoyment and a spider web against danger."[11] Despite this, it is likely that an asymptomatic male with gonorrhea using a condom would be less of a risk to a female sexual contact than the same male not using a condom. In addition, Bolch and Warren[12] noted an antigonococcal effect of one of the vaginal foams used as a spermicidal agent. This obviously would have some protective action for the women.

Besides the loss of the protective roles of the barrier forms of contraception, there has been concern about the direct influence of contraceptive methods upon the incidence of pelvic infection. Clinical data seem to support the concept that the minority of untreated women exposed to the gonococcus develop salpingitis. Fiumara has stated that women who use oral contraceptives are at greater risk of developing gonococcal salpingitis.[13] If this is true, it would identify a high risk population that should have more frequent screening examinations for lower genital tract gonorrhea. A possible relationship between the intrauterine contraceptive device and pelvic infection has been suspected by many physicians. Although early studies did not confirm an increased incidence of pelvic infections with these intrauterine foreign bodies, there have been a number of isolated observations that suggest that such a relationship in fact does exist. Eschenbach and Holmes have found a statistically significant increase in the number of patients with serious pelvic infections among intrauterine device wearers.[4] In addition, I have been aware of occasional serious and life-threatening pelvic infection due to the Group A beta hemolytic streptococcus in intrauterine device users. Besides this, some unilateral tubo-ovarian abscesses have been seen in intrauterine device patients. This unilateral disease seems more common among intrauterine device users. The mechanism is not known, but the relationship seems real. These potential factors must be weighed in the evaluation of office patients with the symptomatology of fever, pelvic or abdominal pain, or an adnexal mass. Some of these masses may be inflammatory in origin.

MICROBIOLOGY OF THE LOWER GENITAL TRACT IN ASYMPTOMATIC SEXUALLY ACTIVE WOMEN

A common example of clinician confusion is the search through the clinical microbiology report of endocervical or vaginal cultures for the presence of pathogens to confirm the diagnosis of salpingo-oophoritis. It has been thought that the presence of such gram negative aerobes as *E. coli* can be equated with infection. There is no good modern basis for this supposition, and evaluation of the vaginal bacterial flora of asymptomatic women, prior to the insertion of an intrauterine device[14] or at the time of uterine removal with vaginal hysterectomy[15, 16] revealed many potential pathogens (Table 1.2). A striking observation of all of these studies was the large number of anaerobes recovered, over 70% of the specimens in a recent study.[16] In fact, one recent study of the endocervical anaerobic bacterial flora of "normal" women found many anaerobes, and no differences in the types of isolates from these women could be found when compared to the endocervical cultures of patients with symptomatic pelvic infection.[17] This indicates that the recovery of anaerobic organisms or other "pathogens" from endocervical cultures is not a discriminating laboratory test for the presence of a pelvic infection. Does the recovery of any bacterial species have clinical significance? I believe there can be an affirmative answer when either of two species is recovered. The isolation of the aerobic group A beta hemolytic streptococcus from the lower genital tract is not always associated with clinical disease. However, since this organism has been

TABLE 1.2

Bacteria Recovered from the Endocervix or Vagina of Asymptomatic, Sexually Active Women

	Gram positive	Gram negative
Aerobes	*Streptococcus viridans*	*Escherichia coli*
	Enterococci	*Proteus*
	Beta streptococcus, not A or D	*Aerobacter aerogenes*
	Coagulase positive staphylococcus	*Klebsiella*
	Coagulase negative staphylococcus	*Pseudomonas*
	Diphtheroids	*Mima polymorpha*
	Lactobacilli	
	Bacillus subtilis	
Anaerobes	*Peptostreptococcus*	*Bacteroides* species
	Peptococcus	*Bacteroides fragilis*
	Clostridium, not perfringens	Fusobacteria
	Clostridium perfringens	
	Propionibacterium acnes	

related to severe pelvic infections, particularly in women utilizing an intrauterine contraceptive device, the discovery of this streptococcus on culture is an indication to me for systemic antibiotic therapy. In addition to this aerobe, *N. gonorrhea* isolation has significance for the clinician. Its presence is not always associated with clinical evidence of upper genital tract disease, even in the absence of systemic antibiotic therapy, but aggressive treatment is indicated so that the possible complications of acute salpingitis can be avoided.

PROPER MICROBIOLOGIC TECHNIQUES FOR THE ISOLATION OF *N. GONORRHEA*

The microbiologic isolation of *N. gonorrhea* requires knowledge of both the host environment and the specific growth requirements of this organism. In a clinical setting, the most frequent site of sampling for this organism is the endocervix, a location that is rich in other bacteria. Any microbiologic sample from this site will contain a multiplicity of organisms. This is an important fact to keep in mind, because organisms competing for the nutrients of the culture media may successfully implant and overgrow, so that *N. gonorrhea* present at the culture site will not survive in the laboratory. This has required two major modifications in culture techniques. First, specific media are utilized, rich in glutamine and carboxylase. Next, the samples are placed in a carbon dioxide-rich environment, so that the most favorable setting is available for the growth of *N. gonorrhea*. To reduce the problem of competing organisms, the antibacterial agents vancomycin and colistimethate, plus the antifungal agent nystatin have been added. As a result, few species other than *N. gonorrhea* can survive on these media. To be certain that colony growth is due to *N. gonorrhea*, oxidase and sugar fermentation tests can be applied to the colonies, as well as microscopic evaluation of the morphology of a gram stain from the bacterial colonies.

With this theoretical knowledge, many practical problems remain for the clinician. He must determine the microbiologic technique that works best for him in his own office environment. Most of the patients who need to be tested for the presence of this organism will be seen in clinics and private offices, far removed from the hospital microbiology laboratory. Transportation may be a critical item in the successful isolation of this organism, for it does not survive in an unfavorable environment for long periods. Nearly all of the studies with transport media demonstrate fewer recoveries of *N. gonorrhea* with increasing time intervals. The most popular and rational microbiologic strategy has been the use of direct specimen plating and incubation by the clinician prior to transport to the laboratory. A number of commercial systems, including Trans-grow, are available for this purpose. Many of the systems have a short shelf life which is increased by refrigeration storage. It is important for the physician and office staff to allow these culture tubes to warm to room temperature before use. The gonococcus, which survives so well in the human host, may not tolerate the chill of the cold medium plate. The crucial ingredient for success still seems to be to minimize the time between specimen collection and the laboratory receipt of the sample. Although the endocervical smear has been downgraded as a diagnostic technique in asymptomatic women, the presence of gram negative intracellular diplococci should have significance for the clinician and result in treatment before the culture report returns in patients with symptoms. However, the absence of gram negative intracellular diplococci does not eliminate the possibility of gonorrhea.

When the clinician has decided upon the appropriate microbiologic system, the next decision is the site for specimen collection to isolate the gonococcus. A number of large scale clinical trials have been performed to provide a basis for choice in this area. These studies indicate that the endocervix is the best single site for culture collection, and that a combination of an endocervical sample and rectal sample provided the highest yield of positive cultures.[18] These results have to be viewed within the framework of clinical practicality for the physician. On our own service at the LAC-USC Medical Center, the added yield of positive cultures by rectal sampling has not been high enough to make us routinely utilize this site in our diagnostic screening maneuvers. Every physician must be aware of the finding by Schroeter and Lucas that one-third of the gonococcal treatment failures were discovered only by rectal culture.[18] For this reason, the rectum, as well as the endocervix, is always sampled as a test of cure 7 to 14 days after the completion of therapy. It is important for the physician to obtain a complete history of the patient's sexual practices. If the woman is practicing rectal intercourse, then rectal cultures are indicated. If she is practicing fellatio, oral pharyngeal cultures should be done. There is one final practical note for specimen collection. The commonly used vaginal lubricants contain preservatives that can be bactericidal to the gonococcus. It is important to avoid their use prior to the obtaining of a specimen.

WHAT POPULATION SHOULD BE SAMPLED?

The physician's decision about the population of women to be sampled must acknowledge the current state of flux that still exists in this area. There was a major drive in the 1960's, with considerable government support, for universal screening of women of child-bearing age. This was based upon the presumptions that the male who had gonorrhea was symptomatic while the woman usually was not. The goal was the discovery and treatment of this large reservoir of asymptomatic females. Recently, a number of clinical observations have opened this observation to doubt. Contemporary studies indicate that infective males may be asymptomatic[19] and, more important, that infected females may have symptomatology.[20] These observations may have some implications for future outpatient gynecologic practice. Rather than the random screening of the entire office patient population, the physician may be able to selectively culture all females of child bearing age with the symptomatology of a vaginal discharge, abnormal uterine bleeding, or urinary tract symptomatology suggestive of a cystitis. One recent study indicated a high yield of positive gonococcal cultures in that population group.[20] I still believe that universal microbiologic screening for this pathogen in sexually active women is the best medical goal, but decisions on the cost-yield ratio of such a screening survey still have to be made. Even if the costs of universal screening are prohibitive, certainly symptomatic patients need to be screened.

The most important impact of these new observations is the significance of the asymptomatic male. As a specialty, Obstetrics-Gynecology has directed all of its efforts towards the improvement of health care for women, and has tried to implement this by restricting the practice of individual specialists to women. In the area of pelvic infection control, this is clearly not an acceptable policy. Our goals should be to prevent re-infection of the treated female by the asymptomatic male, and we must implement in some way the discovery and treatment of such contacts.

A recent development of some interest to the practicing gynecologist has been the finding that there is some immunologic response to exposure to the gonococcus, which might obviate the problem of obtaining a culture. A number of tests methods have been devised to measure serum immunoglobulin response to the gonococcus, utilizing a latex agglutination test. To date, there have been serious shortcomings with this method. Some patients, seen early, with a positive culture for *N. gonorrhea* have a negative test. A different problem is seen in women who have had gonorrhea in the past but who presently are culture negative. Many of these women will have a positive serologic test for gonorrhea. These false negative and false positive results severely restrict the practical application of these serologic tests for gonorrhea. Perhaps a more significant clinical observation is the realization that the presence of these antibodies is insufficient for protection against recurrent disease.[21]

MICROBIOLOGIC EVALUATION OF OTHER POTENTIAL PATHOGENS

In addition to the gonococcus, the presence of other "pathogens" will on occasion need to be evaluated by the clinician. Previously mentioned studies have shown no difference in bacterial flora of the endocervix between asymptomatic and symptomatic women, so that this site should not be used for microbiologic evaluation for organisms (other than the group A beta hemolytic streptococcus). The alternate site, the peritoneal cavity, sampled through the posterior cul de sac, has been shown to be free of bacteria in asymptomatic women.[5] This clearly defines our study population, i.e. those patients with clinical evidence of acute salpingitis. In these patients, in the absence of a cul de sac mass, the vagina should be prepped with an iodine solution, and the peritoneal cavity entered through the posterior cul de sac with a long spinal needle for aspiration. Chow *et al.* have utilized only the needle and have added sterile saline without preservative to lavage the peritoneal cavity and permit the reaspiration and collection of a fluid sample.[5] Eschenbach and Holmes have used a large bore #14 needle and have inserted polyethylene tubing through this for peritoneal cavity aspiration.[4] In symptomatic women, cultures for the gonococcus, aerobes, and anaerobes, as well as a gram stain of the exudate should be performed. This requires some minimal microbiologic materials to be present and available in the office setting.

Minimal microbiologic equipment is needed to adequately equip a gynecology office. There should be a microscope with a satisfactory oil immersion lens, and fresh material should be available for the gram stain. Sterile tubes of a transport medium and sterile oxygen-free tubes should be present for the transport of appropriate specimens to the hospital laboratory for aerobic and anaerobic cultures. If possible, fresh media for the culture of *N. gonorrhea* should be present in the office. Specimens should be transported on a frequent basis, if necessary, during normal office hours.

The exact role of *Mycoplasma* organisms in pelvic infections remains confused and unclear at present. Mycoplasma can be a "pathogen," on occasion, for it has been recovered in pure culture from a Bartholin's abscess,[10] and has been isolated along with other organisms from tubo-ovarian abscesses.[22] In addition, the effectiveness of tetracyclines in the treatment of patients with salpingo-oophoritis suggests that these organisms may have clinical significance. Mycoplasma can frequently be isolated from the endocervix and vagina of sexually active women.[23] Indeed, the multiplicity of male sexual partners seems to increase the recovery rate of this organism from the lower genital tract of females. However, recovery from the lower genital tract does not have the same significance as recovery of the gonococcus. In addition, the complexity of the culture techniques makes it unlikely that either the clinician or the laboratory will employ these isolation techniques at present. If more convincing cause-and-effect evidence of pathogenicity is produced, then changes in future office practice modes will be required.

The incidence of herpes genitalis has reached epidemic proportions. In fact, in many office practices this is the most common veneral disease seen. The clinician usually can recognize the clustered outbreak of vesicles visually on examination. Laboratory confirmation is seldom needed, but can be provided by viral isolation, the presence of multinucleated giant cells on Pap smear, or increase of herpes titer in the blood. On practical grounds for the office gynecologist, evaluation of the Pap smear is the most frequently employed laboratory technique.

SYPHILIS

Any review of sexually acquired pelvic infections in women would be incomplete without a discussion of syphilis. This disease, usually acquired during sexual intercourse, has a limited impact upon pelvic organs and may not be associated with any apparent symptomatology. However, if untreated, it can have disastrous effects in later years upon such vital organ systems as the cardiovascular or central nervous system. The detection of the early phases of this disease by physicians is an important responsibility, for these serious complications can be prevented by appropriate antimicrobial therapy. In addition, there are significant numbers of patients contracting this disease: approximately 25,000 cases of infectious syphilis were reported in the United States in fiscal year 1972. Although this is a large number of cases, it does represent a much smaller population of women than are presently reported with gonorrhea infections. Patients with syphilis will be seen on occasion in an outpatient setting by gynecologists. Because of this, it is important that physicians have a clear understanding of the diagnostic alternatives available to them in such patients.

The microbiologic testing techniques for the detection of syphilis are limited. To date, no system has been devised for the recovery and maintenance of these spirochetes on artificial media. The only direct testing available for clinicians is the dark field examination of the exudate from the visible lesions of primary syphilis for the presence of spirochetes. This examination should be done, if the physician is confronted by a vulvar or vaginal lesion that could be a "chancre." Any lesion, particularly one that causes the patient no discomfort, should be evaluated. Just prior to the collection of a specimen, the surface of the lesion should be abraded and the resulting surface serum collected on a microscope slide. Most physicians will recognize these lesions at the time of pelvic examination in their office, but few will have access to laboratory facilities and personnel necessary for the adequate performance of a dark field examination. This should be available through any approved hospital equipped with an adequately staffed laboratory. The patient should be seen near the hospital laboratory, prior to any antibiotic therapy, to have the test done in conjunction with trained laboratory personnel. The limited time span of these visible lesions, which are frequently asymptomatic, makes this test one that is not commonly performed by the practicing gynecologist.

These restrictions on direct microbiologic testing have caused the gynecologist to look to other host responses to the spirochete *Treponema pallidum* for the diagnosis of syphilis. There is evidence that infection due to this pathogen elicits the production of multiple antibodies. These can be characterized by one of two basic antibody types.

Nonspecific antibodies (reagins) can be identified in patients with syphilis. These antibodies are directed against the lipoidal antigen of the treponema or the lipoidal antigen that results from the interaction of the host and *T. pallidum*. These non-specific tests have usually been referred to as the serologic test for syphilis. The test procedures are of two general types, the flocculation, exemplified by the Venereal Disease Research Laboratory slide test (VDRL), or the complement fixation test, of which the Kolmer is the prototype most commonly used today. There is a time sequence in the development of these antibodies, which is visually characterized in Fig. 1.1.[24] This time sequence must be kept in mind when evaluating the laboratory tests of patients who have had unprotected sexual exposure. These tests are reproducible laboratory techniques, easily performed and quantitated. They have a major disadvantage, related to the non-specific nature of the reagin. They are sometimes positive in patients who do not have syphilis, and estimates of the proportion of false positive tests have run as high as 40%. These troublesome diagnostic problems are more frequently seen in women, and a

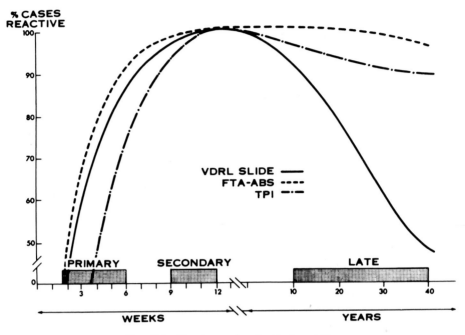

Fig. 1.1. Serology of untreated syphilis

persistent false positive test is often associated with serious connective tissue immunologic disease. (Table 1.3).[25-29] Because of the importance of differentiating patients with positive non-specific antibodies, the physician should be aware of the more specific syphilis tests.

There are a number of tests available to test for specific anti-treponemal antibodies. The *T. pallidum* immobilization test (TPI) was the first devised, but has generally been discarded because it is difficult to perform in such a way that reproducible results can be obtained. The Reiter-protein complement fixation test (RPCF) uses the non-pathogenic Reiter strain of treponema as the antigen. It is a simple test to do in a clinical laboratory but has the double disadvantage of being reactive in only 50% of patients with late syphilis and having a percentage of falsely positive test results in normal patients. Currently, most of the direct treponemal antibody testing is the Fluorescent Treponemal Antibody Absorption (FTA-ABS) test. This test is reactive in most cases of syphilis, and has very few false positive tests. Table 1.4 shows a comparison of the reactivity of different antibody tests during the various stages of syphilis.[30] Although not usually an office procedure, a spinal tap may be performed in patients with a positive VDRL and positive FTA-ABS to determine the presence of neurosyphilis.

How should the practicing physician interpret all these test procedures in their evaluation of patients? Every patient exposed to sexually contacted disease should have a screening reagin test performed. Fortunately for the physician, most laboratories report a positive result as the highest dilution of the patient's serum that gives a positive test. Utilizing the data graphically portrayed in Figure 1.1, it is apparent that titers can be negative, low, or occasionally high (1:32 or higher) in

TABLE 1.3

Development of Connective Tissue Immunologic Disease in Patients with Chronically False Positive Test for Syphilis (Five Combined Series)

	Patients	
	No.	%
Combined series	658	100
Females	483	73
Patients with systemic lupus erythematosus	48	7
Patients with other connective tissue immunologic diseases	122	19

TABLE 1.4

Reactivity of VDRL, TPI, and FTA-ABS Tests during Various Stages of Syphilis

Diagnosis	Number of patients tested	Percentage reactive		
		VDRL	TPI	FTA-ABS
Primary syphilis	191	78	56	85
Secondary syphilis	270	97	94	99
Late syphilis	117	77	92	95
Latent syphilis	954	74	94	95
Normal	384	0	0	1

primary syphilis, are commonly high in secondary syphilis, and are variable in late syphilis. False-positive reactors usually have VDRL titers of 1:8 or below. Gynecologists in their office practice must be prepared to deal with the circumstance of a positive VDRL test in a patient with no clinical findings nor history of previous syphilis. To eliminate the possibility of a laboratory error, the VDRL test should be repeated. If it is still positive with the quantitative titer unchanged and the patient still has no clinical evidence of disease, the patient either has latent syphilis or a false positive test. The patient should be subjected to the more specific treponemal test, the FTA-ABS. If this is negative, the patient has a false positive test for syphilis. The prognosis for patients with false positive reactions varies greatly. Acute reactors have been defined as those women whose reagin test reverted to normal in less than 6 months. These women have a favorable prognosis. Those women whose positive reagin test persisted for over 6 months are termed chronic reactors. Approximately one-fourth of these chronic reactors have been reported to have serious underlying disease (Table 1.3). Because of the concern of the adequacy of therapy for central system syphilis in patients allergic to penicillin, a spinal tap is recommended for those patients with no lesions, a positive VDRL, and a positive FTA-ABS.

DIAGNOSIS OF SEXUALLY ACQUIRED DISEASES ON THE BASIS OF HISTORY AND PHYSICAL FINDINGS

There have been great changes recently in our understanding of the presenting signs and symptoms of women infected with gonorrhea. When programs were instituted by the Public Health Service in the 1960's to control the epidemic of gonorrhea, a number of assumptions were made. It was assumed that the male with gonorrhea was always symptomatic and would seek medical aid. Because of this, only symptomatic males were cultured and treated, and efforts were then implemented to find and treat their female sexual contacts. On the other hand, the woman with lower genital tract disease was assumed to be always asymptomatic. Tremendous money and effort were expended to screen large populations of women, so that asymptomatic carriers could be detected and treated before they infected susceptible males or developed upper genital tract disease themselves. The incidence of reported gonorrhea in males and females seemed to support this concept, for more males than females were reported (Table 1.1). Recent studies have indicated that some modification in this analysis of the epidemiology of gonorrhea is indicated. Evaluation of males culture positive for the gonococcus has demonstrated a significant percentage free of symptomatology.[19] The tacit belief that male symptomatology will result in their entry into the medical care system for diagnosis and treatment is not always correct. In addition, there has been a growing awareness that many women with lower genital tract gonorrhea are symptomatic.[20] A recent study of a population of women seen in an emergency room setting showed an increase in the number of positive cultures for gonorrhea among sexually active women with the complaints of a vaginal discharge, abnormal uterine bleeding, or lower urinary tract symptomatology.[20] In an office setting where routine cultures for gonorrhea are not feasible, these patients represent a high risk population that should be microbiologically screened for this disease. Certainly, any patient named as a contact by a male with gonorrhea should be cultured and treated, whether symptomatic or not.

The physician, in his office, attempts to detect pelvic inflammatory disease on the basis of history and physical findings. Findings that normally increase diagnostic suspicion that acute salpingo-oophoritis is present include lower abdominal pain, increased vaginal discharge, an elevated temperature, and marked tenderness of the pelvic organs on bimanual examination. Recent reports of laparoscopy evaluations of patients with clinically suspected pelvic inflammatory disease have cast some doubt on the accuracy of our evaluations in these women.[31] One laparoscopic study of 814 women who were suspected of having salpingitis on clinical grounds revealed visual confirmation of acute salpingitis in only 532, or 65%. Even more disturbing was the visual evaluation of patients with symptomatology and subsequent categorization as visually normal, nongonococcal salpingitis, and gonococcal salpingitis (see Fig. 1.2). The tremendous overlap of these three groups casts great doubts on our ability as clinicians to make the diagnosis of salpingo-oophoritis on clinical grounds.

There is another side to this evaluation that suggests that the office gynecologist need not eliminate his history and physical examination in his attempt to discover acute salpingo-oophoritis. The quoted study utilized a hodge-podge of symptomatology in the patients submitted to laparoscopy.[31] All patients had sudden onset of lower abdominal pain, and in addition had to have two or more symptoms and signs, which included abnormal vaginal discharge, fever, vomiting, menstrual irregularities, urinary symptoms, proctitis symptoms, marked tenderness of the pelvic organs on bimanual examination, palpable adnexal mass or swelling, and

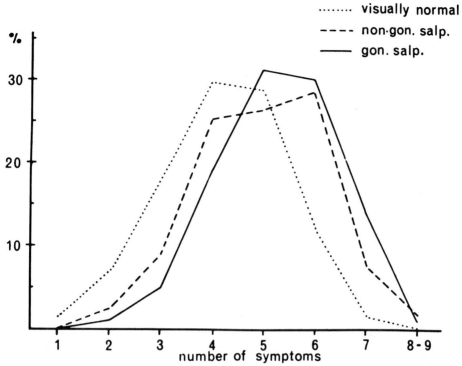

Fig. 1.2. Laparoscopy evaluations of 814 women; percentage distribution of number of symptoms and signs out of 9 registered.

erythrocyte sedimentation equal to or greater than 15 mm per hour. Many of the symptoms chosen were nonspecific and could be related to other pelvic or gastrointestinal pathology. In fact, there was evidence in the study that some of the signs and symptoms were more discriminating for the physician (Table 1.5). In addition to this, there has been a concern that the very strict criteria for the laparoscopic diagnosis of salpingitis may not detect early endosalpingitis in these patients.[32] I believe these concerns are legitimate. Since upper genital tract disease due to the gonococcus is an endosalpingitis, it is possible that laparoscopic evaluation of the surface of the fallopian tubes might not demonstrate discrete changes. Certainly, the more frequent isolation of the gonococcus from ground up portions of tubes[3] rather than by peritoneal surface culture would support this possibility.

With this background, there are acceptable guidelines of practice for the physician seeing outpatients. The office gynecologist should suspect acute salpingo-oophoritis in patients with lower abdominal discomfort, fever, and tenderness or masses on palpation of the adnexa on pelvic examination. These are the patients in whom a gram stain of endocervical secretions for gram-negative intracellular diplococci should be performed, plus needle culdocentesis of the cul de sac. If gram-negative intracellular diplococci are seen in the endocervical smear or if white cells and bacteria are found in the peritoneal fluid obtained by needle

TABLE 1.5

Visual Diagnosis

Clinical findings on admission	Acute salpingitis (n = 623)		Normal (n = 184)		Value
	No.	%	*No.*	%	
Bimanual examination					
Marked tenderness only	573	92	160	87	<0.05
Palpable mass or swelling	308	49.4	45	24.5	<0.001
Erythrocyte sedimentation rate > 15 mm/hour	473	75.9	97	52.7	<0.0001
Abnormal vaginal discharge	394	63.2	74	40.2	<0.001
Fever (>38° C)	205	32.9	26	14.1	<0.001

culdocentesis, then antibiotic therapy is indicated. This approach will not yield a 100% diagnostic accuracy rate, but it should provide appropriate care for the majority of women. In addition to these patients with symptomatology, there are women who should be suspected of having pelvic inflammatory disease. This includes those women with a unilateral adnexal mass who are currently utilizing or have recently employed an intrauterine device.

DIAGNOSIS OF PELVIC INFLAMMATORY DISEASE ON THE BASIS OF LABORATORY FINDINGS

Although many laboratory tests are nonspecific in patients with sexually acquired infections, some results demand physician intervention. The discovery of gram-negative intracellular diplococci on endocervical smear has significance and should require antibiotic treatment. A positive endocervical, rectal, or oropharyngeal culture for the gonococcus is meaningful and requires appropriate antibiotic therapy. The endocervical recovery of the Group A beta-hemolytic streptococcus is an indication for antibiotic therapy. The culture of organisms from cul de sac aspiration in patients with pelvic symptomatology or the positive physical finding of adnexal masses is abnormal and the physician should respond with antibiotic therapy. Some physicians have been impressed with the significance of the sedimentation rate in the management of patients with salpingo-oophoritis.[33] They believe it relates to the presence of active inflammatory disease and is an indication for operative intervention in patients who remain febrile, despite what seems to be appropriate antibiotic therapy.

TREATMENT OF PATIENTS WITH SEXUALLY ACQUIRED PELVIC INFECTIONS

The starting point of therapy for the office practice of gynecology should be the treatment of uncomplicated gonococcal infections in the woman. This group should include those women named as sexual contacts of culture-positive males, as well as culture-positive women who have no clinical evidence of upper genital tract disease. The recommended treatment regimens reflect a number of considerations. *N. gonorrhea* remains quite susceptible to penicillin and other antibiotics, so long as the therapeutic level reached at the infection site exceeds the minimal inhibitory concentration of the organism. Prolonged therapy does not seem to be necessary to achieve a clinical cure. In addition to these microbiologic considerations, most of these patients are relatively asymptomatic and may not be motivated toward prolonged courses of therapy. Finally, no reported series has indicated that antibiotic combination regimens are more effective than single antibiotics in the care of these women. Because of this, all of the treatment regimens, with the exception of the one involving tetracycline, are focused upon therapy that can be completed within one office visit. Table 1.6 contains the regimens currently recommended by the United States Public Health Service (1974).[34] Physicians are cautioned to use no less than the recommended dosages of antibiotics. There can be toxic reactions to the antibiotics used. Most of the accumulated data deal with penicillin reactions. Table 1.7 notes the serious reaction rates in large numbers of patients receiving outpatient penicillin therapy for gonorrhea.[35] In addition to an allergic reaction to penicillin, there is evidence that a small percentage, approximately 0.04%, can have severe central nervous system symptomatology, including a temporary psychosis due to a reaction to the procaine.[35]

A follow-up culture, both endocervical and rectal, is required 7 to 10 days after

TABLE 1.6

Treatment of Asymptomatic Women Who Are Sexual Contacts of Culture Positive Males or Who Have a Positive Endocervical Culture for Neisseria gonorrhea

Drug regimen of choice: Aqueous procaine penicillin G, 4.8 million units intramuscularly, divided into at least two doses and injected at different sites at one visit, along with 1 g of probenecid, by mouth, just before the injections.

Alternative regimens:

A. Patients in whom oral therapy is preferred: Ampicillin, 3.5 g by mouth, along with 1 g of oral probenecid, administered at the same time. There is evidence that this regimen may be slightly less effective than the recommended intramuscular aqueous procaine penicillin G.

B. Patients who are allergic to the penicillins or probenecid:

1. Tetracycline hydrochloride, 1.5 g given orally initially, followed by 0.5 g by mouth four times daily for four days (total dose, 9.5 g). There is no evidence that newer tetracyclines are clinically more effective than tetracycline hydrochloride and all tetracyclines are ineffective as single dose therapy.

2. Spectinomycin hydrochloride, 2.0 g intramuscularly, in one injection.

TABLE 1.7

Comparative Frequency of Anaphylactic Reactions at Five-Year Intervals

	Year of study				
	1969	1964	1959	1954	1954–1969
Total patients treated	27,673	21,922	25,550	19,510	94,655
Anaphylaxis, total	11	10	27	4	52
Mild	6	4	18	—	28
Moderate to severe	5	6	9	4	24
Death	0	1	0	0	1
Anaphylaxis, total:					
rate per 1,000 patients treated	0.40	0.46	1.06	0.21	0.55
Anaphylaxis, moderate to severe:					
rate per 1,000 patients treated	0.18	0.27	0.35	0.21	0.25

therapy. If either or both of these culture site samples are positive for *N. gonor-rhea* and there is good evidence on the basis of an accurate history that the patient has been a treatment failure to either penicillin or tetracycline, and not a re-infec-tion then spectinomycin should be used for therapy. This is based upon the obser-vation that *N. gonorrhea* isolates from treatment failures of penicillin or tetracy-cline have high minimum inhibitory concentrations (MIC's) to either of these drugs, but have MIC's to spectinomycin that are equivalent to those found with culture-positive asymptomatic women.[36]

If the office gynecologist discovers other sites of infection due to the gonococcus, then alternative regimens may be necessary. Pharyngeal gonorrhea in women practicing fellatio is more difficult to treat than anogenital gonorrhea. The ampicillin and spectinomycin regimens are usually ineffective. All such patients should have a reculture of the oral pharynx for gonorrhea after the initial therapy and, if positive, they should receive 9.5 grams of tetracycline as recommended in Table 1.6.

There is one new and revolutionary aspect to the treatment of the woman infected with the gonococcus. Some effort must be made definitely to establish therapy for the male sexual partner. In the past, we have relied upon male symptomatology to bring the male patient into the health care system. It is obvious that males who are asymptomatic and infective will be missed by this dependence. These asymptomatic males are capable of infecting previously adequately treated females. Male treatment must be stressed, and some workable referral system must be established so that this goal can be reached.

In addition to gonorrhea, these asymptomatic women may have been exposed to syphilis. All sexually active patients who are evaluated for gonorrhea should have a serologic test for syphilis performed. If they are serology negative and have incubating syphilis, one recent study indicates that the aqueous procaine penicillin therapy is sufficient for cure.[37] Repeat serologic tests are not necessary. If other treatment regimens are used, a followup serologic test for syphilis should be performed in 3 months. If positive, the appropriate therapy requires a different clinical approach than the one followed for the patient with gonorrhea. There must be an additional evaluation of the specificity of the positive reagin test, which can be accomplished by the use of FTA-ABS testing. If this more specific syphilis testing is positive, then the extent of the disease must be established. Specifically, the physician needs to know if the central nervous system is involved, for then a larger dose antibiotic therapy will be indicated. Antibiotic therapy for syphilis is based upon the twin observations that these spirochetes are exquisitely susceptible to penicillin, but more prolonged exposure to the antibiotic is required. Table 1.8 lists alternate treatment regimens for the patients with syphilis.[38] After treatment, the patient should be followed with periodic VDRL tiers. This serum VDRL test usually becomes negative 6 to 12 months after treatment of primary syphilis and 12 to 24 months after treatment of secondary syphilis.[39]

TREATMENT OF UPPER GENITAL TRACT DISEASE IN PATIENTS CULTURE POSITIVE FOR GONORRHEA

There are usually many clinical signs that the patient has upper genital disease related to the gonococcus. Although these women will often have some symp-

TABLE 1.8

Alternate Treatment Regimens for Syphilis

Penicillin: The drug of choice. For primary or secondary syphilis, a single intramuscular injection of 2,400,000 units of benzathine penicillin G. Alternatively, procaine penicillin G, 600,000 units intramuscularly daily for 8 days, or procaine penicillin G with 2% aluminum monosterate, 2,400,000 units intramuscularly, with two subsequent 1,200,000 units dosages given at 3-day intervals. For the patient with a positive spinal fluid, the choices are benzathine penicillin G, 3,000,000 units weekly for 3 weeks, or 600,000 units of aqueous procaine penicillin G daily for 15 days. Other antibiotics for the penicillin-allergic patient:

Tetracycline: For primary or secondary syphilis, 2 g a day for 15 days. For the patient with a positive spinal fluid, 2 g a day for 30 days. This drug is not recommended for a pregnant woman.

Erythromycin: For primary or secondary syphilis, the propionyl sulfate salt, 2 g a day for 15 days. This drug has not been well evaluated in the patient with a positive spinal fluid.

TABLE 1.9

Suggested Outpatient Treatment Regimens for the Patient with Gonococcal Salpingitis

Tetracycline: 1.5 g of tetracycline hydrochloride, given as a single oral loading dose, followed by 500 mg orally, four times a day for 10 days.

Penicillin: Aqueous procaine penicillin G, 4.8 million units intramuscularly, divided into at least two doses and injected at different sites at one visit, or 3.5 g of oral ampicillin. Oral probenecid, 1 g, is given along with either intramuscular penicillin or oral ampicillin. These initial doses are followed by 500 mg of oral ampicillin, four times daily for 10 days.

tomatology, including lower abdominal discomfort, pelvic pain, and fever, the majority of women seen early in an outpatient setting will have mild symptomatology and will not have all of these signs. Although endocervical and cul de sac cultures are indicated, the finding of gram-negative intracellular diplococci should suggest *N. gonorrhea* and dictate therapy.

The philosophy of antibiotic care for women suspected of having a gonococcal salpingitis is based upon few observations. There simply have been few prospective controlled comparative antibiotic studies. The suggestion is that the minimum therapy should be sufficient for the control of the gonococcus, but the treatment schedule should be longer than for the uncomplicated lower genital tract gonorrhea. Table 1.9 presents the 1974 treatment recommendation of the United States Public Health Service. In this group of patients, it is important to get repeat endocervical and rectal cultures for gonorrhea 7 to 14 days after therapy, for the rectal culture will delineate one-third of the treatment failures. If the patients fail to respond to therapy, re-evaluation is necessary to see whether other pathology is present or whether a different treatment regimen is needed for cure. This may include alternative antibiotic coverage or drainage of a pelvic abscess. The most important treatment obligation is to ensure adequate antibiotic treatment of male sexual partners so that reinfection will not occur.

UPPER GENITAL TRACT DISEASE, NOT GONORRHEA

There is increasing evidence that many women with acute salpingitis have organisms other than the gonococcus as the pathogen. This requires some alternative treatment strategies, tempered with the realization that women with nongonococcal salpingitis usually cannot be distinguished clinically from patients with a gonococcal salpingitis. In these women, the majority have mild symptomatology when first seen.

In the outpatient microbiologic evaluation of patients with salpingitis, endocervical cultures for *N. gonorrhea* and the group A beta-hemolytic streptococcus should be obtained, in addition to a cul de sac aspiration for *N. gonorrhea* and aerobic and anaerobic culture.

Treatment of these women requires that a number of important decisions be made. First, the physician must judge if therapy as an outpatient is indicated for the patient. On our own service, any patient with evidence of a pelvic abscess or suspected pelvic abscess is admitted to the hospital, for we believe that operative intervention should be carried out under anesthesia in the operating room. In addition, the patient with severe symptomatology and little evidence of toleration of oral medication should be admitted to the hospital. The best outpatient treatment regimen for patients with nongonococcal salpingitis has not been established by prospective study. Some preliminary data by Eschenbach and Holmes suggest that tetracycline may have a more favorable clinical response than ampicillin alone.[4] In the patient with a treatment failure as an outpatient, culture results should be considered in further antibiotic therapy. An organism of frequent concern is *Bacteriodes fragilis*, and alternative therapy may include coverage for this organism. There is no evidence that steroids given concomitantly with antibiotics change the prognosis for these patients. The heavy weight of clinical evidence suggests that recurrent episodes of salpingo-oophoritis are due to reinfection and are not a chronic infection. Our therapeutic goal should be appropriate length of therapy for the female and treatment of the male partner, rather than prolonged therapy of the female for chronic infection.

THE RELATIONSHIP OF UPPER GENITAL TRACT DISEASE TO THE INTRAUTERINE CONTRACEPTIVE DEVICE

Although the preliminary statistical data suggested no increased incidence of pelvic inflammatory disease in patients utilizing an intrauterine device, a number of investigators have suggested that such a relationship exists. Wright and Laemmle found a five-fold increase in the salpingitis rate among intrauterine device patients,[40] while Noonan and Adams indicate that intrauterine device users exposed to gonorrhea are more likely to develop salpingitis.[41] Eschenbach and Holmes have also found this relationship.[4] A number of studies have demonstrated a sometimes lethal combination of pelvic infection due to the group A beta-hemolytic streptococcus among intrauterine device wearers. In addition, we have been impressed with the discovery of unsuspected unilateral pelvic inflammatory disease in patients with an intrauterine device in place. A recent report also notes a relationship between the intrauterine device and pelvic actinomycosis.[42] Because of these observations, there are a number of important considerations in these intrauterine device patients. Patients suspected of having salpingo-oophritis should be screened for the group A beta-hemolytic streptococcus, including a gram stain of the endocervical excretions. If there are numerous gram-positive cocci, penicillin rather than tetracycline should be the drug of choice. The presence of an adnexal mass should alert the physicians to the possibility of a unilateral tubo-ovarian abscess. Although previous studies indicated that intrauterine device patients with salpingitis could be treated with the device in place, Eschenbach and Holmes feel that consideration of removal of the device should be a part of therapy. This is particularly true in the period following therapy, so that the greater risk of future salpingitis among IUD users will be avoided. This point will need the clarification of future prospective study.

REFERENCES

1. United States Public Health Service reports.
2. Westrom, L, Effect of Acute Pelvic Inflammatory Disease on Fertility, Am. J Obstet Gynecol., *121:*707, 1975.
3. Curtis, AH, Bacteriology and Pathology of Fallopian Tubes Removed at Operation, Surg Gynecol Obstet, *33:*621, 1921.
4. Eschenbach, DA, and Holmes, KK, personal communication.
5. Chow, AW, Malkasian, KL, Marshall, JR, and Guze, LB, Acute Pelvic Inflammatory Disease and Clinical Response to Parenteral Doxycycline, Antimicrob Agents Chemother, *7:*133, 1975.
6. Thadepalli, H, Gorbach, SL, and Keith, L, Anaerobic Infections of the Female Genital Tract: Bacteriologic & Therapeutic Aspects, Am J Obstet Gynecol, *117:*1034, 1973.
7. Swenson, RM, Michaelson, TC, Daly, MJ, and Spaulding, EH, Anaerobic Bacterial infections of the Female Genital Tract, Obstet Gynecol, *42:*538, 1973.
8. Ledger, WJ, Gee, CL, Pollin, P, Nakamura, RM, and Lewis, WP, The Use of Pre-reduced Media and a Portable Jar for the Collection of Anaerobic Organisms from Clinical Sites of Infection, Am J Obstet Gynecol, in press.
9. Gorbach, SL, and Thadepalli, H, Clindamycin in Pure and Mixed Anaerobic Infections, Arch Intern Med *134:*87, 1974.
10. Russell, FE, and Fallon, R, Mycoplasma and the Urogenital Tract, Lancet *1:*1295, 1970.
11. Fiumara, NJ, Letter to the Editor, New Eng J Med *285:*972, 1971.
12. Bolch, OH, Jr, and Warren, JC, In Vitro Effects of Emko on *Neisseria gonorrhea* and *Trichomonas vaginalis*, Am J Obstet Gynecol, *115:*1145, 1973.
13. Fiumara, NJ, Modern-age Complications of VD: Proceedings International Venereal Disease Symposium, Pfizer Laboratories, St. Louis, 1971, p. 33.
14. Willson, JR, Bollinger, CC, and Ledger, WJ, The Effect of an Intrauterine Contraceptive Device on the Bacterial Flora of the Endometrial Cavity, Am J Obstet Gynecol, *90:*726, 1964.
15. Ledger, WJ, Sweet, RL, and Headington, JT, Prophylactic Cephaloridine in the Prevention of Post-operative Pelvic Infections in

Premenopausal Women Undergoing Vaginal Hysterectomy, Am J Obstet Gynecol, *115:*766, 1973.
16. Ledger, WJ, Gee, CL, and Lewis, WP, Guidelines for Antibiotic Prophylaxis in Gynecology, Am J Obstet Gynecol, *121:*1038, 1975.
17. Gorbach, SL, Menda, KB, Thadepalli, H, and Keith, L, Anaerobic Microflora of the Cervix in Healthy Women, Am J Obstet Gynecol, *117:*1053, 1973.
18. Schroeter, AL, and Lucas, JB, Gonorrhea—Diagnosis and Treatment, Obstet Gynecol, *39:*274, 1972.
19. Handsfield, HH, Lipman, TO, Harnisch, JP, Tronca, E, and Holmes, KK, Asymptomatic Gonorrhea in Men, New Eng J Med *290:*117, 1974.
20. Curran, JW, Rendtorff, RC, Chandler, RW, Wiser, WL, and Robinson, H, Female Gonorrhea: Its Relation to Abnormal Uterine Bleeding, Urinary Tract Symptoms and Cervicitis. Obstet Gynecol *45:* 195, 1975.
21. Kearns, DH, Seibert GB, O'Reilly, R, Lee, L, and Logan, L, Paradox of the Immune Response to Uncomplicated Gonococcal Urethritis, New Eng J Med *289:*1170, 1973.
22. Mardh, PA, and Westrom, L, Tubal and Cervical Cultures in Acute Salpingitis with Special Reference to *Mycoplasma hominis* and T-strain Mycoplasmas, Brit J Vener Dis *46:*179, 1970.
23. McCormack, WM, Almeida, PC, Bailey, PE, Grady, EM, and Lee, YH, Sexual Activity and Vaginal Colonization with Genital Mycoplasmas, JAMA *221:*1375, 1972.
24. Drusin, LM, The Diagnosis and Treatment of Infectious and Latent Syphilis. Med Clin N Am *56:*1161, 1972.
25. Miller, JL, Brodey, M, and Hill, JH, Studies on Significance of Biologic False-positive Reaction, JAMA *164:*1461, 1957.
26. Knight, A, and Wilkinson, RD, The Clinical Significance of the Biological False Positive Serologic Reactor: A Study of 113 Cases, Can Med Ass J *88:*1193, 1963.
27. Harvey, AM, and Shulman, IF, Connective Tissue Disease and the Chronic Biologic False-positive Test for Syphilis (BFP reaction), Med Clin N Am *50:*1271, 1966.
28. Putkenon, T, Jokinen, EJ, Lassus, A, and

Mustakallio, KK, Chronic Biologic False Positive Sero Reactions for Syphilis as a Harbinger of Systemic Lupus Erythematosus, Acta Dermatol Vener *47:*83, 1967.

29. Taffanilli, DL, Wuepper, KD, and Bradford, IL, Fluorescent Treponemal-Antibody Absorption Tests: Studies of False-positive Reaction to Tests for Syphilis, New Eng J Med *276:*258, 1967.

30. Deacon, WE, Lucas, JB, and Price, EV, Fluorescent Treponemal Antibody-absorption (FTA-ABS) Test for Syphilis, JAMA *198:*624, 1966.

31. Jacobson, K, and Westrom, L, Objectivized Diagnosis of Acute Pelvic Inflammatory Disease, Am J Obstet Gynecol *105:*1088, 1969.

32. Rees, E, and Annels, EH, Gonococcal Salpingitis, Brit J Vener Dis *45:*205, 1969.

33. Charles, D, Personal communication.

34. Gonorrhea—CDC recommended treatment schedule, 1974.

35. Rudolph, AH, and Price, EV, Penicillin Reaction among Patients in Venereal Disease Clinics, JAMA *223:*499, 1973.

36. Kaufman, RE, personal communication.

37. Schroeter, AL, Turner, RH, Lucas, JB, and Brown, WJ, Therapy for Incubating Syphilis: Effectiveness of Gonorrhea Treatment, JAMA *218:*711, 1971.

38. Sparling, PF, Diagnosis and Treatment of Syphilis, New Eng J Med *284:*642, 1971.

39. Schroeter, AL, Lucas, JB, Price, EV, and Falcone, VH, Treatment for Early Syphilis and Reactivity of Serologic Tests, JAMA *221:*471, 1972.

40. Wright, NH, and Laemmle, P, Acute Pelvic Inflammatory Disease in an Indigent Population, Am J Obstet Gynecol *101:*979, 1968.

41. Noonan, AS, and Adams, JB, Gonorrhea Screening in an Urban Hospital Family Planning Program, Am J Public Health *64:*700, 1974.

42. Schiffer, MA, Elquezabal, A, Sultana, M, and Allen, HC, Actinomycosis Infections Associated with Intrauterine Contraceptive Devices, Obstet Gynecol *45:*67, 1975.

2

VULVOVAGINITIS

DALE BROWN, JR., M.D.

RAYMOND H. KAUFMAN, M.D.

The predominant symptoms of the several entities classified as vulvovaginitis are abnormal discharge and pruritus. Clinically, the discharge may be excessive in amount, altered in color and consistency, frothy, malodorous, or "cheesy." The pruritus varies from mild to severe, and is associated with an uncontrollable urge to scratch. Krantz[1] believes that any change that interferes with normal separation and regeneration of prenerve endings and Markel discs near the surface of the skin, which are constantly shed during regrowth of the skin, may induce the sensation of pruritus. The warmth and moisture of the vulva and the rubbing together of the opposing surfaces of the skin often give rise to readily apparent changes.

To recognize the abnormal secretions usually associated with vulvovaginitis, one must first be familiar with the features of normal vaginal secretions. Women with good estrogen levels, without vaginitis or cervicitis, have a white or slate-colored secretion, often referred to as being of an epithelioid or curdy consistency. A curdy secretion does not flow, as does the runny, milky, or creamy homogeneous secretion observed in trichomoniasis and *Haemophilus vaginalis* vaginitis. A test of the acidity of vaginal secretions is highly informative. When the pH is within the normal range of 3.8 to 4.2, the possibility of certain infections is virtually eliminated.

Malodorous vaginal secretions are usually indicative of trichomoniasis or *H. vaginalis* vaginitis. However, an occasional woman with apparently normal secretions, having normal pH, complains of an objectionable odor. In such a patient, the offensive odor may also be partially attributable to increased activity of the apocrine gland system and poor hygiene. Lactobacilli or diphtheroids usually predominate in the normal vagina. When viewed in wet mounts, they appear as large rods.

VULVOVAGINAL CANDIDIASIS

Candidiasis now comprises approximately half of all the vaginitides. *Candida albicans* is most often the infecting organism, although *C. tropicalis*, *C. pseudotropicalis*, *C. krusei*, *C. stellatoida*, and *C. guilliermondi* may be responsible in some cases. It has been found that *C. tropicalis* is not only a common causative agent, but is also more likely to be associated with chronicity and recurrence than *C. albicans*.[2]

It appears that susceptibility of the individual plays a much more prominent role in the development of candidiasis than chance contamination of the vagina by candidal organisms. It is primarily a disease of the childbearing years, appearing in 15 to 20% of patients in late pregnancy, as opposed to an estimated 4 to 6% of nonpregnant patients.[3] In fact, pregnancy is the most common predisposing factor, the severity of the disease sometimes increasing throughout gestation. The pronounced increase in the glycogen content of the vagina during pregnancy provides a favorable environment for rapid growth of the candidal organisms. Patients who take oral contraceptives are seemingly more susceptible, since cyclic administration of estrogen and progesterone will produce a vaginal environment similar to that observed during pregnancy.[4] In addition, thinning of the vaginal wall consequent upon the progestational agents may lead to a higher degree of susceptibility to infection.

The vast majority of premenarcheal and postmenopausal patients who develop vaginal candidiasis either have recently taken antibiotics or estrogens or will be found to have diabetes. Since the introduction of antibiotics, the incidence of candidiasis has increased several-fold. The mode of action of these drugs in precipitating the disease remains debatable; such theories as reduction of phagocytosis of the candidal organisms or reduction of antibodies to candidal organisms have been postulated. A heavy concentration of candidal species, particularly in the intestinal tract, may serve as a continuous source of infection and reinfection of the vagina. Because of the low incidence of diabetes, this disease is of little significance to the gynecologist in the overall picture of vaginal candidiasis. Patients with nondiabetic glycosuria, lovers of sweets, and debilitated patients are also predisposed to candidiasis.

The presence of a factor X, possibly related to the susceptibility of mucocutaneous tissues to allergenic or endotoxic substances derived from the cells of the candidal organisms, is probably related to the degree of irritative reaction. Seelig[5] found that patients with recurrent candidal infections had lower antibody titers and also diminution of the candidacidal properties of their blood serum.

Not all women who harbor a candidal species in the vagina have clinical evidence of the disease. Vulvar pruritus is the cardinal symptom of candidiasis, being reported by approximately 90% of the patients. Erythema of the vulva is the sign most often observed and, next in order, edema of the labia minora (Fig. 2.1). Excoriations, produced by scratching, are often present. An abnormal redness of the vagina is observed in only about 20% of patients with candidal infection. Thrush patches are present in only 20% of nonpregnant, as compared to 70% of pregnant patients (Fig. 2.2). The pH of the vaginal secretions is usually between 4.0 and 4.7. Odor is not a characteristic of vaginal secretions incident to candidiasis.

Demonstration of filaments (pseudohyphae) is necessary for the diagnosis of candidiasis. This may easily be accomplished by microscopic examination of slides containing vaginal secretion mixed in 10 to 20% potassium hydroxide (Fig. 2.3). The predominance of lactobacilli in a case of vulvovaginitis with pruritus is strong evidence of candidiasis.

Candida is recoverable from the stool and oral cavity of 75% of women with this infection. In contrast, only 25% of those with negative vaginal cultures are found to have positive stool or oral cultures.

Gentian violet is one of the oldest and most reliable treatments for candidiasis; it

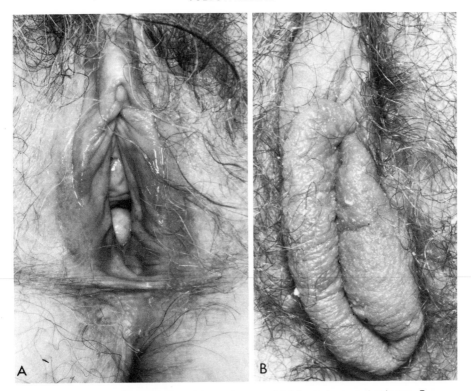

Fig. 2.1. A, Candidiasis with erythema of labia majora and minora. B, Candidiasis with severe edema.

may, however, cause a severe chemical irritation, even though applied in solutions of 1 to 2%. The most effective yet safe treatment available is the use of vaginal nystatin tablets, one inserted into the vagina twice daily for a minimum of 15 days, or Miconazole cream (Monistat) nightly for two weeks.[6, 7] Other medications, such as vaginal candicidin (Vanobid and Candeptin) and chlordantoin (Sporostacin), appear to be less effective.[8, 9] Occasionally, corticosteroids applied topically are justified to reduce inflammatory reactions and relieve itching until the candidacide has taken effect. Currently, the prevention of reinfection is a problem. It is likely that most recurrent infections are endogenous in origin. For chronic or recurrent infection, the use of continuous therapy for 3 to 4 weeks, even during the menstrual period, as well as intravaginal candidacides at bedtime for 7 to 10 days before each menstrual period, have been recommended. Intravaginal candidacides with any course of an antibiotic therapy are recommended. Nystatin or amphotericin B given orally to inhibit growth of intestinal organisms have also been suggested. The efficacy of this method in preventing reinfections is highly debatable. When nystatin is taken orally, it is not absorbed from the intestinal tract and consequently has no direct beneficial effect upon vulvovaginal candidiasis. Some observers believe the discontinuance of oral contraceptives adds to the cure rate. It has been found that cleansing of the preputial folds and application of a candiacidal agent reduces the reinfection rate. Although it is strictly conjectural, the patient's

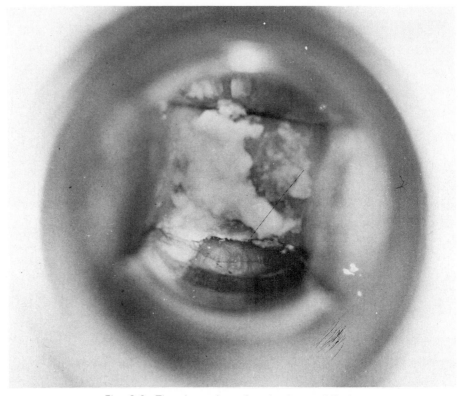

Fig. 2.2. Thrush patches of vagina in candidiasis.

intake of carbohydrates should possibly be limited. After all known predisposing factors have been eliminated and all precautions taken against reinfection, patients with obstinate disease must use prophylactic vaginal candidacides every 2 to 3 days for an indefinite period.

PRIMARY CUTANEOUS CANDIDIASIS OF THE VULVA

This disease, which is relatively rare in the United States, is favored by warm, humid climates in which maceration and other changes in the skin provide a good environment for growth of the fungus. Obese patients seem particularly susceptible.

Primary cutaneous lesions involve chiefly the labia majora and the genitocrural folds, the perianal region, and the inner thighs. The lesions are usually extensive when first observed by the physician. They tend to be moist, weeping, and beefy red in appearance, with rather precisely defined scalloped edges (Fig. 2.4). Older, larger lesions are characteristically associated with smaller, discrete satellites, thus offering a clue to the diagnosis (Fig. 2.5). Budding forms and pseudohyphae of candidal organisms can be demonstrated in scrapings placed in 20% potassium hydroxide. Mere isolation of the organisms, however, does not prove that the patient has cutaneous candidiasis; the diagnosis is justified only after careful correlation of the clinical and laboratory findings. Differentiation between

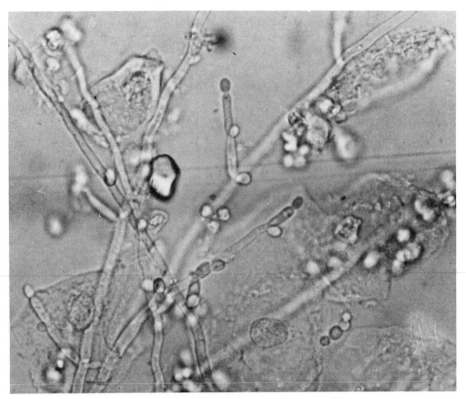

Fig. 2.3. Spores and filaments in candidiasis under high power magnification.

trichophyton infections causing tinea cruris and primary cutaneous candidiasis may be made microscopically, since the presence of hyphae alone suggests a tineal infection.

Treatment for this condition consists of topical applications of amphotericin B or nystatin.[10] In the weeping stage, a lotion is preferable to creams or ointments. Application of Castellani's paint or 1 to 2% gentian violet affords rapid relief, although prolonged use of these agents may cause untoward effects. To ensure their effectiveness, all other preparations must be used daily for 14 days or longer.

DIABETIC VULVITIS

Diabetes is a powerful predisposing factor in candidiasis, yet it is of little overall significance in the general problem, since only 1 to 2% of the general population has diabetes. Vulvovaginal candidiasis, however, may prove to be a major problem to women with diabetes, for the disease in many of these patients may develop into a chronic and resistant vulvitis. Diabetes should be considered in any patient with chronic or recurrent candidiasis, or in any patient who acquired the infection before puberty or after menopause.

We believe the term "diabetic vulvitis" is useful for a special variety of vulvar dermatitis that arises only in diabetic patients. It frequently persists long after the

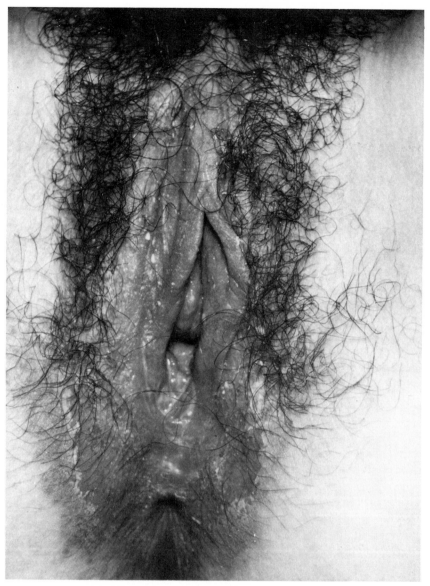

Fig. 2.4. Primary cutaneous candidiasis, with well defined scalloped edges.

fungus which initiated its development has been eradicated. It must be assumed that bathing of vulvar tissues with glucose-laden urine, as well as elevated glucose levels in body fluids and tissues, stimulate and contribute to candidal growth. Widespread chronic vulvitis in diabetes develops from a multiplicity of factors, some of which are only indirectly related to the diabetes. Unquestionably, the severity and extent of this infection depend to some extent upon the duration of poorly controlled diabetes and pruritus, the duration of untreated candidal and bacterial infections, the vigor of scratching, and the patient's individual susceptibil-

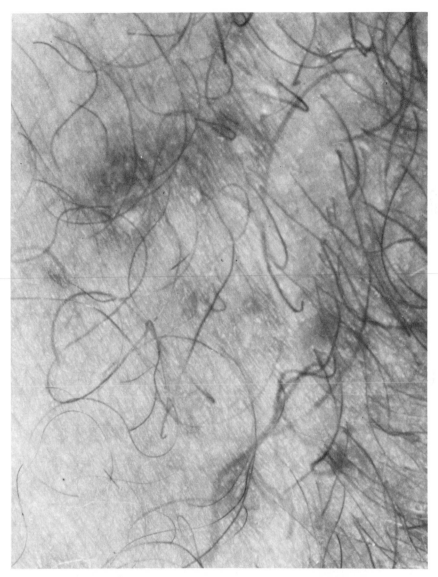

Fig. 2.5. Satellite lesions of primary cutaneous candidiasis.

ity to the allergenic and endotoxic substances produced by the fungi and bacteria. Fully developed vulvitis may persist for months or years after the diabetes has been controlled and all the fungi eradicated. This is probably based on the well developed, widespread chronic neurodermatitis perpetuated by an uncontrollable scratch-itch reflex.

The symptoms of diabetic vulvitis consist of chronic pruritus, irritation, burning, dysuria, and dyspareunia. Clinically, the involved tissues are practically always edematous, and typically a diffuse bright red. Thrush patches may be found in the vestibule and vagina. Superficially, a grayish-white film over the vulva is occasionally observed, or the vulvar skin may have a glazed or shiny appearance. Excoriations in the natural folds of the skin are frequently associated (Fig. 2.6).

In addition to treatment for the diabetes and topical applications for associated candidiasis, the pruritus must be controlled by the topical use of corticosteroid preparations, such as 0.025% fluocinolone acetonide cream (Synalar), 0.05% flurandrenolone cream (Cordran), and 1% hydrocortisone cream (Cortef). Tranquilizers are sometimes helpful and necessary to break the scratch-itch reflex, which is often an acquired nervous habit. Supplemental vitamins, especially the B complex, have been recommended by Parks.[11]

TRICHOMONIASIS

The causative agent of vaginal trichomoniasis is the unicellular protozoan flagellate, *Trichomonas vaginitis*. Infection with this organism does not involve the vagina alone, but also Skene's ducts and the lower urinary tract in women, and the lower genitourinary tract of men. Since the majority of patients acquire the disease through sexual intercourse, it should be considered a venereal disease. Vulvar contact between homosexuals is sometimes a mode of transfer, as well as vulvovaginal contamination by inanimate objects such as douche nozzles, bath towels, and wet bathing suits. These possibilities, however, are remote.

Currently, trichomoniasis comprises approximately 10% of all vaginal infections. The disease is observed primarily in women with relatively normal estrogen

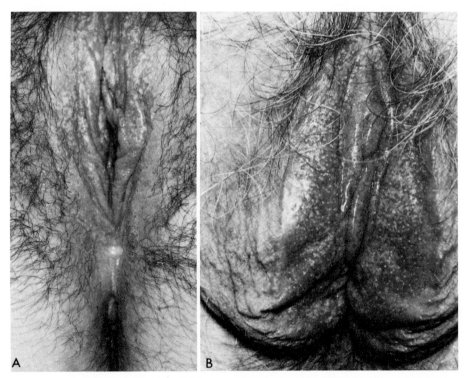

Fig. 2.6. A, Diabetic vulvitis, excoriated areas. B, Glazed, shiny appearance of skin.

levels. It is prone to be slightly worse immediately after menstruation, and can be most acute during pregnancy.

According to the severity of the infection, trichomoniasis may be classified as asymptomatic, chronic, or acute. A vaginal flora having a pH of 3.8 to 4.2, and consisting predominantly of lactobacilli and only a small number of living trichomonads, is believed to indicate an asymptomatic or carrier stage of the infection. The majority of patients in this group give a clearcut history of past clinical disease and, subsequently, almost all experience exacerbations.

Patients whose vulvovaginal tissues exhibit no distinct gross changes yet who have an excessive amount of malodorous vaginal secretion of an abnormal consistency, with an elevated pH and containing large numbers of trichomonads, are regarded as having the chronic type of trichomoniasis. This is the most common variety. In some patients, the chronic state is maintained (and the acute stage prevented) by the frequent use of acid or medicated douches.

An abnormal discharge, gross tissue reactions in the vagina or vulva or both, and irritative manifestations, particularly pruritus, edema, and erythema, characterize the acute stage of the infection. Under the microscope, actively motile organisms, usually moving in the direction of the flagella, are clearly visible in a wet mount saline solution of the vaginal secretion (Fig. 2.7). In a relatively unsuitable environment, the trichomonads frequently assume a spherical shape. These forms have been referred to as pseudocysts, although trichomonads do not under any circumstance form cysts.

The cardinal symptom of the disease is a discharge. This varies in amount, at times being voluminous. The amount often depends upon both the natural tissue reaction from the infection and the hygienic practices of the individual patient. The color of the discharge is greenish in only 10% of patients; occasionally it is yellow, though it is more often gray.[12] This is contrary to the apparently prevalent opinion that most, if not all, trichomonal infections are accompanied by a green discharge. Frothiness is present in the discharge of approximately 10% of the patients (Fig. 2.8). Abundant frothiness points to trichomoniasis or, less often, to an *H. vaginalis* vaginitis. The odor from trichomoniasis is probably more offensive than that of any other vaginal infection.

A diffuse redness is the only gross change apparent in the vaginal tissues of approximately two-thirds of the patients with the acute stage of the disease. The strawberry vagina, the result of edematous and ecchymotic papillae projecting through the discharge, is alluded to as the usual type, although this picture is found in less than 10% of patients (Fig. 2.8).

In a small but definite percentage of patients, a pseudomembrane forms over the vagina. This pseudomembrane is thin and gray in color and cannot be wiped away. It may appear as small, discrete lesions, or may cover the entire mocusal surface of the vagina. In most such conditions, the papillae are swollen.

Occasionally, a patient with severe vaginitis may be suspected of having trichomoniasis, yet no trichomonads can be detected on wet mount preparations. One may find, however, a large number of polymorphonucleocytes and immature basal and parabasal epithelial cells. Since it is most likely that the toxicity of the secretions has caused complete immobility of the trichomonads, re-examination after 48 to 72 hours is in order.

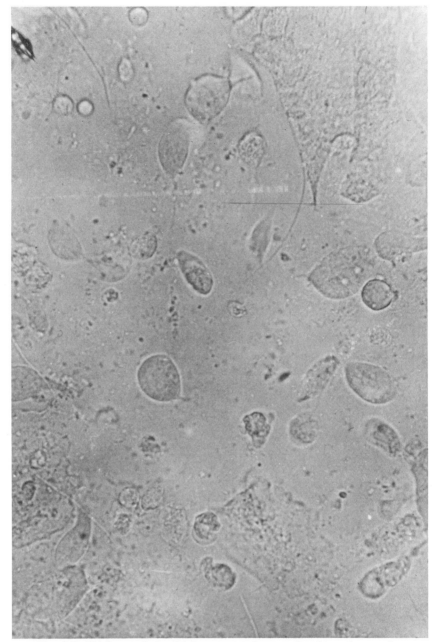

Fig. 2.7. Trichomoniasis: high power microscopic view of secretions, showing multiple trichomonads.

Cultures for diagnosis of the infection are seldom warranted. If culturing is necessary, however, the simplified Trypticase serum technique of Küpferberg is highly suitable.

Urinary symptoms incident to a urethrocystitis solely from the effects of *T.*

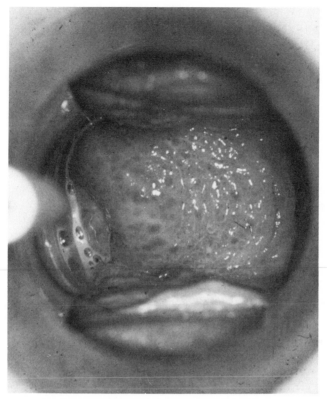

Fig. 2.8. Frothy discharge with trichomoniasis; also ecchymotic papillae.

vaginalis infection are observed fairly often in patients with or without vulvovaginal trichomoniasis. A mild abacturic pyuria accompanied by demonstrable trichomonads in a clean voided or catheterized specimen of urine is often attributed to this infection. This is definitely assured if the urinary symptoms and trichomonads disappear upon treatment for the infection.

Probably fewer than 20% of men harboring the organism have signs or symptoms of trichomoniasis. The diagnosis of the disease in men can be made by collection of the first 5 to 30 ccs, of an early morning specimen of urine; the trichomonads will appear as spherical in shape. At times, only the flagellum will exhibit motion. These organisms have been referred to as pseudocysts.

It is imperative that both sexual partners have simultaneous and identical treatment. Metronidazole (Flagyl) given to both in a dosage of 500 mg every 12 hours for 5 days has been the most successful regimen in our experience. The drug may be contraindicated for patients with some types of blood dyscrasias and disease of the central nervous system. It is also suggested that the drug be withheld during pregnancy, especially the first trimester, although no detrimental effect upon the mother or unborn child has yet been reported following its administration during this time. Treatments with topical agents have been largely ineffective. They are still used, however, for the patient who is extremely sensitive to drugs, perhaps during pregnancy, or for those with blood dyscrasias or diseases of the central nervous system. For these exceptional patients, topical agents such as furazolidone nifuroxime (Trichofuron) suppositories, or Devegan tablets may be employed. Whatever the topical agent selected, it should be continued for 30 days or longer. Douching with a strongly acid or medicated preparation after coitus with an infected male affords some protection against contracting the infection. Condoms and similar protectives may also be safeguards against the disease.

H. VAGINALIS **VAGINITIS**

Until recent years, any vaginitis or unusual vaginal discharge not readily explained by identifiable agents was termed "nonspecific vaginitis." Probably more than 90% of vaginitides previously classified as nonspecific were in actuality caused by *H. vaginalis*, also sometimes referred to as *Corynebacterium vaginale*.[13] Today, approximately 40% of vaginal infections are a result of *H. vaginalis*.[14] Alertness on the part of physicians to the possibility of such an infection, in addition to the use of available laboratory tests, should lead to a specific diagnosis of practically every case of a discharge or vaginitis observed in current clinical practice.

H. vaginalis vaginitis is essentially nonexistent in premenarcheal subjects. Sexual intercourse is almost surely the method of transmission: a high rate of reinfection of patients whose consorts remain untreated is therefore to be expected. Transmission by inanimate objects, such as douche nozzles, bath towels, and wet bathing suits, is unlikely since the organisms are extremely susceptible to dryness; their viability depends upon the presence of moisture.

The incubation period of the infection is probably 5 to 10 days after inoculation. Once the *H. vaginalis* has been established in the vagina, it will become the prevailing organism, the lactobacilli being largely eliminated during the first week of the infection.

Relatively few patients experience irritative symptoms, such as pruritus or burning. Discharge and malodor are the patient's chief complaints. Often the signs and symptoms are so mild as to escape attention of the patient, although she will admit the necessity of frequent douching for hygiene or will report that the husband has commented about her unpleasant odor.

Any patient whose ovarian activity is normal yet who has a gray, homogeneous, malodorous vaginal discharge with a pH of 5 to 5.5, in which no trichomonads are found, is likely to have *H. vaginalis* vaginitis. The discharge may vary from scant to profuse (Fig. 2.9). Usually it is less abundant than that produced by trichomoniasis and has a less offensive odor. The consistency of the discharge resembles a thin homogeneous flour paste. A frothy discharge is present in approximately 7% of the cases.

H. vaginalis is a surface parasite which does not invade the vaginal wall; therefore gross vulvitis and vaginitis are not a part of the disease. Histologic sections do not show any evidence of an inflammatory or other abnormal reaction.

The diagnosis can be made simply from a wet mount preparation of the discharge in physiologic saline on a glass slide. The typical appearance of clue cells, i.e. epithelial cells which appear to be stippled or granulated, is the *sine qua non*

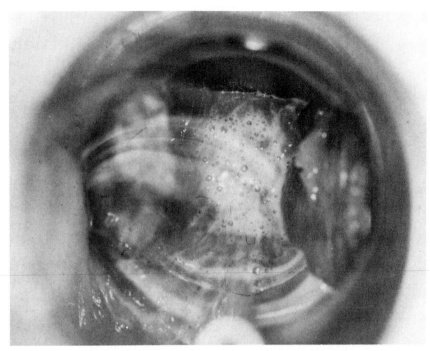

Fig. 2.9. Frothy discharge of *H. vaginalis* vaginitis.

diagnostic feature (Fig. 2.10). Lactobacilli are conspicuously absent. If trichomoniasis is associated, the accuracy of the diagnosis by this method falls to
approximately 50%. *H. vaginalis* is a minute, rod-shaped, gram-negative bacillus
when observed in a gram stained smear.[15-17] Culture of the organism is most
successful with the use of Casman's blood agar plates incubated under increased
carbon dioxide tension for 24 hours at 37°C.[15]

The most effective treatment for *H. vaginalis* vaginitis consists of the administration of Ampicillin, 500 mg every 6 hours for 5 days; Keflex, 500 mg q 6 hours for
6 days, or Anspor, 250 mg q 6 hours for 6 days, is also recommended. Oral
tetracycline administered in doses of 250 mg every 6 hours for 5 days is partially
effective. Sulfonamides inserted intravaginally twice daily for a minimum of 10
days, have also proven successful in many cases. The male consort should also be
treated with systemic medications.

DESQUAMATIVE INFLAMMATORY VAGINITIS

This rarely observed condition, which exhibits the microscopic features of
postmenopausal atrophic vaginitis, affects women with high estrogen levels. No
author reporting on this condition has been able to assign a specific causative
agent.[18, 19] The uniformly poor response to antibacterial agents suggests that
bacterial infection is not primarily responsible. An unidentifiable viral infection has
not been excluded as one of the primary causes, nor has the possibility that the
vagina is undergoing some type of dystrophic process.

The pathogenesis of the atrophic status of the vaginal mucosa is not understood.

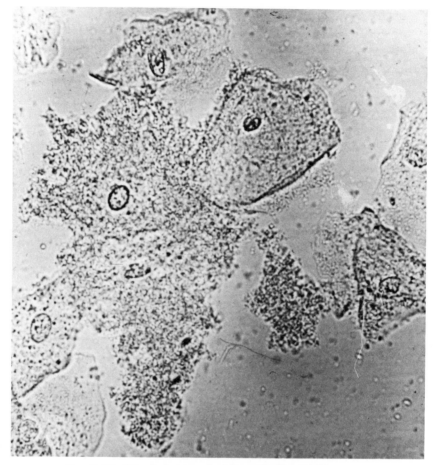

Fig. 2.10. Stippled clue cell of *H. vaginalis* vaginitis.

It may be presumed that basal and parabasal cells in women with high estrogen levels are the result of failure of mucosal proliferation or maturation, or both, accelerating desquamation being produced by the effects of some unknown agent or process.

The high percentage of basal and parabasal cells, as well as pus cells, in secretions of these patients has led to the theory that the etiology may lie in an estrogen deficiency. Relatively few bacteria are present, and lactobacilli are essentially lacking. Histologically, both acute and chronic inflammatory reactions are found, and in some areas of the epithelium superficial ulcerations are present.

Most patients complain of a moderate to copious discharge, usually homogeneous and purulent, although malodor is not a feature. Mild burning and pruritus are the only irritative symptoms reported by a majority of the patients. The pH of the vaginal secretion varies from 5 to 6.8.

Examination will disclose an acute inflammation of all or a part of the upper half of the vagina, especially the opposed surfaces of the posterior fornix and the ectocervix (Fig. 2.11). The margins are usually well delineated, and in some areas

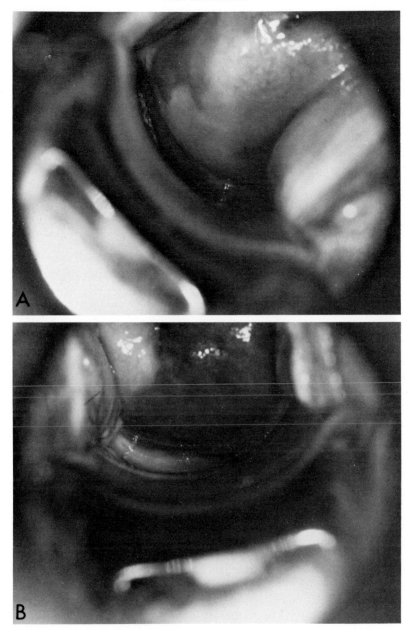

Fig. 2.11. A, and B, Desquamative inflammatory vaginitis. Delineated, inflamed opposed surfaces high in the vagina.

the epithelium may be covered by a grayish pseudomembrane, which peels off when the vagina is wiped. The sites of the inflammatory reaction remain unchanged for an indefinite time.

The diagnosis of this condition is made when a patient is found to have normal ovarian activity, a localized persistent vaginitis, especially in the upper vault, and an abnormal discharge containing a high percentage of immature epithelial and pus cells, the specific cause of which is unknown.

These lesions usually do not heal spontaneously. Sulfonamides and other antibiotics administered systemically or locally have been unsuccessful. Intravaginal cortisone applications have proven most effective.

TORULOPSIS GLABRATA

Although little is known about this fungus, it is believed to be a marginal or weak pathogen producing mild vulvovaginitis in susceptible patients. Approximately 8 of every 100 patients who harbor these organisms report a mild itching and burning sensation and a discharge.

The clinical feature most often observed is an increased vaginal discharge without malodor, having a white or slate color and a consistency less curdy than normal. The pH is usually about 4.5. A mild erythema of the vulva may be apparent.

As a rule, the diagnosis may be made by a wet mount preparation of secretions in physiologic saline. This may reveal spores similar to those of Candida, though usually they are smaller and highly variable in size. Hyphae are conspicuously absent, and pus cells are relatively few in number. Also, in vaginal secretions treated with 20% potassium hydroxide numerous small spores with no hyphae can be discovered. Cultures of the organism may reveal small, smooth colonies without hyphal tips, and will cause gaseous fermentation of both glucose and trehalose.

Torulopsis glabrata responds less favorably to fungicidal agents employed for candidiasis than to gentian violet or commercial compounds containing this chemical. The recurrence rate is high, and some patients appear to be resistant to treatment.

ATROPHIC VAGINITIS

Whether from natural menopause, castration, ovarian destruction from disease, or functional ovarian failure, loss of estrogen is followed by varying degrees of atrophy of all vulvovaginal and uterine tissues. Much has been written about increased susceptibility of the atrophic vagina to infection, yet one rarely finds such infections as candidiasis, trichomoniasis, or *H. vaginalis* vaginitis in an extremely atrophic vagina. If a postmenopausal patient reports an irritating discharge, however, infections from these pathogens should be excluded before the signs and symptoms are attributed to atrophic vaginitis.

Vaginal bloody spotting is probably the most commonly reported symptom of atrophic vaginitis. This may be spontaneous or post-traumatic in origin. The irritative symptoms include dysuria, external burning, pruritus, tenderness, and dyspareunia. Dyspareunia may be the result of either fissuring and ulceration of the vulvovaginal epithelium, or stretching of the deeper inelastic tissues of a stenotic introitus. Occasionally, symptoms of bladder irritability, such as frequency, urgency, and burning may be associated.

On examination, the vagina exhibits a pale erythema, and its folds and rugae have partially or wholly disappeared. In exceedingly rare cases of advanced atrophy, opposed denuded surfaces of the epithelium can agglutinate, producing adhesive vaginitis. This is more often observed following surgical trauma or irradiation. At times, after complete withdrawal of estrogen, masses of granulation tissue are observed in the vagina, especially in the lower half, and perhaps in the vestibule (Fig. 2.12). In severe atrophy, areas of excoriation and fissuring are sometimes present. With extreme shrinkage and retraction of the vagina the urethral mucosa may evert at the meatus, constituting a variety of the urethral caruncle. Distribution of the hair growth over the labia majora and mons becomes sparse, and the hairs become brittle and coarse.

The discharge associated with vaginal atrophy is highly variable, yet seldom profuse. Acidity of the vaginal secretions is diminished, frequently reaching a pH of 7.5, although it usually ranges from 5.5 to 7.

The diagnosis may be made on the basis of the history, the clinical appearance of the vagina, a slight vaginal discharge with a mild to moderate vulvar irritation, and the laboratory findings. A wet mount preparation of a smear will reveal a predominance of parabasal cells and polymorphonucleocytes, with various types of bacteria. Stained smears have a dirty background, as seen in trichomoniasis.

Treatment consists of the administration of estrogens, either systemically or intravaginally. Estrogenic creams may be applied to the vagina nightly for a week to 10 days, or until the symptoms are relieved; the applications are then repeated twice or three times weekly. Vaginal absorption of excessive dosages of estrogens can produce such effects as nausea, vomiting, mastalgia, and uterine bleeding. The use of bacteriocidal agents is rarely necessary.

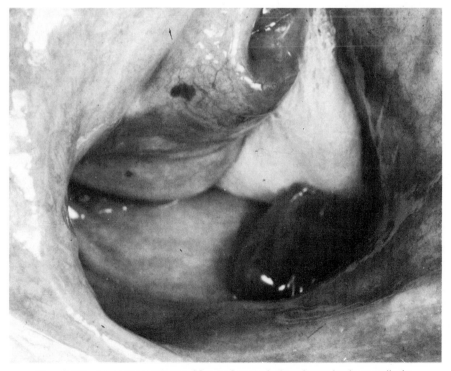

Fig. 2.12. Atrophic vaginitis. Mass of granulation tissue in the vestibule.

HERPES GENITALIS

Herpes genitalis is an acute, herpetic inflammatory disease of the genitalia, caused in most cases by the Herpes simplex virus, type 2. The incidence is much higher than is generally suspected, especially in women with vaginal infections.[20] The majority of patients with primary disease are teenage girls and unmarried women. The mean age of those with primary disease has been 26½ years, and those with recurrent disease, 36½ years.[21]

Once the infection is acquired, generally from a sexual contact,[22] symptoms of a primary attack usually appear within 3 to 7 days. Not all patients have grossly manifest lesions of the primary type, however, since the initial infection may be relatively mild. Subjects who have had extragenital type 1 infections are afforded some degree of protection against the type 2 virus. The heterologous nature of antibodies to herpes simplex viruses may well explain the many milder, even asymptomatic primary infections.

The chief symptoms consist of hyperesthesia, burning, itching, dysuria, and frequently, exquisite pain and tenderness of the vulva. Vulvar dyspareunia makes intercourse unbearable. Occasionally, urinary retention is experienced. The majority of patients have a low grade fever for several days. Primary lesions persist from 3 to 6 weeks. Unless secondarily infected, the majority will heal without any scar formation.

The primary lesions may involve the vestibule, labia minora, periclitoral fissures, the perianal skin, the vagina, and the cervix. They appear as widespread, indurated papules with red vesiculations and ulcerations (Fig. 2.13). Often they coalesce, forming bulbae and large ulcerations, perhaps involving most of the vulva and perianal skin. The persistence of the vesicular stage of the lesions is dependent upon the degree of moisture at the site; those within the labia minora will ulcerate within 24 to 48 hours. Extensive vulvar lesions may be associated with severe inflammatory reaction and varying degrees of edema, particularly in the labia minora and foreskin. Lymphadenopathy is almost always present.

Recurrences represent flareups of latent infection rather than reinfection. The fact that herpes viruses persist in the body in a dormant state and are forever subject to reactivation is no longer debated. On the basis of their studies using animal models, Stevens and Cook[23] believe unequivocally that dormant herpes virus resides in the neurons of the sensory ganglia.

The incidence of recurrent disease is unknown, although it is relatively high. The recurrent attacks are often provoked by specific physical or emotional factors, particularly at premenstrual time. Other contributing factors may be respiratory infections, fever of any origin, digestive or gastrointestinal disturbances, trauma, or exposure to sunlight.

Recurrences appear on the sites of the primary lesions (Fig. 2.14). As a rule, healing takes place within 7 to 10 days, without scar formation. Occasionally, secondary bacterial infection delays healing, giving rise to an inguinal lymphadenitis. Lymphadenopathy, however, is not uniformly associated with recurrent disease, as it is with the primary disease.

The diagnosis of herpes genitalis should always be suspected in the presence of a herpetic or superficial ulcerative condition of the vulvovaginal tissue. Cytological

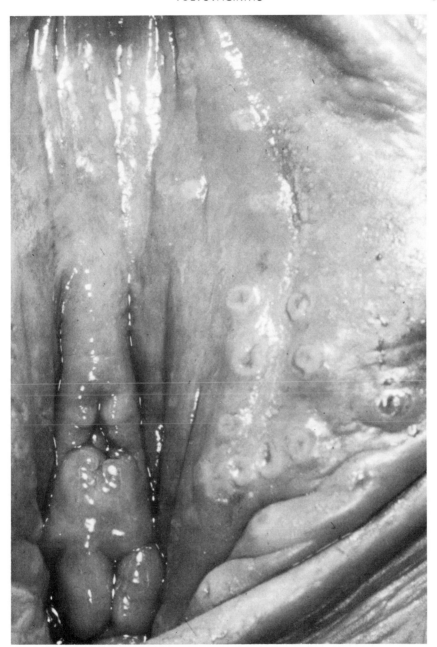

Fig. 2.13. Vesicular ulcerative lesions of primary herpes.

studies may offer confirmatory evidence of herpes simplex infection by enlargement of the nuclei and displacement of the chromatin against the nuclear
membrane. Many of the epithelial cells contain a distinct acidophilic intranuclear
body surrounded by a clear zone. Multinucleated giant cells are usually observed;
their presence in any vaginal smear should always suggest viral disease.

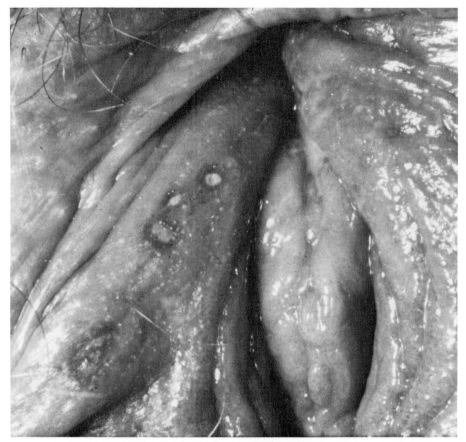

Fig. 2.14. Recurrent herpetic lesions.

Neutralizing antibodies may be demonstrated by serological methods.[24, 25] A rising titer following suspected infection is considered evidence of primary herpetic infection, whereas a high antibody titer in the acute stage, which is sustained at essentially the same level in the convalescent stage, is indicative of a recurrent infection.

The rapid course of this disease is a distinguishing feature from other vesiculoulcerative lesions of the vulva. Herpes zoster, because of its unilateral distribution, its failure to recur in the same site, its longer duration, its larger and more persistent lesions, can easily be differentiated from herpes genitalis. Herpes genitalis, however, has been confused with multiple chancres of syphilis, condylomata, vaccinia, and Behcet's syndrome.

Until recently, no specific therapy has been available for genital herpes virus infections. A promising new approach, however, is the use of photodynamic inactivation of the virus by heterotricyclic dyes, such as neutral red or proflavin.[26-28] The technique of this procedure consists of rupturing and unroofing early vesicular lesions with a sterile needle. Aqueous neutral red, 1% solution, or aqueous proflavin 0.1% solution, is applied liberally to the base of each vesicle; the lesions are then exposed to a cool white 15-watt fluorescent light or 100 watt incandescent light for 15 minutes at a distance of 6 inches. Each patient is then instructed to re-expose the lesions to fluorescent or incandescent light for 15 minutes at 6 and 18 to 24 hours later. The majority of patients who received this treatment reported that their symptoms disappeared within a matter of hours, and the course of the infection was shortened. This therapeutic procedure appears more effective for recurrent than for primary disease. Additional measures such as hot sitz bath, wet dressings, use of Burow's solution diluted to 1 to 20 parts of water, cold milk compresses, or saturated solution of boric acid may afford some relief.

The chief danger from herpes genitalis during pregnancy lies in the fact that it may be transmitted to the child in utero after premature rupture of the membranes or during delivery.[29] A patient with active herpetic lesions whose membranes have been ruptured for less than 4 hours should be delivered immediately by cesarean section.

Because of the recurrence rate and incurability of the disease, its emotional effects upon women and couples, the potential danger to the fetus during pregnancy and delivery, and its possible relationship to the genesis of cervical cancer, this infection is assuming serious consideration in clinical practice.

Controversy has arisen regarding the potential dangers of utilizing photodynamic inactivation to treat herpes virus infections. Work done by Rapp in which hamster kidney cells grown in tissue culture underwent transformation following exposure to photodynamically inactivated virus, making them capable of inducing tumor growth in other hamsters, raised a question as to whether such an inactivated virus would result in cell transformation in the human. Certainly this is a possibility. It is difficult, however, to draw conclusions about events happening in patients on the basis of what happens in immature hamster cells. Also, there is no evidence to suggest that photoinactivation of herpesvirus is more of a hazard than the recurrent herpes infections that are not treated. A characteristic of recurrent herpes lesions is that they occur in the same location. During herpesvirus replication, at least 100 defective particles are produced for each infective one. A continued and repeated assault in the same area with an abundance of defective virus produced under natural conditions may well constitute a greater risk of oncogenesis than infections in which the replication of the virus is cut short by photoinactivation. Thus, we hesitate to condemn a potentially beneficial method of treating a debilitating and potentially dangerous disease on the basis of assumptions arrived at utilizing conditions far removed from those actually seen in the patient.

CONTACT VULVOVAGINITIS

Contact vulvovaginitis is an inflammatory response to a primary irritant or allergenic substance. The majority of such responses are induced by agents intentionally applied for therapeutic or hygienic purposes. Primary irritants, i.e. those that cause an irritative response in the majority of persons upon their first exposure, may include types of vaginal sprays, bubble baths, strong detergents used in cleansing undergarments, synthetic materials used in undergarments, and scented toilet tissue. Nitrofurazone (Furacin) is associated with reactions in approximately 1% of all patients.

A cumulative primary irritation may develop after primary exposure to some varieties of intravaginal medications employed in the treatment of vaginitis. Allergic reactions usually indicate sensitization through previous exposure to an offending substance; in contrast to primary irritant reactions, allergic reactions seldom provoke clinical changes until several days or a week after contact.

Clinically, the response of a primary irritant reaction or allergic reaction may consist of erythema, edema, vesicles or bullae, and weeping. Frequently, erythema and edema are the earliest and only signs observed. Crusting may develop in the drier areas of the body; this is less likely to appear on the vulva. The majority of vulvovaginal reactions of this type do not exhibit the classic eczematoid response. Gentian violet, however, is capable of inciting eczematoid reactions in any patient if applied over a long period of time.

Oleoresins present in poison oak and poison ivy give rise to a reaction within a few hours to several days after contact, usually being transmitted by contaminated hands. This is followed within 24 to 48 hours by vesicles and bullae. An arrangement of the lesions in linear streaks is diagnostic of this condition.

The symptoms of contact vulvovaginitis may consist of varying degrees of tenderness, pain, burning, and pruritus, the last being the principal symptom. In some cases, painful lymphadenitis is associated. Urinary retention is not unusual in severe cases.

The removal of the causative agent is often followed by rapid resolution of the reaction. The use of other agents that may aggravate the eruption, such as antibiotics, should be avoided. Wet compresses, such as Burow's solution (diluted 1:20) or concentrated boric acid solution, may afford immediate relief. After 24 to 48 hours, previously weepy, tender lesions may become dry, less painful, and more suitable for the application of therapeutic creams. Flucinolone acetone (Synalar cream), hydrocortisone acetate (Cortef ointment) or Triamcinolone acetonide (Aristocort) have been proven effective. Antihistamines, such as diphenhydramine (Benadryl), although widely employed in contact dermatitis, leave much to be desired as a treatment for lesions on the vulva.

Reactions induced by a potassium permanganate burn, which formerly were observed relatively often, are now seldom encountered. When present, they appear as multiple, sharply demarcated, deep, punched-out ulcers with a characteristic brownish-black eschar over the base and immediately surrounding the mucosa. Treatment for these lesions consists of washing them with physiologic saline to eradicate the residual potassium permanganate. An analgesic may be given for pain.

In pediatric patients, vulvovaginal reactions may be attributable to poor hygiene such as failure to cleanse the perineal area in the backward direction from the vaginal orifice. At times strong medicated soaps may cause severe contact dermatitis in this age group. Foreign bodies, depending upon their shape, consistency, and chemical constituents may also provoke acute chemical irritations. Usually, the reaction will disappear following removal of the foreign body under anesthesia.

Acknowledgment. All photographs in this chapter courtesy of Dr. Herman L. Gardner.

REFERENCES

1. Krantz, KE, Innervation of the Human Vulva and Vagina, Obstet Gynecol *12:*382, 1958.
2. Gardner, HL, and Kaufman, RH, *Benign Diseases of the Vulva and Vagina*, C. V. Mosby, St. Louis, Mo, 1969.
3. Wilson, DG, Vaginal Candidiasis during Pregnancy, West J Surg Obstet Gynecol *64:*180, 1956.
4. Walsh, H, Hildebrandt RJ, and Prystowsky, H. Candidal Vaginitis Associated with the Use of Oral Progestational Agents, Am J Obstet Gynecol *93:*904, 1965.
5. Seelig, MS, Mechanism by Which Antibiotics Increase the Incidence and Severity of Candidiasis and Alter the Immunological Defenses, Bact Rev *30:*442, 1966.
6. Sloane, MD, A New Antifungal Antibiotic, Mycostatin (Nystatin), for the Treatment of Moniliasis: A Preliminary Report, J Invest Derm *24:*569, 1955.
7. The Clinical Challenge of Candidiasis—a Round Table Discussion, Ortho Pharmaceutical Corportion, Raritan, NJ, May, 1974.
8. LeChevalier, H, Acker, RF, Corke, CT, Haenseler, CM, and Waksman, SA, Candicidin, a New Antifungal Antibiotic, Mycologia *45:*155, 1953.
9. Kittleson, AR, A new class of organic fungicides, Science *115:*84, 1952.
10. Engel, MF, Amphotericin B Lotion in Monilial Intertrigo, Arch Derm *92:*687, 1965.
11. Parks, J, Diagnosis and Management of Vulvar Lesions, Med Ann DC *30:*582, 1961.
12. Gardner, HL, Trichomoniasis, Obstet. Gynecol. *19:*279, 1962.
13. Gardner, HL, and Dukes, CD, New Etiologic Agent in Nonspecific Bacterial Vaginitis, Science *19:*853, 1954.
14. Gardner, HL, and Dukes, CD, *Haemophilus vaginalis* Vaginitis, Ann NY Acad Sci *83:*280, 1959.
15. Dukes, CD, and Gardner, HL, Identification of *Haemophilus vaginalis*, J Bact *81:*277, 1961.
16. Criswell, BS, Marston, JH, Stenback, WA, Black, SH, and Gardner, HL, *Haemophilus vaginalis* 594, a Gam-negative Organism, Can J Microbiol *17:*865, 1971.
17. Criswell, BS, Stenback, WA, Black, SH, and Gardner, HL, Fine Structure of *Haemophilus vaginalis*, J Bact *109:*930, 1972.
18. Gray, LA, and Barnes, ML, Vaginitis in Women: Diagnosis and Treatment, Am J Obstet Gynecol *92:*125, 1965.
19. Gardner, HL, Desquamative Inflammatory Vaginitis: A Newly Defined Entity, Am J Obstet Gynecol *102:*1102, 1968.
20. Rawls, WE, Gardner, HL, Flanders, RW, Lowry, SP, Kaufman, RH, and Melnick, JL, Genital Herpes in Two Social Groups, Am J Obstet Gynecol *110:*682, 1971.
21. Gardner, HL, and Kaufman, RH, Herpes Genitalis: Clinical Features, Clin Obstet Gynecol *15:*896, 1972.
22. Rawls, WE, and Gardner, HL, Herpes Genitalis: Venereal Aspects, Clin Obstet Gynecol *15:*912, 1972.
23. Stevens, JG, and Cook, ML, As quoted in *Hospital Practice*, April, 1972, p. 32.
24. Nahmias, AJ, and Dowdle, WR, Antigenic and Biologic Differences in Herpes Virus Hominis, Proc Med Virol *10:*110, 1968.
25. Plummer, G, Waner, JL, Phuangsab, A, and Goodheart, CR, Type 1 and Type 2 Herpes Simplex Viruses: Serological and Biological Differences, J Virol *5:*51, 1970.
26. Wallis, C, and Melnick, JL, Photodynamic Inactivation of Animal Viruses: A Review, Photochem Photobiol *4:*159, 1965.
27. Friedrich, EG, Jr, Relief of Herpes Vulvitis, Obstet Gynecol *41:*74, 1973.
28. Kaufman, RH, Gardner, HL, Brown, D, Wallis, C, Rawls, WE, and Melnick, JL, Herpes Genitalis Treated by Photodynamic Inactivation of Virus, Am J Obstet Gynecol *117:*1144, 1973.
29. Nahmias, AJ, Josey, WE, and Naib, ZM, Significance of Herpes Simplex Virus Infection during Pregnancy, Clin Obstet Gynecol *15:*929, 1972.

3
CONTRACEPTION

PAUL F. BRENNER, M.D.

DANIEL R. MISHELL, JR., M.D.

Contraception is a temporary method for the prevention of pregnancy used by either or both sexual partners. The number of patients presenting to the physician and the number of contraceptive methods from which to choose are increasing. The social, psychologic, and economic reasons behind the demand by society for contraception are complex, but the reality is that the medical skills of providing highly effective reversible family planning techniques must be mastered by the medical community. The mechanical barrier methods of condoms, diaphragm, and spermicidal preparations and the behavioral methods of coitus interruptus and rhythm are time honored, but a demand for more effective methods not associated with the act of coitus has led to the development of the oral steroid contraceptive and the modification of the intrauterine device. Both of these methods have been accompanied by a myriad of technical and practical problems faced daily by the contraceptive practitioner.

The choice of a general method of contraception is the first decision to be made. In the majority of instances the patient comes to the physician with a particular method in mind and, if all contraindications to the proposed method can be excluded, the decision is quite easy. For those patients undecided, such factors as degree of effectiveness, untoward systemic effects, daily patient responsibility, and interruption of the sexual act are the most important. Each decision for a contraceptive method is one of compromise because there is no available method at this time which is completely effective, free of any systemic reactions, does not require patient supervision, and does not interrupt the sexual act. It is the responsibility of the contraceptive counselor to explain this compromise as well as the advantages and disadvantages of each method and in this way assist the patient in choosing a contraceptive method. When a contraindication to a method selected by the patient exists this should be clearly indicated as well as the alternatives available.

ORAL CONTRACEPTION

The oral contraceptive is the family planning method most frequently chosen by contraceptive users in the United States. Among sexually active women ages 18 to 45 in this country, 30% take the pill.[1] It is the responsibility of the medical community to identify those women for whom the hormonal formulations contained within the pill are contraindicated. Furthermore, for women who are eligible and elect to use oral contraceptives, the physician has a dual obligation to prescribe the medication with the lowest therapeutic dose and the least side effects (medication which promises the greatest patient acceptance), and then to properly monitor the patient while she is using this drug.

Patient Selection

When prescribing oral contraceptives, the physician is constantly balancing benefits versus risks.[2] There are certain situations in which the potential risks of contraception far outweigh the benefits which might be obtained. These absolute contraindications for oral contraceptives include hormone-dependent tumors, impaired liver function, thromboembolic disease, pregnancy, gestational diabetes, congenital hyperlipidemia, and severe heart disease.[3] Cancers of the breast and pelvic organs are the estrogen-dependent neoplasms of concern. Benign breast disease is not a contraindication for the use of oral contraceptives, and perhaps their use may be beneficial. Until there is more information, women with vaginal adenosis whose mothers received diethylstilbestrol during pregnancy should not use the pill. Active liver disease and a history of jaundice or pruritus of pregnancy would contraindicate use of the pill, but a past history of liver disease which is presently inactive with normal liver function does not. Thromboembolic phenomena include a past history of thrombophlebitis, deep vein thrombosis, pulmonary thrombosis, myocardial thrombosis, cerebral thrombosis, and sickle cell disease. It does not include varicose veins or sickle cell trait. Pregnancy and undiagnosed abnormal uterine bleeding which might suggest either a complication of pregnancy or possible genital malignancy negate the use of this medication. Women should not be given oral contraceptives if there is a possibility of pregnancy. The ingestion of oral contraceptives during pregnancy may increase the incidence of congenital limb reduction defects as well as cause masculinization of the external genitalia of the female fetus. There have been recorded cases where a gestational diabetic received oral contraceptives and became overtly diabetic. When the medication was discontinued, the patient remained a diabetic. Gestational diabetics should not be given the pill. Patients who are at increased risk for diabetes mellitus (obesity, delivery of an infant whose birth weight exceeded 4000 g, unexplained stillbirth, previous abnormal blood glucose levels, or family history for diabetes) should be tested for diabetes before starting a steroid contraceptive. An oral glucose tolerance test performed after 3 days of a high carbohydrate diet (6 to 8 slices of bread each day) is a practical means of screening for diabetes mellitus. Overt diabetics may be given oral contraceptives, keeping in mind that their insulin dosage may have to be adjusted. Hyperlipidemia has been correlated with the ingestion of estrogens and therefore congenital hyperlipidemia is an absolute contraindication for the use of any formulation containing estrogen. There are other conditions which are relative contraindications to the use of oral contraceptives. These include migraine headache, severe depression, hypertension, leiomyomata uteri, oligomenorrhea-amenorrhea, and epilepsy.[3]

Most patients who have migraine headaches notice an increased frequency of their attacks while taking oral contraceptives, although an occasional patient reports improvement. A patient seldom develops migraine headaches while taking the pill. Essential hypertension would be an indication to advise a nonhormonal form of contraception, although not an absolute contraindication. Progressive hypertension (malignant) is a high risk malady, and the patient should be strongly urged to avoid endogenous (pregnancy) as well as exogenous increased steroid levels. Uterine fibroids are known to increase in size as circulating levels of estrogen increase. Patients who have oligomenorrhea or amenorrhea prior to starting oral contraceptive therapy have a higher incidence of postpill amenorrhea than those with regular menses. When these medical problems are present it is preferable to counsel the patient to use another form of contraceptive other than the pill. With proper patient selection, 85% of women remain eligible to use the oral contraceptive.

Oral Contraceptive Selection

There are three types of oral hormonal contraceptive formulations available. The most common and most effective is the combination oral contraceptive, where one tablet containing both a gestational and estrogenic agent is taken daily for 21 days. In the sequential type oral contraceptive regimens, estrogen alone is given the first 14 to 16 days and a gestational agent is added to the estrogen for the last 5 to 7 days. This regimen has two major limitations. First there is inconsistent inhibition of ovulation, with a failure rate at least double that of the combination regimen, and second the sequential tablets contain a higher dosage of estrogen and, therefore, are associated with an increased incidence of adverse effects.[4] This type of formulation should not be used as a contraceptive. The third type is the minipill, with which a tablet containing gestagen only is taken by the contraceptive user every single day with the advantage that there are no estrogen effects. The gestagen-only regimen is associated with two major problems. There is frequent disruption of the menstrual cycle with episodes of both irregular bleeding and amenorrhea, and there is diminished effectiveness when compared with other oral contraceptives. The minipill has a use-pregnancy rate of 2 to 8%, probably because of the failure of this therapeutic modality to inhibit ovulation consistently.[3] Therefore, the gestagen-only type of oral contraceptive is rarely indicated and it is the combination form which is the first choice for nearly all women.

The particular combination oral contraceptive formulation to be prescribed is the one containing the lowest effective dose with an acceptable incidence of side effects. Important metabolic aberrations have been associated with exogenous estrogen administration. These alterations include increased serum triglycerides, increased plasma insulin and decreased glucose tolerance, decreased serum amino acids and albumin, and increased serum α-2 and β-globulins, increased coagulation factors, increased carrier proteins in the serum, increased free cortisol, and increased plasma renin substrate.[5] Undesirable symptomatology may result from these alterations of protein, lipid, and carbohydrate metabolism. Although these unwanted symptoms occur with some frequency serious sequelae associated with the use of oral contraceptives are relatively rare. A causal relationship between the use of oral contraceptives and thromboembolism has been established.[6, 7] There is evidence that the increased incidence of thromboembolism is related to the amount of estrogen and that formulations containing 50 μg or less of the estrogen component are associated with a reduced incidence of thromboembolism. Therefore, it is best not to prescribe pills with a greater amount of estrogen unless it becomes necessary to prevent breakthrough bleeding. It is possible that preparations containing less than 50 μg of estrogen have a lower incidence of adverse metabolic effects, but no studies have been undertaken to verify this possible benefit. Formulations containing less than 50 μg of estrogen are probably as effective as the higher dose preparations if taken consistently, but they are associated with a higher incidence of breakthrough bleeding. A few small clinical studies of sub-50-μg estrogen formulations revealed pregnancy rates less than 1 per 100 woman-years, similar to the high dose formulations. However, if a tablet is omitted, the pregnancy rate may be greater than formulations with a greater amount of steroid, as ovulation is more likely to occur when the pill is missed.[8] Definitive randomized studies to determine whether lower dose formulations have an increased pregnancy rate in actual use have not been undertaken. When intermenstrual bleeding occurs, the woman may stop taking these pills and be at risk for pregnancy.

The determination of the lowest effective dose must take into consideration potency as well as actual weight. In this respect, mestranol is less potent than ethinyl estradiol per unit weight,[9] and norethindrone and norethynodrel are the least potent, on an equal weight basis, of the five gestational agents currently in use as a component of oral contraceptives.[10] All four currently available formulations containing less than 50 μg of estrogen contain ethinyl estradiol.

When selecting a combination oral contraceptive the patient should be informed it is possible that formulations containing less than 50 μg of estrogen may have a lower incidence of adverse metabolic effects, but this benefit has not been substantiated. Furthermore, formulations composed of 50 μg of mestranol and 1 mg of norethindrone are the least potent oral contraceptives available that are not associated with an increased incidence of menstrual abnormalities. With this information the physician should probably prescribe preparations containing 50 μg of mestranol and 1 mg of norethindrone and utilize a formulation with a lower dosage of estrogen only for those women who are willing to have an increased risk of irregular bleeding for a possible but unproven metabolic benefit. Oral contraceptives are not prescribed according to a hormonal profile of the patient (estrogen dominant, large breasts and heavy menstrual flow; progesterone dominant, small breasts and scanty flow), as there is no evidence that this procedure causes a higher compliance or a lower incidence of side effects.

For the patient who has been started on the oral contraceptives by another source and is doing well, no effort is made to change the pill to meet the criterion above as long as she is not taking a daily dose of estrogen which exceeds 50 μg. Should the patient presently be taking a larger dose, an attempt should be initiated to reduce the estrogen component to 50 μg in each tablet.

Oral Contraceptives for the Adolescent

Steroid contraception should not commence until regular menstrual cycles are established. At this time the physician need no longer be concerned with iatrogenic premature epiphysial closure or disturbance of the hypothalamic-pituitary-ovarian axis.[11] The young adolescent, aged 12 to 16, has a high incidence of failure with the oral steroids. These individuals frequently forget to take the pills as directed and, in general, are not capable of performing the daily patient monitoring necessary for this method of contraception. Whenever possible other methods, particularly the condom which protects against venereal disease, or the copper intrauterine device, should be used for the young adolescent.

When to Start the Pill—After a Pregnancy

After pregnancy, there is some confusion as to the proper time to begin the pill. If the gestation ends in abortion the first menses is usually preceded by ovulation,[12] and therefore, after termination of a gestation at 12 weeks or less, the oral contraceptives should be started immediately. When a gestation is concluded between 13 and 28 weeks the oral contraceptive should be started 1 week after the termination of the pregnancy. When a pregnancy has progressed more than 12 weeks before being aborted, ovulation usually does not occur for 3 weeks or more and the risk of thromboembolic disease may be lessened by delaying 1 week before commencement of a combination oral contraceptive. For a patient who has given birth after the 28th week, oral contraceptives should be started 2 weeks after delivery. The 2-week delay reflects a compromise in an effort to reduce the incidence of postpartum thrombophlebitis, while initiating contraception before the first expected ovulation. The above statements do not apply to nursing mothers. All steroids are transferred to the breast milk,[3] and the gestagens may increase the incidence of jaundice in the newborn. Therefore it is contraindicated to give steroids to the nursing mother. If a woman who plans to nurse her newborn for a long period of time must have oral contraceptives, it is best to prescribe the mini-pill because this medication does not alter milk production or quality.

Concomitant Use of a Second Method

It is not uncommon when prescribing the pill to ask the patient to use a second contraceptive method, foam or a spermicidal jelly, during the first cycle of use. The rationale for this approach is that the patient may ovulate early in the pill cycle, before hypothalamic suppression occurs. Occasionally, a patient will ovulate before the pills are started and therefore may not have ovulation inhibited the first cycle. A second method offers added protection to this patient. It must be stressed that the effectiveness of the oral contraceptive depends on the patient taking the medication properly and that a second concomitant method is a poor substitute for patient counseling. It is necessary to use a second method during the initial cycle of oral contraceptive use.

Having identified those women for whom there are either absolute or relative contraindications for the pill and having dispensed an oral contraceptive with the lowest dosage which is both effective and associated with an acceptable level of side effects, the contraceptive practitioner still has a most important responsibility remaining—proper patient monitoring.

Breakthrough Bleeding

Breakthrough bleeding reflects insufficient estrogen stimulation to maintain the lining of the uterus. Bleeding occurring at any time during contraceptive tablet ingestion is not an indication to double the number of pills taken per day but rather to finish the cycle at the present dosage. If the uterine bleeding is too heavy, then stop the pills and consider the bleeding as an episode of menses in terms of timing future contraceptive therapy. In the next cycle increase the dosage of estrogen. Breakthrough bleeding is not considered a reason to switch to a sequential formulation. If an increase from 50 µg to 80 µg fails to eliminate the untoward bleeding, then one must individualize the therapy trying various formulations, avoiding preparations with 100 µg of ethinyl estradiol. When faced with a problem of abnormal uterine bleeding in a contraceptive user, the physician must always be cognizant of the possibility of an underlying organic cause, particularly in the older patient.

Amenorrhea

Failure of the oral contraceptive user to have withdrawal bleeding is another clinical example of insufficient estrogen priming or excessive gestagen suppression of the endometrium. If the failure to bleed unduly concerns the patient the dose of estrogen in each tablet may be increased or the amount of gestagen reduced. If the patient does not mind being amenorrheic and can be relied upon to take her medication correctly she can continue at the same dosage. Pregnancy must be excluded by proper testing, as it may be dangerous to ingest the pills when pregnant.

Postpill Amenorrhea

Postpill amenorrhea of 6 months duration or longer deserves investigation and should not simply be assumed to be the aftereffects of the pill. Postpill amenorrhea in association with galactorrhea should be investigated immediately. A number of women with this problem will be found to have pituitary tumors. The incidence of postpill amenorrhea is higher in patients who have menstrual cycle irregularities prior to starting oral contraceptive therapy than in those with regular menses.[13]

Missed Tablets

Whenever one or more tablets have been omitted the patient should be instructed to use another method for the remainder of the cycle. If bleeding has not occurred she should finish her tablets; however, should bleeding occur consider this a menses and start a new full package of tablets on the 5th day of cycle.

Nausea, Emesis, Breast Engorgement

There are several side effects, including nausea, emesis, and breast engorgement, which result from the estrogen component of the oral contraceptive. If these problems occur and are persistent this is an indication to change to a formulation containing less estrogen.

Weight Gain

There are two possible mechanisms of action to explain increased weight in oral contraceptive users. The first is fluid and electrolyte changes and the second nitrogen retention.[5] The literature is most confusing in attributing a specific component of the pill to weight gain, and most likely both components contribute to fluid retention while the progestational agent is most responsible for alteration in nitrogen balance. While some weight gain may be tolerable, the patient who gains in excess of 10 pounds should be advised to discontinue the pill and select another form of contraception.

Acne, Hirsutism

The five gestational agents presently incorporated into oral contraceptives are 19-nortestosterone derivatives, which have slight androgenic activity. Of these norethynodrel, which has a double bond in the 5–10 position of the A ring, is the most estrogenic. The gestagen increases sebum production, and the estrogen inhibits it. Therefore, patients with acne and/or hirsutism should be treated with formulations containing norethynodrel, as this formulation possesses the least androgenic activity and therefore will be least likely to exacerbate the acne and/or hirsutism.

Leg Pain, Chest Pain, Headache, Shortness of Breath

Thromboembolic disease is a life-threating situation. Both retrospective and prospective studies have indicated that estrogen is one factor which increases patient risk for this most serious process. If the patient using oral contraceptives has clinical evidence of deep vein thrombosis there is no question but to stop the steroid medication and to begin appropriate therapy without delay. Any oral contraceptive user presenting with leg pain must be examined with the diagnosis of deep vein thrombosis in mind. All pill users complaining of chest pain, with or without evidence of deep vein thrombosis, should stop the oral contraceptive therapy. An electrocardiogram, chest x-ray, and lung scan must be considered in order to clarify the possibility of a pulmonary embolus. Pulmonary emboli can occur without clinical evidence of deep vein thrombosis. Sudden onset of chest pain and persistent chest pain are ominous symptoms which are in themselves indications for immediately stopping hormonal therapy. Similarly, headaches which are of sudden onset or of a persistent nature are an indication to stop oral contraceptive regimens until their relationship, if any, to the therapy can be ascertained. Nowhere in the monitoring of pill users is clinical judgment more important than for those women who complain of leg pain, chest pain, shortness of breath, or headaches. The possibility of thromboembolic phenomena must always be considered. If there is any uncertainty it is best to act in behalf of patient safety and discontinue the medication until any possible relationship between the oral contraceptive and the symptomatology can be decided.

Elective Surgery

Any estrogen-containing formulation should be terminated 1 month prior to planned surgery to lessen the incidence of postoperative thrombophlebitis.

Monilia Vaginitis

While some oral contraceptive users develop leukorrhea consistent with monilia vaginitis, only a small number will have altered carbohydrate metabolism. Should the monilia infection either fail to respond to appropriate therapy or reoccur, then an elevation in blood glucose levels should be excluded. Although several reports indicate an increase of vaginitis, particularly moniliasis, in pill users, one prospective study has shown that contraceptive steroids do not cause an increased incidence of monilia vaginitis.[14]

Other Symptoms

There are many other untoward effects which have been reported by women using the pill. These symptoms include nervousness, irritability, fatigue, alopecia, and pruritus. If the symptomatology is marked then the patient should be advised to discontinue the medication. Oftentimes, when the complaints are less bothersome, either reassurance or changing preparations is all that is necessary. An etiology for these symptoms other than the steroid ingestion must be excluded. The patient presenting with any of the above symptoms may be indirectly attempting to relate that she really does not wish to take the pill, and appropriate questioning will clarify the problem. Many of these so-called minor side effects will disappear if the patient is reassured and is willing to continue the therapeutic regimen.

Patient Monitoring

Before starting a woman on oral contraceptives, at the conclusion of the first few cycles of medication, and at least annually thereafter the patient should be properly screened. This evaluation includes a history, breast examination, blood pressure, weight, abdominal examination, pelvic examination, Papanicolaou smear, and SMA 12. This is a minimum in terms of both the number of times the patient is seen and the laboratory tests utilized.

When to Conceive

When the decision is made to stop the oral contraceptives for a planned pregnancy the patient will often inquire how long she should wait before attempting to conceive. There is an increase of chromosomal aberrations in specimens from spontaneous abortions occurring in the first few cycles after discontinuing oral contraceptives. There is no evidence for an increased incidence of abortion in these cycles. The patient should also be advised that there may be a delay in the return of ovulation. Whether or not to delay conception in the first few cycles after stopping the pill remains controversial.

Rest Period

Approximately one-fifth of all oral contraceptive users who discontinue their medication do so on the advice of their physician. The rationale is to give the patient a rest period from the steroid therapy of several months every few years to lower the incidence of untoward metabolic effects. It should be stressed that there is no scientific basis for this decision and there is a high incidence of unwanted pregnancy. There is no evidence that the rest period offers any advantage to the oral contraceptive user, and this practice must be discouraged.

The Age to Stop the Oral Contraceptive

There is a definite decline in a woman's fertility between the ages of 40 to 45 and a rather marked decline in the next 5 years. Past the age of 40 the woman's need for a potent ovulatory suppressor decreases, the possibility that steroid medication may confuse the clinical appearance of organic pelvic disease increases, and her risk for thromboembolic disease increases. For these reasons women who are 40 or older should be encouraged to cease using oral contraceptives and select some other method, including sterilization. This is not an absolute dictum, and individualization of advice is mandatory. Should the patient elect to continue the oral contraceptives into her late forties, at age 50 they should be stopped and one month later the serum level of follicle-stimulating hormone should be determined. Until the level of this protein hormone exceeds 40 to 50 milli-International Units per ml, indicating ovarian failure, some form of contraception must be recommended.

INTRAUTERINE CONTRACEPTIVE DEVICE

The intrauterine contraceptive device (IUD) is one of the older methods of contraception. Although used only by an estimated 8% of women, the intrauterine device has shown the greatest percentage increase in selection by contraceptive users of this country in the last 5 years, and is now selected as frequently as the oral contraceptive among wives of obstetricians.[1]

Patient Selection

There are definite contraindications to the placement of an intrauterine device. These include pregnancy, pelvic infection (septic abortion or postpartum endometritis, pelvic inflammatory disease, or tubo-ovarian abcess in the past 3 months), distortion of the uterine cavity (congenital anomaly or submucus fibroid), a uterine cavity sounding <5 cm in depth, carcinoma of the endometrium, or a history of abnormal uterine bleeding. Anemia must be considered at least a relative contraindication to the use of an IUD.

Device Selection

At present there are three intrauterine devices available for use in the United States, the loop, double coil, and copper 7. Distribution of the Dalkon Shield has been stopped by its manufacturer. The Lippes Loop and Saf-T-Coil have a mechanism of action which depends on their size and shape. The Copper 7 is smaller and serves as a carrier system for an additional contraceptive agent. The plastic devices without copper have the advantage that they do not require periodic removal and reinsertion and the disadvantages of a greater amount of blood loss when compared to copper IUD's.[15] The copper devices are associated with much less pain during and after their insertion. They are especially suitable for nulliparous women who have a high incidence of removal for pain with other devices.[16, 17] In selecting an intrauterine device for the multiparous patient, the greater blood loss associated with the loop and Saf-T-Coil must be balanced against the need for periodic removal of the copper-containing devices.

Method of Insertion

A bimanual examination is performed first, with special attention to the size and position of the uterus. Evidence of pregnancy, pelvic infection, and irregularity in the shape of the uterus are specifically considered. A speculum examination is performed next, and a Papanicolaou smear is obtained. Using sterile gloves, the

IUD is placed inside the inserter. A tenaculum is applied to the upper lip of the cervix and the uterine cavity[13] sounded to determine its depth. If the cavity is less than 5 cm insertion should not be attempted. The IUD, contained within an inserter, is placed in the uterine lumen to a depth previously determined from the sound and the IUD is released. The tenaculum is held under constant tension during the insertion to ensure as straight an alignment of the uterus as possible; marked tension causes vagal reflex. The placement of the IUD may be effected by two methods. The first is the expulsion method, wherein the IUD is dislodged from a fixed inserter by a forward motion of the plunger. Intrauterine devices that are contained within an inserter sheath with a fixed hood, such as the loop, must be placed by this method. The second, the withdrawal method, involves retraction of a mobile hood on the inserter approximately 10 cm so that it does not limit the placement of the IUD. The inserter containing the IUD is then used as a sound and is inserted into the uterine cavity until the top of the fundus is reached. The plunger is then held fixed with the first finger and thumb of one hand and the inserter sheath is retracted with the third and fourth fingers of the same hand over the plunger. This ensures a consistent high fundal position. After insertion, all instruments are removed and the patient is again examined bimanually to ascertain any evidence for malplacement of the device. When possible, the withdrawal method is preferred as this allows the device to be placed at the top of the fundus irrespective of the depth of the uterine cavity.

These methods allow for the insertion of most devices. Occasionally, a uterus is so sharply flexed that with a rigid inserter and plunger placement of the device is not possible. In these instances a copper device may be used with a malleable loop inserter, which has been separately sterilized, to achieve proper placement.

Timing of Insertion

Whenever possible it is preferable to insert an intrauterine device during the egress of menses. This is done not because it is technically easier to perform the procedure at this time but because the patient will be less concerned with any increased bleeding which might occur. And one is less likely to be placing an IUD in an early pregnant uterus if insertion is coordinated with the menstrual flow.

With respect to the insertion of an IUD subsequent to a recent gestation, the IUD should be inserted immediately after a first trimester abortion[18] and 2 weeks after a second trimester abortion. Postpartum, a delay of 6 weeks is recommended in order to minimize the risk of both uterine perforation and increased expulsion. Both these events occur with greater frequency when placement of an intrauterine device is undertaken soon after delivery.[19]

Concomitant Use of a Second Method

It is helpful for the patient to use a supplemental method of contraception for the first month after insertion of an intrauterine device. This method should not be one that may cause either uterine bleeding or pelvic pain. IUD users are instructed to use foam for the initial month only. If the patient is presently using oral contraceptives without bleeding problems but wishes to change to an IUD, she is advised to continue the oral medication, if there is no other contraindication, for the first month of use of the device. Use of the combination of these two methods for any other reason or for any longer period of time is not advised. It only compounds and confuses the diagnostic possibilities of untoward reactions.

Patient Followup

The patients are routinely re-examined at 3 months postinsertion and annually thereafter. Breast and pelvic examinations, cytosmear, and complete blood counts are performed at the yearly visits. More frequent visits are necessitated for the investigation of any untoward reaction the IUD user may experience.

Perforation

Perforation of the nonpregnant uterus with an IUD is estimated to be 1 per 1,000 insertions with the loop and 1 per 350 insertions with the Copper 7. When it occurs it is usually at the time of insertion. The dangers to the patient include possible bowel obstruction, bowel perforation, pelvic infection and formation of multiple dense adhesions. Extrauterine closed devices must be removed as soon after detection of the ectopic location as possible, as they place the patient at risk for a bowel obstruction. The Dalkon Shield should be removed immediately, as very dense adhesions of the pelvic and/or intestinal structures form around it. The copper-bearing devices must be quickly removed as the copper is most tissue-reactive and one copper device has been reported to have perforated a loop of bowel. In the past physicians were less committed to early retrieval of the ectopic loop or double coil unless specifically requested by the patient. Recently, however, there have been reports of extrauterine loops surrounded by dense adhesions, pelvic infections, and bowel injury. Thus it is now recommended that all extrauterine IUD's be removed soon after the diagnosis is established.

The availability of devices with a straight vertical limb has led to another complication, cervical embedment. In an apparent attempt by the uterus to expel a device of this design, occasionally the vertical stem of the device is pushed into the wall of the cervix. As a result the device is embedded deep into the cervix or, in the extreme case, the device actually perforates through the cervix, usually the posterior lip. The risk of cervical perforation with the copper 7 is 1 per 500. When examining wearers of copper IUD's, the cervix must be palpated very carefully with this possible problem kept in mind. If an embedded device is detected it is recommended to remove it as follows. Under paracervical block the cervical canal is dilated. Frequently, the dilator as it impinges upon the junction of the vertical and horizontal limbs of the device will dislodge the device from the wall of the cervix and then the device can be removed through the cervical canal. Should the dilator fail to dislodge the device then a narrow forceps should be used for this purpose. The procedure of extracting the device through the cervical wall is not advised. This needlessly damages tissue and creates a direct fistulous tract for the entrance of bacteria into the endometrial cavity. If the patient desires another IUD she is asked to wait at least 60 days before reinsertion and a device of a different design is selected.

Expulsion

When the intrauterine device is found in the vaginal vault or the tip of the device is visualized on speculum examination or palpated during bimanual examination, the diagnosis of a partial or complete expulsion is confirmed. This possibility must also be considered for every patient who indicates that she or her partner feel the tip of the device, or who complains of pelvic pain or increased bleeding, or who believes the string suddenly feels longer. In all of these situations the cervical canal should be sounded in an attempt to palpate the tip of the device with the end of the sound if the device is not seen or palpated manually. If the device is found to be partially expelled it is not capable of rendering the contraceptive effect it was intended for and it must be removed. Some 20% of IUD expulsions are unnoticed by the users, and it is estimated that one-third of all pregnancies occurring in IUD users follow an unnoticed expulsion.[3] Younger age, low parity, and small devices are all factors associated with an increased frequency of expulsion. A patient indicating that the IUD remains her first choice as a contraceptive method after an expulsion may have the same device inserted again. Should this be expelled, a third insertion may be performed as a final attempt to provide this method of contraceptive for the patient.

Missing Strings

A rather frequent complaint of IUD users is inability to locate the strings, particularly during the period just after insertion. A speculum examination may be all that is necessary to visualize the strings. When the strings are not detected, the possibilities are that the device has been completely expelled unnoticed by the patient, that the device and strings are located within the uterine cavity, or that the device has perforated the wall of the uterus. Any suggestive signs or symptoms of pregnancy should be investigated with appropriate tests. If pregnancy is excluded, further diagnostic procedures should proceed as follows. The uterine cavity should be sounded with the possibility of detecting the device by this method. If the device is located and the patient desires removal, an attempt is made to remove the device with a hook or endometrical biopsy instrument, which is usually successful. Should this fail the device is preferably removed by hysteroscopy or, if this technique is not available, the device should be removed by dilatation and blind instrumentation. In those instances where the device is not located by the sound, an X-ray of the abdomen and pelvis is obtained. A device not seen by roentgenography is assumed to have been completely expelled unnoticed by the user. If the device is seen in the pelvis, then either by placing a sound in the uterus and taking anteroposterior and lateral x-ray views of the pelvis or by a hysterogram it is determined whether the device is intra- or extrauterine. The intrauterine located device may be left in place if desired by the patient or else removed as described above. Ectopically located devices in the cul-de-sac may be retrieved by colpotomy. The other ectopically situated devices may be removed by laparoscopy or else by laparotomy.

Strings Too Long

This complaint may originate from either sexual partner, and the strings can be cut shorter. Trimming strings to the external os frequently results in the retraction of the strings within the endometrial cavity with the concomitant problem of missing strings. It is not recommended to trim the appendages of the device shorter than 1 inch, as very short strings, although visible, may act as rigid needles. The complaint of the IUD strings being too long should alert the physician to the possibility of partial expulsion of the device and the appropriate investigation conducted.

Pregnancy

Although a highly effective method, most intrauterine devices are associated with a 1 to 2% pregnancy rate per year. When pregnancy occurs after the IUD has been removed, intentionally or unintentionally, the pregnancy may be managed irrespective of the previous presence of the IUD. When pregnancy occurs with the IUD still in situ then the device should be removed if the threads are visible. If the threads are not visible and the patient elects to continue the pregnancy, the device may be left in place if it is not a Dalkon Shield. In pregnancy, IUD's are not situated within the amniotic cavity or in direct association with the fetus.[3] They should not be considered a danger to the fetus, although the incidence of abortion is increased.[20] The one exception to this management is the Dalkon Shield. If this device cannot be removed easily the pregnancy should be terminated. There is a hazard of pelvic infection associated with this device which is sometimes fatal. In contrast to other devices the Dalkon Shield has a multifilament tail which allows bacteria to enter the uterine cavity by a wick-like activity.[21] Thus, it is recommended that all Dalkon Shields be removed if associated with pregnancy.

The IUD user who has an accidental pregnancy with the device in utero must be advised that there is a 50% chance for spontaneous abortion. There is an increased opportunity for an ectopic pregnancy. This is not to be interpreted to mean that the IUD is a causative factor for ectopic pregnancy. The Comparative Statistical Program, having accumulated 244,000 woman-months of IUD experience, revealed that the IUD prevents intrauterine pregnancy at a rate of 97–98% and that the IUD prevents ectopic pregnancy at a rate of 90%. The patient pregnant with an IUD has a 1:20 chance of an ectopic pregnancy.[3] In summary the IUD is effective in preventing ectopic pregnancy but not as effective as it is in preventing intrauterine gestations. Patients with therapeutic abortions should have the evacuated products examined histologically to ascertain that an intrauterine gestation was present.

Bleeding and Pain

The most common reason for terminating the use of the intrauterine device is bleeding and pain. These events account for more than 50% of all terminations.[3] That the symptoms are related to the device is determined by first excluding all other causes. Pelvic examination, sounding the cervix, and appropriate laboratory tests are undertaken. Depending on the patient's age, further procedures to exclude malignancy may be required. If the device is believed to be the offending agent, the decision whether to remove the device or leave it in situ will depend on the severity of the symptoms and the length of time since the device was inserted. In the first 3 months increased bleeding (number of days) and cramping are rather common, and the patient should be advised accordingly at the time of insertion. If the pain can be controlled by mild (non-narcotic) analgesics and if the device was inserted less than 3 months before or if the pain is associated only with menses and can be controlled with the same analgesics, then the patient is encouraged to continue using the IUD. It is not reasonable to mask pelvic pain with narcotics, and rather than this choice the device should be removed. Similarly, if excessive bleeding occurs which does not result in anemia and which occurs in the first 3 months of IUD use or occurs once a year or less often, then the patient is again reassured and encouraged to continue using the IUD. Abnormal uterine bleeding of a greater magnitude than described above should be considered an indication for removal of the IUD.

Blood Loss

Blood loss may be a rather insidious problem for the users of intrauterine devices. Marked alterations in hemoglobin concentration and iron stores may occur and yet the patient or physician may be unaware of this change. It has been reported that IUD users have significantly greater average menstrual blood loss when compared to a control group of noncontraceptive users, while the selectors of the oral contraceptive have a marked reduction in average menstrual blood loss when compared to the same controls. In a normal menstrual cycle about 35 ml of blood are lost. Oral contraceptive users lose about 20 ml of blood each cycle, while in women wearing a coil or a loop, about 70 to 80 ml of blood are lost and in those wearing a Copper T, 50 to 60 ml are lost per cycle.[22] Nevertheless, studies have shown that hemoglobin and hematocrit levels are unaltered for nearly all IUD users. The contraceptive counselor should determine hemoglobin concentrations annually in users of the IUD and prescribe supplemental iron when it is indicated.

Infection

There are three reasons to suspect that an intrauterine device can be the source of a bacterial infection, which may invade the upper genital tract. First, IUDs of the preantibiotic era were associated with serious pelvic infections and their sequelae. Second, the endocervical mucus, which is known to harbor bacteria, must be traversed in the insertion of the device. Third, most IUDs have an appendage which potentially is a conduit from the nonsterile vagina to the endometrial cavity. Transfundal culture studies revealed that the endometrial cavity was nearly always sterile even with the loop in place, provided more than 24 hours had elapsed since insertion, and was always sterile more than 1 month after loop insertion.[23] Culture of the threads in utero indicated that they did not serve as a conduit for the passage of bacteria, with the important exception of the multifilament tail of the Dalkon Shield. Breaks in the sheath of the tail have been demonstrated in 34% of Dalkon Shields recovered from patients.[21] Bacteria situated between the filaments may gain entrance to the endometrial cavity through these breaks, and it is therefore best that these devices be removed from all patients, nonpregnant as well as pregnant. It appears that the risk of initiating an upper genital tract infection after insertion of a loop is slight, and this risk is limited to the first month after insertion of the device. If pelvic inflammatory disease occurs in a wearer of an IUD later than 30 days after insertion, it is unlikely that the device is the initiating offender. Therefore, treatment with antibiotics should begin without removal of the device, unless a tubo-ovarian abscess is present. Should an abscess be present or should the patient fail to respond at any time in the course of antibiotic therapy (ampicillin 0.5 g every 6 hours for 10 days) then the patient should be hospitalized, the device removed, and increased antibiotic therapy begun.

Neurovascular Sequelae

Symptoms of syncope, diaphoresis, pallor, weakness, lethargy, tachycardia, and convulsions have all been noted to occur during or immediately after IUD insertion and, more rarely, after removal of an IUD.[24] These symptoms occur most frequently in nulliparous women and with the insertion of a rigid device. The use of a smaller copper device has reduced the incidence of these side effects to less than 1%. Either pain or direct uterine stretch reflexes may initiate this vagal response. Most often the symptoms subside before any therapy is prescribed. Occasionally, removal of the device may be necessary to alleviate the vagal symptomatology, and very rarely atropine, 0.1 mg administered intravenously, may be necessary. Most important, these reactions may be delayed in their appearance after the insertion procedure and, therefore, it is necessary to retain the patient for observation for at least 30 minutes after the insertion of the device.

Method of Removal

Most often removal of the intrauterine device is accomplished quite easily by gentle traction on the appendage. Removal may be performed at any time in the menstrual cycle with the appropriate warning being given that the patient no longer has contraceptive protection until a new method is initiated. Infrequently one may encounter difficulty in removing an IUD. This should be heeded as a warning signal and all efforts to remove the device stopped, as the device may be embedded in the wall of the uterus or may have perforated the uterus. A hysterogram should be performed to ascertain whether the device is penetrating or perforating the uterine wall. Perforating devices must be removed under direct vision as outlined under the section "missing strings." If the device is within the endometrial cavity firmer traction may be applied to the appendage or the device may be removed by instrumentation, preferably the hysteroscope.

SPECIAL SITUATION: CONTRACEPTION FOR THE PATIENT WITH SIGNIFI-CANT CARDIAC DISEASE

The selection of a contraceptive method for the cardiac patient presents a rather difficult compromise. The danger of a pregnancy in these women must be balanced against an additional crisis created by the undesired side effects of a contraceptive method.[25] The homeostatic mechanisms of these patients are already severely challenged and a contraceptive crisis may be all that is needed to precipitate an acute, life-threatening situation. The following recommendations are offered: (1) Formulations containing 50 μg or more of estrogen (combination oral contraceptive, combination parenteral contraceptives, sequential oral contraceptives, the "morning-after" pill) should be strictly avoided. (2) Conventional methods of contraception (diaphragm, condom, foam) may be offered with careful consideration of their lowered use effectiveness. (3) Insertion of an intrauterine contraceptive device with antibiotic treatment poses little risk. If the intrauterine contraceptive device is selected for the cardiac patient she should receive prophylactic antibiotics for at least 72 hours to prevent septicemia and subacute bacterial endocarditis. A reasonable therapeutic regimen would be 1.2 million units of Procaine Penicillin and 0.5 g of streptomycin given intramuscularly 1 hour before the time of insertion and penicillin VK 250 mg orally every 6 hours for 3 days. If the patient has a prosthetic cardiac valve she should continue the streptomycin every 12 hours for six doses.

CONDOM

The National Fertility Society in 1970 surveyed the family planning method used by married women living with their husbands. The use of condoms, 14.2%, was third only to oral contraceptives, 34.2%, and sterilization of either partner, 16.3%.

The theoretical effectiveness of the condom, 2.6 pregnancies per 100 woman-years, compares very favorably with some of the intrauterine devices currently being used and, except for local irriation and (very rarely) allergy, the condom is free from systemic or local effects. The drawbacks to the use of condoms relate to the necessity of patient monitoring of the method and interference with coitus. These two factors render the condom an inconvenient method and account for the relatively poor use-effectiveness, 17 pregnancies per 100 woman-years, when compared to either the oral contraceptive or the IUD.

It is important to provide proper instruction for the use of condoms which include (1) apply the condom before attempting vaginal penetration, (2) cover the entire length of the erect penis with the condom, (3) leave a reservoir to retain the ejaculate, (4) use adequate lubrication to prevent tearing of the condom or vaginal irritation, and (5) hold the condom against the base of the penis and withdraw the penis and condom simultaneously before the penis becomes flaccid.[26]

There is a specific situation where the condom is the method of contraception of first choice. This is for the woman with multiple sexual partners. Here the risk of veneral disease is high, and the condom is the contraceptive method which offers maximum protection for the user as well as his partner against venereal disease.

DIAPHRAGM

The diaphragm has a favorable theoretical effectiveness, 2.5 pregnancies per 100 women-years similar to that of the intrauterine device and condom. This contraceptive method is free of untoward systemic effects and does not have to involve coital interference. On the other hand, the practical efficacy of the diaphragm relies heavily on proper patient monitoring of the method, which requires both a high degree of motivation and some manual dexterity in mastering the technique of insertion. It is the problems related to these latter factors which explain the use effectiveness of 18 pregnancies per 100 woman-years of use of the diaphragm.[26]

The properly fitting diaphragm will fit just posteriorly to the symphysis pubis and deep into the cul-de-sac so that the cervix is completely covered and preferably behind the center of the membrane. The largest diaphragm which fills this space comfortably is selected. If too small a diaphragm is selected, there is a possibility of pregnancy. The arching diaphragm is preferable for those women with an anteverted uterus.

The fittings are performed with the diaphragm and not the rings. In this manner, the patient learns proper placement and amount of jelly to use, avoids insertion of the diaphragm with the membrane arched in the wrong direction, and allows for instruction in palpating the cervix behind the membrane. The patient is instructed in the necessity of placing the spermicidal jelly in the center of the diaphragm as well as along the edge. This affords the added protection of having a spermicidal agent over the cervix. The patient at least twice removes and inserts the diaphragm and is examined vaginally by the instructor after each insertion to ascertain proper placement. The patient is taught that if the diaphragm is correctly situated, the upper edge is posterior to the symphysis as determined by palpation, the cervix is behind the diaphragm as determined by palpation, and the diaphragm is not uncomfortable when the patient is walking.

The patient is instructed to leave the diaphragm in place for a minimum of 8 hours following coitus. Another instillation of spermicidal jelly into the vagina is indicated when the diaphragm has been placed more than 6 hours prior to coitus. An additional placement of spermicide is recommended for each coitus which occurs before the diaphragm is removed. Highly motivated, correctly fitted, and properly instructed patients find the diaphragm an acceptable means of contraception.

Having attempted to answer the most common questions pertaining to the contraceptive methods commonly available one cannot help but be aware of the temporal relevance of this work. There continues to be clinical testing of new dosages for the hormonal preparations already available. More important are the development of other routes of administration of these formulations, including intravaginal rings, intrauterine devices, subdermal implants, and long acting injectibles. An impressive number of new IUDs are being tested, as well as an intracervical device. The amount and diversity of research and development presently being undertaken with respect to contraception will continue to expand the magnitude and complexities of the services offered by the practitioner of contraception.

REFERENCES

1. Westoff, CF, The Modernization of U.S. Contraceptive Practice, Fam Plan Perspect 4:9, 1972.
2. Hellman, LM, The Oral Contraceptive in Clinical Practice, Fam Plan Perspect, 1:13, 1969.
3. Mishell, DR, Jr, Current Status of Contraceptive Steroids and Intrauterine Device, Clin Obstet Gynecol 17:35, 1974.
4. Feldman, JG, and Lippes, J, A Four-year Comparison between the Utilization and Use-effectiveness of Sequential and Combined Oral Contraceptives, Contraception 3:93, 1971.
5. *Human Reproduction, Conception and Contraception*, Hafez, ESE, and Evans, TN, Eds., Harper and Row, New York, 1973.
6. Vessey, MP, and Doll, R, Investigation of Relation between Use of Oral Contraceptives and Thromboembolic Disease: A Further Report, Brit Med J 2:651, 1969.
7. *Oral Contraceptives and Health: An Interim Report from the Oral Contraceptive Study of the Royal College of General Practitioners*, Pitman Publishing, New York, 1974.
8. Preston, SN, A Report of a Collaborative Dose-Response Clinical Study Using Decreasing Doses of Combination Oral Contraceptives, Contraception 6:17, 1972.
9. Delforge, JP, and Ferrin, J, A Histometric Study of Two Estrogens: Ethinyl-Estradiol and its 3-Methyl-ether Derivative (Mestranol): Their Comparative Effect upon the Growth of the Human Endometrium, Contraception 1:57, 1970.
10. Greenblatt, RB, Progestational Agents in

Clinical Practice, Med Sci *10:*37, 1967.

11. Frisch, RE, and Nagel, JS, Prediction of Adult Height of Girls from Age of Menarche and Height at Menarche, J Ped *85:*838, 1974.

12. Vorherr, H, Contraception after Abortion and Post-partum, Am J Obstet Gynecol *117:*1002, 1973.

13. Shearman, RP, Secondary Amenorrhea after Oral Contraceptives: Treatment and Follow-up, Contraception *11:*123, 1975.

14. Spellacy, WN, Zaias, N, Bahi, WC, and Birk, SA, Vaginal Yeast Growth and Contraceptive Practices, Obstet Gynecol *38:*342, 1971.

15. Israel, R, Shaw, ST, and Martin, MA, Comparative Quantitation of Menstrual Blood Loss with the Lippes Loop, Dalkon Shield and Copper T Intrauterine Devices, Contraception *10:*63, 1974.

16. Mishell, DR, Jr, Israel, R, and Freid, N, A Study of the Copper T Intrauterine Contraceptive Device (TCu 200) in Nulliparous Women, Am J Obstet Gynecol *116:*1092, 1973.

17. Roy, S, Cooper, D, and Mishell, DR, Jr, Experience with Three Different Models of the Copper T Intrauterine Contraceptive Device in Nulliparous Women, Am J Obstet Gynecol *119:*414, 1974.

18. Boyd, EF, Jr, and Holstrom, EG, Ovulation following Therapeutic Abortion, Am J Obstet Gynecol *113:*469, 1973.

19. Tietze, C, Contraception with Intrauterine devices, Am J Obstet Gynecol *96:*1043, 1966.

20. Lewit, S, Outcome of Pregnancy with Intrauterine Devices, Contraception *2:*47, 1970.

21. Tatum, HJ, Schmidt, FH, and Phillips, DM, Morphological Studies of Dalkon Shield Tails Removed from Patients, Contraception *11:*465, 1975.

22. Hefnawi, F, Askalani, H, and Zaki, K, Menstrual Blood Loss with Copper Intrauterine Devices, Contraception *3:*133, 1974.

23. Mishell, DR, Jr, Bell, JH, Good, RG, and Moyer, DL, The Intrauterine Device: Bacteriologic Study of the Intrauterine Cavity, Am J Obstet Gynecol *96:*199, 1966.

24. Conrad, CC, Ghazi, M, and Kitay, DZ, Acute Neurovascular Sequelae of Intrauterine Device Insertion or Removal, J Reprod Med *11:*211, 1973.

25. Brenner, PF, and Mishell, DR, Jr, Contraception for the Woman with Significant Cardiac Disease, Clin Obstet Gynecol, *18:* 155, 1975.

26. Bernstein, GS, Conventional Methods of Contraception: Condom, Diaphragm and Vaginal Foam, Clin Obstet Gynecol *17:*21, 1974.

4

ASPIRATION ABORTION IN AN OFFICE SETTING

ALAN J. MARGOLIS, M.D.

SADJA BREWSTER GOLDSMITH, M.D., M.P.H.

INTRODUCTION

Physicians involved in women's health care are aware of the recurrent problem of unwanted pregnancy. The need for abortion services in the United States is likely to rise to 1 to 2 million procedures per year, or over 500 abortions per 1000 live births. First-trimester aspiration abortions can be seen as relatively simple minor surgical procedures which are suitable for a well equipped office setting. Such procedures should be available locally at a reasonable cost in all rural as well as urban communities.

SAFETY AND FEASIBILITY OF THE OFFICE SETTING

There is ample evidence that first trimester abortions can safely be performed outside the hospital operating room. The Joint Program for the Study of Abortion (JPSA)[1] showed that aspiration abortions performed in clinics had somewhat fewer complications than those in hospitals. Such clinics have provided counseling, contraception, and the abortion procedure at low cost in a reassuring, informal atmosphere. A well equipped medical office can function in the same way. Data comparable to the JPSA study are not available for abortion in the doctor's office. However, since the United States Supreme Court decision of January, 1973, makes first trimester abortions legal in any location, it is clear that increasing numbers are being carried out in the office setting. A review of 1973 mortality figures from the State of California[2] and the Abortion Surveillance Unit of the Center for Disease Control[3] show a sustained low death rate which testifies to the safety of first trimester abortions in various settings.

PROS AND CONS OF THE OFFICE SETTING FOR ABORTION

There are advantages to the patient and physician in performing early abortions in the office. The patient benefits from the lower cost and greater privacy of the office setting as compared to the hospital. She will be in a more familiar and reassuring environment, helped by people who can be selected for their empathy and reassurance. She can be cared for in one visit. The doctor is able to schedule cases for his/her convenience, avoiding the delays of the operating room. Many doctors choose to see abortion patients at special times in their office because of the longer time they and their staff may spend with this group.

Problems of the office setting include the need for the purchase, maintenance, and sterilization of equipment to perform abortions. If substantial difficulties arise during a procedure, it is less convenient to be in an office than a hospital with its backup services. However, serious problems are rare if patients are adequately screened (see below), and if there is a plan for the transfer of the patient to a hospital in an emergency.

CONTRAINDICATIONS TO OFFICE ABORTION

While most women with early pregnancies can be aborted in the office, an occasional patient requires hospitalization. Some women demand or obviously need a general anesthetic because of intense anxiety and inability to tolerate the abortion procedure under local anesthesia. Individuals with musculoskeletal deformities may be acutely uncomfortable in the lithotomy position. Abnormalities of the vagina, cervix, or uterus may require too much manipulation to be tolerable by the conscious patient. A history of allergy to local anesthetics may make paracervical block unwise.

Well controlled chronic diseases (diabetes, blood dyscrasias, epilepsy, or rheumatic or congenital heart disease) are generally not contraindications to local anesthesia or office abortion. However, if any of the foregoing problems are acute, the patient may require hospitalization. In addition, any patient with a serious systemic illness requiring steroids, antibiotics, anticoagulation, or close observation should be hospitalized for abortion.

EQUIPMENT FOR OFFICE ABORTION

Vacuum Sources

A standard pump for abortions, generating a vacuum of 60 to 70 torr, is extremely convenient and generally used for abortion procedures. Alternate nonelectric sources of vacuum, such as the specially adapted 50-ml syringe, are occasionally used for very early first trimester abortions (up to 7 weeks from last menstrual period (LMP) or menstrual regulation procedures. However, a standard pump with at least a 500-cc receptacle should be available as a backup to the syringe, in case the volume of blood and tissue obtained makes the use of the syringe awkward or time consuming.

A basic tray for first trimester abortions should include the following sterile instruments:

Bivalve speculum
Ring forceps and cotton balls (to cleanse the cervix and vagina with povidone-iodine solution)
Tenaculum (single tooth or atraumatic)
10-ml syringe and a 22-gauge 3½ inch spinal needle (for the paracervical block)
Malleable uterine sound

Tapered cervical dilators (Pratt, Hanks, or Hawkins-Ambler)
Small, sharp curette
Polyp forceps

Suction cannulas and connecting tubing are available in various sizes and types: flexible or stiff, plastic or metal, straight or curved. We favor the use of flexible Karman cannulas for early procedures because they require minimal cervical dilation and may lessen the risk of uterine perforation. A 6-mm cannula can be used in pregnancies up to 9 weeks from last menstrual period; an 8-mm cannula can be used up to 11 weeks from LMP. The flexible cannulas are also available in 10-mm diameter size. For a more advanced gestation, a wide-mouthed 12-mm stiff plastic cannula is advisable to permit the passage of fetal parts and the larger placenta.

Laminaria can be inserted to eliminate forcible dilation of the cervix when a cannula of 9 to 12-mm in diameter is to be used. The prior insertion (8 to 24 hours in advance) of a laminaria causes the cervix to dilate and soften without significant pain. A cannula of 12 mm can then be introduced without difficulty.

EMERGENCY EQUIPMENT AND PLANS FOR TRANSPORTATION OF THE PATIENT

The following emergency equipment should be immediately available in or adjacent to the procedure room:

An oxygen tank with measuring gauge and flow valve
A face mask with positive pressure ventilation bag
An oropharyngeal airway
A low pressure suction machine or device to aspirate secretions from the mouth and pharynx
The equipment to instill intravenous fluids, including a plasma expander
Appropriate drugs for parenteral treatment of uterine atony (methylergonovine), hypotension (a pressor amine), or the side effects of local anesthesia (a barbiturate or diazepam).

The transfer of a patient to the hospital involves notification of the emergency room or admissions department, a call for an ambulance, and appropriate safeguards during movement (maintenance of the airway and intravenous fluids). All office personnel must know their role in evacuation of the patient, and an occasional drill is helpful. A written outline of the steps involved in the move to the hospital, including important telephone numbers, should be posted for quick reference.

EVALUATION OF THE PATIENT BEFORE ABORTION—COUNSELING

Women generally need and welcome an opportunity to discuss their pregnancy and the decision for abortion with an empathetic and objective person. This can be the physician or a doctor's assistant or counselor whose personality and training has prepared her/him for preabortion counseling. The counselor will generally review the woman's life situation at the moment—her feelings about the pregnancy, the abortion decision, her partner, and her future life plans. Some women wish and need extensive discussion about these subjects, and others require minimal time. The counselor should also explain the abortion procedure—its discomforts, safety, duration, and technique, as well as postabortion directions. After this discussion, the patient can review an information sheet (Appendix 1) and sign a consent form (Appendix 2).

Future plans for contraception should always be discussed in counseling, and prior contraceptive problems should be reviewed. Male and female sterilization may be explored as an option. If the partner is present, it is desirable to have him participate in this discussion in order to make contraception a mutual decision and responsibility. Women should also be offered the opportunity for further counseling postabortion, either at the doctor's office or through referral if this seems appropriate.

MEDICAL HISTORY

A self-administered medical history form is convenient and effective in the evaluation of abortion patients (Appendix 3). The preabortion history should cover the following areas:

Acute illness requiring hospitalization for abortion

Conditions indicating a need for preliminary care, such as cardiac disease requiring antibiotic prophylaxis, gonorrhea or pelvic inflammatory disease requiring immediate treatment and delay of abortion in some cases

Allergies to local anesthetics, analgesic agents, or antibiotics

Current drug usage

Last menstrual period, menstrual history, dates of coitus if known, and recent withdrawal from oral contraceptives—for assessment of the duration of pregnancy

Past contraceptive use and contraceptive problems, screening questions for contraindications to oral or intrauterine contraception, future plans for birth control or sterilization

Prior pregnancies including a history of uterine fibromyomata, uterine anomalies, cervical dysplasia or cervical stenosis, which may affect abortion techniques. (A past history of cesarian section, myomectomy, adnexal surgery, or postpartum hemorrhage does not generally affect the abortion technique.)

PHYSICAL EXAMINATION

After a brief general physical evaluation (vital signs, heart, breasts, and abdomen), a thorough pelvic examination should be performed. A speculum exam without lubricant should first be done to obtain an endocervical culture for gonorrhea and vaginal/cervical cytology if necessary. The bimanual examination will reveal the size of the uterus, its position, and any possible abnormalities such as a bicornuate or arcuate uterus, fibromyomata, or adnexal masses.

Evaluation of the duration of pregnancy requires considerable experience in correlating weeks from last menses with uterine size in women of varying parity. Findings on the bimanual examination are influenced by the thickness and tone of the abdominal wall and the position of the uterus. Uterine depth as measured by a sound cannot be consistently correlated with weeks of gestation—the products of conception may interfere with fundal sounding, and an unwanted perforation may occur with the sound. Since it is important to make office abortions as safe as possible, the less experienced clinician should limit such procedures to women whose pregnancies are less than 10 weeks from LMP, and the experienced physician should not go beyond 12 weeks from LMP.

Diagnosis of the very early gestation also requires experience. Patients requesting "menstrual regulation" before the pregnancy test is positive need a careful review of the signs and symptoms of early pregnancy, including minimal uterine softening or enlargement and breast tenderness or fullness. Such careful screening is important so that nonpregnant women can avoid the discomfort and expense of uterine aspiration in most cases.

LABORATORY TESTS FOR ABORTION

Pregnancy Test

Patients should be told to bring a first morning urine specimen at the time of their preabortion evaluation. Pregnancy tests can be conveniently run in the office with any of the reliable 2-minute slide test reagents. Such testing is important whenever the physician is not certain that the pelvic findings indicate an intrauterine pregnancy.

Test for Anemia

A hemoglobin or hematocrit determination can be done in the office and should be routine for abortion patients whose pregnancies are over 8 or 9 weeks from LMP. Women with 10 grams per cent of hemoglobin or less should generally be aborted in a hospital with blood banking facilities. In pregnancies of 8 weeks or less from LMP, blood loss from an abortion procedure under local anesthesia approximates the loss during a menstrual period, 30 to 50 ml.

Rh Determination

An Rh determination should be performed on every abortion patient who is more than 6 weeks from LMP. If the woman is Rh negative, she should be advised to have Rh immune globulin because of the risk of sensitization after abortion (Appendix 4). Some doctors only test for the Rh D factor, and omit tests for the Du factor, Rh antibodies, and the minor crossmatch before giving Rh immune globulin. This policy results in the administration of some unnecessary immune globulin, but has no risk and may be less expensive for the majority of women.

Data are currently being gathered on the efficacy of a decreased dose of Rh immune globulin for first trimester abortion patients. The present recommended dose is calculated to be effective for the average patient at term, at which time the potential for red cell infusion is far greater than in the first trimester.

Gonorrhea Culture

A cervical culture for gonorrhea should be obtained before the abortion procedure, as 1 to 8% of sexually active gynecologic patients may be carrying the gonococcus. Ideally the culture should be done 2 to 3 days in advance so that results are obtained and treatment given prior to abortion. However, many busy abortion services have found that cultures taken at the time of abortion are satisfactory if results are obtained in 48 hours and treatment is given immediately. The foregoing applies to the asymptomatic patient without an obvious infection. If a purulent cervicitis is found at the time of abortion, it is wise to treat the patient with high dose antibiotic therapy, appropriate for gonorrhea, before the procedure.

PREABORTION MEDICATIONS AND THE PARACERVICAL BLOCK

Analgesia and mild sedation are helpful before an abortion procedure. A variety of orally administered narcotics and sedatives are convenient and often used. Drugs given intravenously have the advantage of immediate effect and shorter duration. The intravenous injection of 25 to 50 mg of meperidine combines pain relief with some sedation. Alphaprodine (20 to 30 mg) given subcutaneously gives a similar effect. Diazepam (5 to 10 mg) given intravenously is useful in the highly anxious patient.

Much of the discomfort of aspiration abortion comes from stimulation of the internal os by dilation and passage of the aspirating cannula. Fortunately these sensations can be dulled significantly by small amounts of local anesthetic solution. The diffuse network of nerves innervating the uterus can be blocked using a 1% solution of lidocaine without epinephrine. Anesthetic, 3 ml, is injected just beneath the vaginal epithelium at each of four sites—3, 5, 7, and 9 o'clock—at the juncture of the cervix and the vagina. A small amount of anesthetic can also be placed at the tenaculum site to relieve awareness of the pressure of that instrument. Rapid diffusion of the anesthetic permits nerve blockade if one waits 2 or 3 minutes after injection. Increases in anesthetic volume do not significantly increase the degree of anesthesia but do increase the likelihood of an adverse reaction manifested by paresthesias, vertigo, muscle irritability, and convulsions.

ASPIRATION TECHNIQUE

After a careful pelvic examination, the appropriate size cannula is selected (see above) for duration of gestation and uterine size. The cervix may need minimal dilation if a 6-mm flexible cannula is used. Tapered dilators (or prior insertion of a laminaria) should be used before the insertion of larger cannulas. The cannula should then be introduced to the fundus and withdrawn slightly. After suction is established the cannula is moved within the uterus to aspirate all parts of the cavity. A combination of rotary and gentle to and fro motion is generally effective. Amniotic fluid is seen in the cannula and tubing, followed by placental tissue, decidua, fetal parts and blood. Occasionally placental tissue or fetal parts jam the openings of the cannula or are seen in the cervical os, where they can be removed with uterine or polyp forceps. When the uterus is empty, the aspirate consists solely of frothy blood, and the uterine walls are felt to be closely applied to the cannula.

When a Karman cannula is used, curette-like sensation occurs as the empty uterus contracts.

Many clinicians use a small curette at the end of aspiration to check for complete evacuation. This instrument is often valuable to detect submucous fibromyomata or uterine anomalies and to remove retained tissue in these instances. There is controversy over the routine use of a curette after aspiration because of its potential for perforation or damage to the myometrium. Some clinicians prefer to use only flexible instruments, e.g. the Karman cannula, up to 9 to 10 weeks from LMP.

An intrauterine contraceptive device (IUD) can be inserted immediately after the abortion without discomfort owing to the existing cervical dilation and the paracervical block. A variety of studies from abroad[4, 5] on postabortal IUD insertions have shown no higher proportion of bleeding problems or infection among postabortal women with an IUD. However, several recent U.S. studies not related to abortion[6, 7] indicate that pelvic infection may be increased 5 to 9 times in IUD users compared to matched controls not using the IUD. The increased risk of endometritis or salpingitis, especially in the woman with several partners, should be carefully explained to any woman contemplating IUD use, along with instructions to seek immediate treatment for the symptoms of infection.

An example of a brief operative note for abortion procedures is found in Appendix 5.

Immediately after the abortion, the operator should examine the aspirated tissue for its amount and for identification of the placenta. The villous structure of the early placenta is most easily identified when the tissue is suspended in saline in a shallow glass plate. Embryonic parts are rarely seen before 9 to 10 weeks from LMP but should be identified thereafter.

When placental tissue is not found, the following possibilities should be considered: (1) the patient may not have been pregnant, in which case the total volume of aspirated material is generally very scant, (2) in a very early abortion or in the aspiration of tissue destined for inevitable abortion, the placenta may be too small or macerated to be seen without a microscope, (3) the aspiration may have been incomplete, with the placenta remaining in the uterus, (4) there may be an ectopic gestation with only decidual tissue in the uterus.

In these circumstances another pregnancy test should be run immediately. In situations (1) and (2), the test will probably be negative, in which case rapid microscopic tissue examination will clarify the matter and careful followup is all that is needed. In situations (3) and (4), the pregnancy test will probably be positive, and an immediate repeat aspiration is necessary (see below, ectopic pregnancy).

Aspirated tissue should be sent for microscopic evaluation by a pathologist to detect hydatidiform mole or choriocarcinoma, which may not be grossly evident in early abortion specimens.[8]

POST ABORTION INSTRUCTIONS, MEDICATIONS, AND THE USE OF ANTIBIOTICS

A written list of instructions and advice with emergency telephone numbers is important. Specific information for future reference (Appendix 6) will enable the patient to help herself more effectively and to avoid needless anxiety and unnecessary physician consultations.

Suggested times for resumption of intercourse, douching, and the use of vaginal tampons may vary depending on the advisor's medical viewpoint but should be specified.

If a woman has chosen oral contraception, she should begin the cycle within 24 hours of abortion. If an IUD has not been inserted at the time of the procedure, it can safely be placed at a checkup 2 weeks postabortion. Barrier types of contraception (condom or diaphragm) should be used immediately and regularly because ovulation returns rapidly after early pregnancy termination.

The abortion patient may be given a prescription for small amounts of oral analgesics and uterotonics such as methylergonovine.

Most clinicians do not routinely use antibiotics after abortion because of the low incidence of infection and the questionable efficacy of prophylactic antibiotics in many medical areas. However, a recent study by Hodgson et al.[9] discussed the prophylactic use of tetracycline in a large abortion clinic with a resultant decrease in reports of major and minor complications. Tetracycline was given in amounts designed to eradicate the gonococcus—1.5 g 2 hours before the procedure and 0.5 g every 6 hours to follow for 4 days. The question of whether such antibiotic usage is justified is still being debated, and more studies are needed, adequately controlled and in various patient groups.

EARLY COMPLICATIONS OF FIRST TRIMESTER ABORTIONS

Perforation of the Uterus

The softened pregnant uterus is occasionally perforated during an abortion procedure by a sound, a dilator, the aspiration cannula, or a curette. Perforation should be recognized by the passage of an instrument unusually far into the uterine cavity, or by the appearance of omentum or bowel in the cannula or at the cervix. The JPSA report[1] shows a perforation rate of 4 per 1000 suction procedures. It has been noted that perforations are more likely to occur during difficult dilations of the cervix or if a retroverted uterus is not recognized by the operator. Whenever the diagnosis of perforation is suspected or confirmed the patient should be hospitalized for observation and prepared for possible laparotomy.

If the perforation occurs with a sound or dilator prior to aspiration, the procedure should be suspended at that point. The majority of such perforations heal without surgical intervention, but the possibility of laceration of the uterine artery and subsequent serious internal or vaginal bleeding should be considered. The abortion can be performed 1 or 2 weeks later in a hospital setting.

If perforation occurs during suction curettage, significant injury to bowel or omentum is more likely. If the cannula is introduced to an unusual depth with vacuum applied or if bowel or omentum appear in the cannula, the patient should be transferred to a hospital and prepared for laparotomy.

Laparoscopy has been used to diagnose the extent of intra-abdominal injury after suspected perforation. With this technique laparotomy can be avoided if unnecessary or performed more promptly if indicated. In some cases the abortion can be completed under laparoscopic visualization.

Bleeding

Blood loss is small in the uncomplicated aspiration abortion, owing to rapid and complete evacuation of the uterus. Bleeding is increased if the abortion time is prolonged owing to inexperience of the operator and uncertainty as to when the uterus is empty. Bleeding can also occur when the pregnancy is further advanced than originally diagnosed, so that the tissue cannot pass through the cannula. In this instance it is often wise to use intravenous oxytocin after further dilating the cervix, and then the uterus can be evacuated by a larger cannula and ovum forceps.

On rare occasions the uterus fills with blood within the hour after aspiration. The patient complains of severe pelvic pain, vaginal bleeding is heavy, and the uterus is enlarged and tender. Reaspiration of the uterus should be promptly performed; there may be retained tissue with a significant amount of clotted blood within the uterus. Subsequently the uterus contracts well and further bleeding is minimal.

Hypotension

Immediately after an abortion done under local anesthesia, patients may complain of cramping, faintness, or nausea. They may have bradycardia and hypotension, a syndrome also commonly seen after IUD insertion. This problem can be treated with leg elevation, oxygen, and the occasional use of a vasopressor agent.

Ectopic Pregnancy

Whenever immediate inspection of aspirated tissue does not reveal placenta, the physician should consider an ectopic implantation. Another pregnancy test should be obtained at once. If this test is positive and an immediate repeat aspiration fails to produce placenta, the patient should be hospitalized for further evaluation, including culdocentesis if indicated, curettage under anesthesia, laparoscopy, and/or laparotomy. If the repeated pregnancy test is negative, the uterus seems empty, and there are no adnexal masses, the patient may be sent home, but she should be warned of a possible ectopic pregnancy, followed closely, and re-evaluated in a few days with another pregnancy test and pelvic examination. Rapid microscopic examination of the aspirated tissue will help to distinguish between decidua and nonpregnant endometrium.

Patients who become pregnant using an intrauterine device are a high risk group for ectopic pregnancy; there is an increased ratio of ectopic to uterine pregnancies in these women owing to the IUD's protection against uterine implantation. Tietze and Lewit[10] have reported a 4 to 5% rate of ectopic pregnancies among all pregnancies occurring with an IUD; Vessey and colleagues[11] reported an 8.9% rate.

LATE COMPLICATIONS AND SEQUELAE OF ABORTION

During the week following abortion, the patient is at greatest risk to develop complications related to retained products of conception. Postabortion bleeding is often intermittent and less in amount than an average menstrual period. Moderate increase in flow can be treated by an oral ergot derivative. Should the patient report heavier bleeding, she should be examined promptly. If the uterus is soft and enlarged, bleeding is significant, or there is any tissue in the cervix or vagina, a repeat aspiration is indicated. Sharp curettage should be avoided in order to minimize the occurrence of uterine synechiae.

Endoparametritis has an incubation time of 2 to 5 days. Such infection will be manifested by pain in the lower abdomen and fever. Because retained tissue may have been the nidus for the infection, reaspiration of the uterus is often helpful. The initial choice of antibiotic can be ampicillin or tetracycline. A patient manifesting pelvic peritonitis or toxic symptoms should be hospitalized for parenteral antibiotics and close supportive care.

Continued pregnancy is signaled by the absence of postabortion vaginal bleeding as well as a continuation of symptoms of pregnancy. Failure to aspirate the products of conception can be related to uterine perforation or the production of a false passage. In these cases, repeat aspiration can be performed in 2 to 3 weeks. A failure can also occur when the pregnant horn of a bicornuate uterus is not identified.

The late sequelae of abortion that have created the greatest concern are those affecting subsequent wanted pregnancies—possible increased risk of spontaneous abortion in the second trimester, premature birth, or neonatal mortality. These problems have been attributed to damage to the cervix at the time of dilation or too vigorous curettage of the basal layers of the endometrium. The current trend in the United States to perform abortions earlier, with minimal dilation of the cervix, should lessen the potential for future problems.

The most extensive data on the effect of induced abortion on subsequent pregnancies has come from Hungary and has been recently reviewed by Tietze and Dawson.[12] They showed evidence that the percentage of infants weighing less than 2,500 g at birth and mortality in the first week of life tended to increase with pregnancy order regardless of prior abortions, and with number of prior abortions regardless of pregnancy order. These data are under continuing evaluation.

The World Health Organization and the National Institutes of Health are currently sponsoring collaborative studies to evaluate the effect of induced abortion on subsequent wanted pregnancies.

MENSTRUAL REGULATION

Aspiration of the uterus shortly after a missed period, before currently standard pregnancy tests are accurate, has been called menstrual regulation (extraction or induction) or endometrial aspiration. The technique used in these procedures is similar to that outlined in this chapter, with the use of a 5- or 6-mm flexible cannula. The operator must examine the aspirated tissue carefully and send it for microscopic examination in order to know whether or not a pregnancy was indeed present and terminated successfully. Because of the occasional difficulty in aspirating the very small implantation site, there is a continued pregnancy rate of 2 to 5% in these cases. A repeated pregnancy test at a 2-week followup visit is strongly advised.

The advantage of menstrual regulation is the immediate relief that it affords the anxious woman whose life circumstances may make a delay for the confirmation of pregnancy very stressful. The disadvantages of the procedure are its expense, its discomfort, and its small risk of continued pregnancy, uterine perforation, or infection. If a practitioner chooses to offer this procedure before the diagnosis of pregnancy is confirmed, his/her patients should be fully informed of the pros and cons involved. Patients should be informed that the likelihood of pregnancy is only 50% when a period has been delayed by a week, and that it rises to 85% by the end of a second week past the missed period. At that point a pregnancy test on a concentrated urine specimen should be diagnostic so that the aspiration procedure need not be performed unnecessarily.

The concept of "menstrual regulation" was being developed prior to the 1973 United States Supreme Court decision legalizing abortion. Since that decision, it seems less necessary to perform uterine aspiration before the diagnosis of pregnancy. However, in countries where legal and social attitudes make overt abortion unacceptable, "menstrual regulation" may be important as a method of birth prevention and as a means to introduce the use of contraception.

CONCLUSION

Abortion in an office setting has the advantage of being confidential, convenient for doctor and patient, and relatively inexpensive compared to a hospital-based procedure. A substantial need for accessible and inexpensive abortion care is likely to continue in our society, until there is a marked improvement in contraceptive techniques, such as a postcoital pill without significant side effects.

At present, contraception reduces the frequency of abortion but does not eliminate it. Tietze[13] estimates that after 5 years of a liberalized abortion law, 17 to 23% of abortions will be repeat procedures if women are using a method as effective as the pill. Greater numbers of repeat procedures will be necessary if couples use simpler methods (condom or diaphragm) in an effort to avoid the side effects of the pill or IUD.

Health professionals must make pregnancy testing, counseling, and abortion available in all communities so that women with unwanted pregnancies can receive prompt care. Our goal should be to have 95% of abortions performed in the first trimester, with over half of these in the first 8 weeks from LMP.

Appendix 1

EARLY ABORTION BY VACUUM ASPIRATION

An abortion procedure is the termination of an early pregnancy by vacuum aspiration of the lining of the uterus. This information sheet will explain the procedure and some of its complications.

Before the abortion you will be given a pill or injection to make you more comfortable during the procedure. The doctor will go over your medical history and will examine your heart, breasts, abdomen and pelvic region. You will be given a test for gonorrhea at this time.

During the abortion a counselor/medical assistant will be with you in the room at all times. You can also have a partner or friend in the room with you, if you like.

The doctor will give you a local anesthetic (numbing medicine) in your cervix which will make you more comfortable during the procedure. Many women do not feel the local anesthetic being given since this area does not have many pain nerves. The doctor will then enlarge the opening into the uterus with small instruments if necessary—this is called dilation of the cervix. The doctor then inserts into the uterus a small plastic tube attached to a vacuum pump. The tube is moved within the uterus for about 3 minutes in order to remove all pregnancy tissue by the suction process. At the end of this time you may experience menstrual-like cramping as the uterus contracts down to its normal size. The doctor then checks to make sure that all the tissue has been removed, with a small instrument called a curette. After this, the pregnancy tissue is examined by the doctor and sent to a laboratory for further analysis. In most early abortions we do not see the embryo/fetus because it is too small, but we always check for the presence of placental tissue (afterbirth).

After the abortion, you will rest on the examining table for a time. Your doctor and counselor will give you written followup instructions, and will help you choose a good method of birth control. You will be given a return appointment for a checkup. You will then get dressed and go to our recovery room or waiting room, have some refreshments, and wait until you are entirely recovered and ready to leave with a friend.

There are certain complications that can arise during and after an abortion:

Infection of the uterus and other pelvic organs (fallopian tubes, ovaries, and abdominal cavity) may occur after an abortion. The signs of infection are fever, pain, and irregular or excessive bleeding—this is discussed in your followup information sheet which you will receive today. Infection is treated with antibiotics and rest. A pelvic infection may result in a lowering of your future fertility, so it should be treated promptly and thoroughly.

Heavy bleeding may occur after an abortion procedure. This problem is treated with medicines, antibiotics, and/or reaspiration of the uterus to remove any retained tissue that is causing the bleeding.

An early pregnancy is occasionally missed during the abortion procedure, so that the woman remains pregnant afterwards. This is a rare complication. If you continue to have symptoms of pregnancy after the abortion, we will recheck you promptly.

On rare occasions an instrument can perforate through the uterus into the abdominal cavity. In this case the woman may need to be hospitalized for observation and possibly for abdominal surgery.

You will be given a telephone number to reach the doctor should these or any other complications occur. Your followup appointment is important to check for any complications as well.

Appendix 2

READ AND BE CERTAIN THAT YOU FULLY UNDERSTAND BEFORE YOU SIGN

Consent to Early Abortion

I hereby direct and request _____, M.D. or his/her associates to perform an ASPIRATION ABORTION under paracervical block anesthesia. If any unforeseen condition arises or is discovered in the course of the abortion calling in his/her medical judgement for procedures in addition to or different from those contemplated, I further request and authorize him/her to do whatever he/she deems medically necessary.

I am__days beyond my normal menstruation, and I have had a *positive pregnancy test*.

I understand that the purpose of this procedure is to terminate my pregnancy, but that no warranty or guaranty has been made to me as to the results of this procedure. It has been explained to me that in some instances pregnancy is not terminated by this procedure and, if that happens, further treatment or procedures will be necessary.

I understand that there are alternate methods of treatment, including a hospital abortion now or later in my pregnancy, or continuation of the pregnancy.

I also understand that the procedure is carried out by suction aspiration of the contents of the uterus.

I further understand that the *risks* involved include perforation of the uterus with possible damage to abdominal organs, or hemorrhage, or infection, or low blood pressure after the procedure, or an allergic reaction to local anesthesia, or failure to terminate the pregnancy, or emotional reactions. If the procedure leads to any of these or other complications, I understand that I may need further medical care, including hospitalization and/or surgery; I agree to seek such care promptly upon the appearance of any unusual symptoms.

I hereby release the aforementioned physician and associates from any and all claims arising out of or connected with the above procedure, or any resulting complications or expense.

I have read the above and I fully understand the contents of each paragraph. I have also read and fully understand the information sheet entitled Early Abortion by Vacuum Aspiration.

Date _____   Patient's signature _____

_____
Witness

YOU MUST GIVE *INFORMED* CONSENT.   ASK QUESTIONS UNTIL YOU UNDERSTAND ALL OF THIS FORM.

Appendix 3

MEDICAL HISTORY FOR ASPIRATION ABORTION

Date_____

Name_____   Age___ Birth Date_____

Occupation_____   Address _____

Telephone_____   Blood Type_____
                                                   (Rh + or −, if known)

What was the first day of your last normal menstrual period?

Have you had a pregnancy test?   Results   Date

Are your cycles regular (25–35 days apart?) Yes   No. Irregular_____
                                                                    (comment)

Do you have very heavy periods?___Severe cramps? _____

Total number of: Pregnancies_____Live births___Living children _____

                  Miscarriages___Induced abortions _____

What problems did you have with prior pregnancies, births, or abortions?_____

What methods of birth control have you or your partners *ever* used in the past?

What problems have you ever had with any of these birth control methods?

What birth control methods (if any) have you used since your last normal period?

Did you stop the pill just before your last period?_____

What method of birth control would you like to use after the abortion?_____

Do you want more information on female or male sterilization?_____

Answer the following questions by writing YES or NO on each line after each question. If you answer YES, please write details. We will review your answers with you.

Have you ever had any serious illness in the past?_____

Are you taking any medicine, drugs, tranquilizers, etc.? _____

Have you ever been hospitalized except for pregnancy?_____

Have you ever had an operation? (Cesarean section, appendectomy, D&C?)_____

Have you ever had a blood transfusion?_____

Have you ever had an allergic reaction to a medicine? (rash, hives, etc.?)_____

Are you allergic to penicillin? _____

Are you allergic to local anesthetic?_____

Where do you go when you are sick (doctor, clinic, hospital?)_____

Have you ever had an abnormal Pap smear? _____

When did you last have a Pap smear? (month and year) _____

Have you ever had any of the following conditions? Answer YES or NO on the line after each question. If you answer YES, please give details.

Allergies (asthma, eczema, hives, hay fever) _____

Anemia (low blood)_____

Breast lump or tumor _____

Diabetes _____

Epilepsy_____

Fainting or loss of consciousness _____

Heart disease (rheumatic fever or other problem)_____

High blood pressure_____

Infected or clotted veins _____

Varicose veins _____

Hepatitis (liver disease)_____

Kidney problems (bladder or urine infection)_____

Migraine headaches _____

Sickle cell anemia_____

Ovarian cyst or tumor _____

Pelvic infection (in uterus, ovaries, or tubes) _____

Vaginal infections_____

Gonorrhea (clap) _____

Syphilis _____

Other significant illness (What?)_____

Has any member of your family had diabetes, high blood pressure, heart disease, or any inherited disease?_____

Comments: _____

Physical examination: Ht. __Wt. __ B.P. _____

   Skin _____

   ENT _____

   Neck _____

   Heart _____

   Lungs_____

   Breasts _____

   Abdomen _____

   Pelvic: Vagina and vulva _____ Cervix _____

           Uterus _____ Size (weeks)_____

                                  Consistent with dates: Yes __No__

           Adnexa_____ Rectovaginal_____

Diagnostic impression: _____

Treatment plan: _____

_____ M.D.

                        Signature of physician

Appendix 4

TEST FOR THE Rh FACTOR FOR WOMEN WHO HAVE AN ABORTION

When you come in for your abortion procedure you will have a simple blood test to determine the Rh factor of your blood. We do this to find out whether you are Rh positive or Rh negative.

About 12% of people are Rh negative. That is, they *do not* carry on their red corpuscles the Rh substance which the other 88% of people have. An Rh negative woman who is bearing an Rh positive pregnancy may become sensitized to the Rh factor if she has an abortion.

In the simplest terms, approximately five drops of Rh positive blood are enough to sensitize a woman and affect all subsequent Rh positive babies she might deliver. This small amount of blood can get into the blood stream during the course of a routine abortion. If this occurs, the blood is recognized as a foreign substance and the woman's system produces antibodies to it just as antibodies are protectively produced against measles or chickenpox. If another Rh positive pregnancy occurs, the antibodies attach themselves to the fetal blood cells and weaken them. The weakened cells live but a short time and as they disappear the fetus gradually becomes more and more anemic.

A small injection of Rh immune globulin given into the hip or arm within 72 hours of abortion will effectively prevent this risk of sensitization from abortion. The only known side-effect is a welt at the site of the injection. This procedure is for your protection in the future if and when you want to have a baby.

Appendix 5

VACUUM ABORTION OPERATIVE NOTE

Date of operation _____

Weeks of estimated gestation (based on LMP)

RH type _____

Hemoglobin _____

GC culture _____

Contraceptive plans: ☐IUD ☐Pill ☐Diaphragm ☐Other _____

Analgesia: _____

Anesthesia: ☐General ☐Paracervical block 1% Xylocaine __ml

Uterus: size __weeks gestation

             ☐Ant ☐Mid ☐Post

             Sound __cm

Dilation to: __Pratt or __Hegar

Cannula: __mm

Tissue volume: ☐ small ☐ mod ☐ large (for gestation)

Villi seen: ☐ + ☐ – molar degeneration: ☐ + ☐ –

Embryo: ☐none ☐incomplete ☐complete ☐probably complete

Blood loss: __ml Perforation: ☐ + ☐ –

Special findings or problems: _____

_____

IUD: (specify type and size) _____

_____

                             Signature

Appendix 6

EARLY ABORTION—INSTRUCTIONS FOR AFTER YOUR PROCEDURE

1. You should go home to rest after the procedure. Do not overdo today. You may resume work or normal activities tomorrow. You should have a thermometer at home.

2. You will probably have some bleeding off and on for the next 10 to 14 days. Don't be surprised if it varies from very light to moderately heavy; your bleeding will probably increase with increased exercise and decrease with rest.

3. It is extremely important to report the following problems to us if they occur:
   excessive bleeding (heavier than the heaviest day of your period)
   chills and fever of over 100 degrees
   prolonged abdominal pain
If any of these problems occur, take your temperature and call us at the following number:

4. You may use Tampax in 3 days, and you may bathe or shower daily.

5. You should not have sex relations for a week following the procedure, so that you will not become infected. When you begin to have sex, have your partner use a rubber until your followup visit with the doctor.

6. If you wish to start the birth control pill, start it tonight or tomorrow. If you wish the IUD or the diaphragm, we will fit you at your followup visit.

7. Your next menstrual period should begin 4 to 6 weeks from the day of your procedure. If you take the pill, it will begin after you complete the first package.

8. Your followup visit is very important to you and should not be cancelled or postponed.

REFERENCES

1. Tietze, C, and Lewit, S, Joint Program for the Study of Abortion (JPSA): Early Medical Complications of Legal Abortion. Stud Fam Plann 3:97, 1972.
2. State of California Department of Health, Therapeutic Abortion in California, a Biennial Report Prepared for the 1974 Legislature.
3. Center for Disease Control, Abortion-related Mortality, 1972–1973—United States, Morbidity and Mortality, Weekly Report 24:no. 3, 1975.
4. Andolsĕk, L, Experience with Immediate Post-abortion Insertions of the IUD, in Lewit, S, ed., Abortion Techniques and Services, Excerpta Medica, Amsterdam, 1972, p. 63.
5. Nygen, K-G, and Johannson, EDB, Insertion of the Endouterine Copper-T (T Cu 200) Immediately after First Trimester Legal Abortion. Contraception 7:299, 1973.
6. Faulkner, WL, The Association between the Use of the Intrauterine Device and the Development of Acute Pelvic Inflammatory Disease. Presented at the annual EIS conference, April 1975, Center for Disease Control, Atlanta, Georgia.
7. Targum, SD, and Wright NH, Association of the Intrauterine Device and Pelvic Inflammatory Disease. A Retrospective Pilot Study. Am J Epidem 100:262, 1974.
8. De Cherney, AH, Silverman, BB, and Mastroianni, L, Jr, Abortion and Unrecognized Trophoblastic Disease, New Eng J Med 285:407, 1971.
9. Hodgson, JE, Major, B, Portmann, K, and Quattlebaum, FW, Prophylactic Use of Tetracycline for First Trimester Abortion. Obstet Gynecol 45:574, 1975.
10. Tietze, C, and Lewit, S, Evaluation of Intrauterine Devices: Ninth Progress Report of the Cooperative Statistical Program. Stud Fam Plann, no. 55, 1970.
11. Vessey, MD, Doll, R, Johnson, B, and Peto, R, Outcome of pregnancy in women using an intrauterine device. Lancet 1:495, 1974.
12. Tietze, C, and Dawson, D, Induced Abortion: A Factbook. Reports on Population/Family Planning, Nov. 14, 1973.
13. Tietze, C, The "Problem" of Repeat Abortions. Fam Plann Perspect 6:148, 1974.

5

THE ANTENATAL DETECTION OF GENETIC DISORDERS

MITCHELL S. GOLBUS, M.D.

INTRODUCTION

The most significant advance in clinical genetics in the last 15 years has been the advent of the prenatal diagnosis of genetic defects. Prior to this innovation genetic counseling was limited to the passive role of providing families or individuals with risk figures for future offspring. Although this form of counseling is effective in helping the involved family make decisions about reproduction, its effect is to reduce the incidence of genetic disease only minimally, and that, by restricting reproduction. It does not aid the counselees to have a healthy family. With the onset of prenatal diagnosis, genetic counseling assumed new dimensions. The family which was unwilling to risk reproduction on the basis of the risk figures could now have their own children without fearing the birth of a child with a specific serious genetic disease.

Starting at the turn of the century a number of scientific and technical advances have culminated in the ability to provide prenatal diagnosis (Table 5.1). At the present state of our knowledge, the birth of a genetically handicapped child can be avoided only when prenatal diagnosis is coupled with selective abortion. Therefore, in addition to the advances delineated in Table 5.1, a necessary prerequisite for the widespread application of prenatal diagnosis was the relaxation of restrictions on performing elective therapeutic abortions. That this relaxation has occurred is testified to by the over one million elective abortions being done annually in the United States for socioeconomic indications. This general availability of abortion services removed a large deterrent to the wider use of prenatal diagnosis.

TECHNICAL FACETS

Currently, prenatal diagnosis of most genetic defects requires amniocentesis. It should be emphasized that the amniocentesis is a procedural endpoint and must be preceded by the careful recording of a family pedigree and appropriate genetic counseling. To do this the counselor must be able not only to verify the diagnosis of previously affected relatives and determine the applicable genetic facts, but also to recognize and deal with the psychosocial implications of the material with which he is dealing. Genetic counseling should include not only discussion of the risk of having a genetically defective infant but also of the dangers of amniocentesis (see

TABLE 5.1

Scientific and Technical Advances Leading to the Development of Prenatal Diagnosis

1900	Reannouncement of Mendelian rules of inheritance by deVries, Correns, and Tschermak
1909	Garrod's concept of inborn errors of metabolism
1949	Barr's discovery of sex chromatin body
1952	First demonstrated specific enzyme defect causing human disease
1953	Beginning of widespread use of amniocentesis in Rh disease
1955	Antenatal sex determination using sex chromatin of amniotic fluid cells
1955	Determination of nutritional requirements for tissue culture of human cells
1956	Tijo and Levan introduce new techniques to cytogenetics and determine human chromosome number is 46
1959	Delineation of chromosome aneuploidy as a cause of human disease
1968	Reports of prenatal diagnosis of chromosome aneuploidy and of an inborn error of metabolism (galactosemia)
1970	Chromosome "banding" techniques described

"Complications") and any reservations about the results that may be obtained. We urge that the husband be present at the counseling session and take part in the decision whether or not to have an amniocentesis. The couple then signs a consent form designed to emphasize the limitations of prenatal diagnosis (Fig. 5.1).

Amniocentesis

The timing of amniocentesis is a function of when amniotic fluid can consistently and safely be obtained, the time required for fluid analysis or cell culture and analysis, and legal/societal limits as to how late in pregnancy therapeutic abortion may be performed. Obtaining amniotic fluid in the first trimester requires a transvaginal approach and is associated with a significant risk of uterine infection and subsequent abortion.[1] Fluids from pregnancies of less than 12 menstrual weeks' gestation contain very few cells, of which only 20 to 30% are viable and, consequently, there is a very low rate of successful cell culture.[2, 3] Fuchs[4] has shown that at 15 menstrual weeks there is an average of 125 cc of amniotic fluid and that this volume increases 50 cc per week for the next 13 weeks. Analysis of our data indicates that the time required for cell culture and analysis is not a function of the gestational age at which the fluid is obtained.[5] Therefore, it is our practice to do amniocentesis at 15 menstrual weeks, which allows sufficient time for repeat amniocentesis in the event of failure to grow the cells and also often allows a diagnosis to be made prior to quickening. There are a number of studies indicating that therapeutic abortions performed after quickening have greater psychiatric sequelae than those performed earlier.[6, 7]

A pelvic examination is done prior to the amniocentesis to ensure that the uterine size is compatible with the dates, to ascertain the state of the cervix, and to agitate the uterus gently so fetal cells that theoretically may have sedimented with the patient on her back are resuspended in the amniotic fluid. In doing the pelvic examination we have discovered two patients who were not pregnant and three patients with an open internal cervical os. After the abdomen is aseptically prepared, 1% xylocaine is used as a local anesthetic. A 22-gauge, 3½ inch-long spinal needle with stylet is used to obtain 18 cc of amniotic fluid. To avoid

Reproductive Genetics Unit and Birth Defects Center
University of California, San Francisco

Consent for Diagnostic Amniocentesis for Genetic Counseling

I, _____ , hereby request and authorize Dr. Mitchell S. Golbus and associates to perform a diagnostic amniocentesis (withdrawal of amniotic fluid through a needle passed into the uterus through the abdominal wall), and to make a prenatal determination of the chromosome constitution and/or biochemical status (relating to _____) of the unborn fetus. It has been explained to me and I understand that:

1. The procedure of amniocentesis involves a small risk to both mother and fetus, and I realize that miscarriage is a possible complication.

2. There is a possibility that insufficient fluid will be obtained or that growing the fetal cells may not be successful, thereby necessitating a repeat amniocentesis.

3. The chromosome and/or biochemical analyses may not be successful.

4. It is possible that the results of the chromosome and/or biochemical analyses may not accurately reflect the status of the fetus.

5. The findings of a normal chromosome constitution or of a normal biochemical status of the fetus does not eliminate the possibility that the child may have birth defects and/or mental retardation because of other disorders.

6. In the case of presently undiagnosed twins, the results provided pertain to only one of the pair.

7. The amniotic fluid also will be examined to determine if the fetus has a defect in the tube enclosing the brain and spinal column. This test is 80% effective in discovering this relatively infrequent fetal abnormality.

This amniocentesis is being performed for the following reasons:_____

_____

Signed:_____

Witness: _____

Date:_____

Fig. 5.1. Patient consent form

contamination of the sample with maternal tissue, the stylet always must be in place when the needle is advanced. One syringe is used to draw the first 0.5 cc of fluid to make sure it is clear of blood; a second syringe is used to obtain the specimen. There were 6 cases among the first 100 we counseled in which sufficient amniotic fluid was not obtained at the first attempt and a second attempt was necessary 1 to 2 weeks later. As we have gained experience we have been able to halve the incidence of "dry taps."

There are a number of reports of fetal injury[8, 9] or increases in Rhesus antibody titre in sensitized pregnancies[10] following amniocentesis in the second half of pregnancy. However, to date there is only one reported instance of severe fatal injury from an early second trimester amniocentesis and that was in a congenitally malformed fetus. It has been suggested that all pregnancies should have placental localization by β-scan ultrasonography prior to amniocentesis,[11] but the value of this procedure is unproved. Although claims have been made that the incidence of "bloody taps" is lower after placental localization,[12] this needs to be tested by alternating patients and not by comparing dissimilar series. The total fetal-placental blood volume at 15 to 16 menstrual weeks is only 15 cc,[13] and the likelihood of causing a 0.1-cc fetomaternal hemorrhage, considered necessary to cause Rh isoimmunization,[14] by amniocentesis is very low. No instance of this occurring has been reported to date. A study of 23 patients who underwent amniocentesis in early pregnancy revealed no immediate fetal heart rate changes following the procedure.

We have on nine occasions (approximately 1% of our series) obtained dark brown amniotic fluid. Five of these instances represented missed abortions, but in four the fetus was living. One of the latter four was aborted at the request of the parents, and the placenta had a clot adherent to 50% of its surface, suggestive of an abruptio placenta. The remaining three pregnancies have continued and reached term with the delivery of normal healthy infants. This indicates that dark brown fluid does not always mean the demise or abnormality of the fetus and may follow an early abruption.

Cell Culture

There are almost as many techniques for amniotic fluid cell culture as there are prenatal detection centers.[15-20] The most important contribution to successful culturing is the skill of the person involved, and most large centers have a success rate of 95% or greater.[5] Our technique is to divide the amniotic fluid into two tubes and centrifuge at 1000 rpm for 7 minutes. The supernatant is decanted and the cell pellet is resuspended in 1 cc of medium. We use Eagle's Minimum Essential Medium with Earle's salts supplemented with 20% fetal calf serum, L-glutamine, penicillin, and streptomycin. The resuspended cells from each tube are plated into a 30-cc plastic T-flask containing 3 cc of medium. The medium is replaced after 4 days, and thereafter the medium is changed three times a week. The emphasis on parallel cultures is to minimize the risk of contamination and loss of a specimen, to allow for verification of any abnormal findings, and for possible identification of abnormalities that arose *in vitro*. Enough cells are obtained in 2 to 4 weeks for cytogenetic studies and in 3 to 6 weeks for biochemical assays.

Verification of Diagnosis

The absolute number of genetically abnormal fetuses that have been prenatally diagnosed and the pregnancies terminated is still small. In order to verify the accuracy of prenatal diagnosis and to further investigate the chromosomal and biochemical abnormalities diagnosed, it is important that the aborted fetal tissue be amenable to study. We have shown that fetal tissue from prostaglandin $F_{2\alpha}$-aborted fetuses can be cultured for cytogenetic and biochemical studies and that the tissue enzymology is relatively unaltered.[21] For this reason we urge that intra-amniotic instillation of prostaglandin $F_{2\alpha}$ be considered as the optimal method for terminating pregnancies in which a genetically abnormal fetus has been diagnosed.

INDICATIONS AND RESULTS

Chromosome Disorders

Chromosomal heteroploidy (deviation from the normal diploid number) is responsible for a substantial segment of birth defects and reproductive wastage.

Sterility, reduced fertility, embryonic or fetal death, stillbirth, and/or congenital malformations may result from an aberration in chromosome number. Each year in the United States 15,000 infants with a chromosome abnormality are born, and there are an estimated 175,000 spontaneous abortions of chromosomally abnormal fetuses.

The incidence of chromosome heteroploidy varies with the population selected for study. A number of surveys have been done on unselected newborns,[22-28] with a total of 149 major chromosomal abnormalities found among 25,106 neonates, an incidence of 0.59%. The incidence rises to 2.2% if the population considered is full term, low birth weight infants,[29] to 5.8% in cases of perinatal death,[30, 31] and to 32.2% of children studied because of a suspected cytogenetic abnormality.[25, 32] Obviously, the size of this last figure will depend on the degree of suspicion required to order a karyotype at different institutions.

The most common indication for prenatal diagnosis is advanced maternal age. The relationship between the incidence of the Down syndrome and maternal age was noted long before the chromosomal etiology of the syndrome was known. Mitchell[33] observed that children with the Down syndrome tended to be born at the end of the sibships, and it was later shown that this increased frequency was related to maternal but not to paternal age.[34, 35] The risk of having a newborn with trisomy 21 rises to 1:250–290 for age 35–39, to 1:80 for age 40–44, and to 1:20 for age 45 or more.[36, 37] The risk of having a newborn with other chromosomal aneuploidies (trisomy 13, trisomy 18, 47,XXY, 47,XXX, or 47,XYY) also rises with increasing maternal age, but to a lesser degree.[38, 39] These increases are all relative, and the risk never becomes statistically great in absolute terms. There is no sharp dividing line above which maternal age should be considered "advanced," but most centers have used either 35 to 40 years as their criterion. We have felt that women over 35 should receive genetic counseling as to the risks of having a child with trisomy 21 and the risks of amniocentesis, but consider the 35–39 age group as a "gray zone." Although more hesitant about performing amniocentesis in this age group than in women over 39 years old, we will if requested.

The second most common indication for prenatal diagnosis is in women who have previously borne a child with trisomy 21. The recurrence risk, both from retrospective studies[40] and prospective prenatal diagnosis studies,[41] appears to be 1–2%, irrespective of maternal age. The chances of having a second chromosomally abnormal child after bearing a child with trisomy 18 or 13 are unknown, but these families usually approach pregnancy fearfully, and we have been willing to offer them prenatal diagnosis in subsequent pregnancies. There has been a recent report of a trisomy 18 fetus diagnosed prenatally in a woman who had previously given birth to a child with trisomy 18.[42]

When one of the parents is the carrier of a balanced chromosomal translocation there is a considerable risk of meiotic nondisjunction leading to a trisomic fetus. While there is also a presumably equal chance of a monosomic fetus, this does not have the same clinical significance in that such a fetus is extremely unlikely to be carried to the stage of viability. The most common example is familial Down syndrome resulting from the translocation of the long arm of chromosome 21 to the long arm of chromosome 14, i.e. t(14q21q). Women who carry this balanced translocation pass the translocation chromosome in such a manner that 10 to 15% of their offspring have the Down syndrome while the comparable risk for men who carry this balanced translocation is 2 to 4%.[43] Other balanced chromosome translocations or inversions may be associated with a significant risk of having aneuploid offspring and are, therefore, an indication for prenatal diagnosis.[44-46]

Antenatal cytogenetic studies may be considered for some other very rare indications. If either parent is a chromosomal mosaic with two cell lines containing different chromosome complements, their risk of having a chromosomally abnormal child is one-half the proportion of their gametes which are abnormal (assuming monosomic zygotes will be spontaneously aborted), and such cases have been reported.[47, 48] Also, if either parent has an unusual karyotype such as 47,XXY or 47,XX,21+ then the pregnancy should be monitored because of the increased chance of chromosomal abnormality.[49, 50]

We occasionally have patients referred to our prenatal detection center because of exposure to irradiation or various teratogens during early pregnancy. It is our feeling that amniocentesis to evaluate chromosomal breaks is not indicated in these instances since the relationship of such chromosomal breaks to anomalous development is unknown, and the failure to find breaks might induce an unwarranted sense of well-being. Another controversial question is whether or not to suggest antenatal diagnosis to parents who are carriers of a balanced D/D translocation. This is the most common translocation in man, occurring in 1:1000 individuals.[51] It is unclear whether the carrier state for this translocation is associated with an increase in meiotic nondisjunction.[52] We have seen two families in which one parent was a D/D translocation carrier and one child with anatomic malformations had been born, who, after genetic counseling, decided they wished to have an amniocentesis. One of these fetuses had a karyotype of 46,XX,t(2q+14q−) with the translocation appearing balanced. No reports of children with a similar karyotype could be found, and it was impossible to predict the effect of this chromosome abnormality on the fetus. The parents elected to continue the pregnancy; an apparently normal infant with the karyotype previously found was delivered at term and has developed normally to age 2.

The results of the first 600 pregnancies monitored in the University of California, San Francisco, prenatal detection program plus those of 15 other centers are summarized in Table 5.2.[42, 45, 53-74] It is noteworthy that in pregnancies studied because of maternal age the percentage of abnormal fetuses found was substantially above what would be predicted by newborn studies. Although any of these pregnancies that might have terminated as late abortions or stillbirths would not have been included in newborn statistics, it is unlikely that this is a sufficient explanation for the discrepancy. It is more probable that the individuals coming to the prenatal detection centers are in some way a selected group and different from the population as a whole.

The results for the pregnancies monitored because of a previous child with trisomy 21 were in the range predicted. The miscellaneous indications were not detailed by all authors, but from those studies which gave the indications and from our own experience, most of these pregnancies were monitored because of a history of children with the Down syndrome elsewhere in the family, previous children with

TABLE 5.2
Cumulative Experience of Prenatal Detection Programs

Indication	Pregnancies studied	"Affected" fetuses found	
	No.	*No.*	*%*
Chromosomal			
Translocation carriers	111	21	18.9
Maternal age > 40 years	759	29	3.8
Maternal age 35–39 years	862	20	2.3
Previous trisomy 21	754	11	1.5
Miscellaneous	403	7	1.7
X-linked diseases	181	82[a]	45.3
Inborn errors of metabolism	155	31	20.0
Neural tube defects	227	20	8.8
Total	3,452	221	6.4

[a] Includes one trisomy 21 fetus.

a chromosomal abnormality, or previous children with congenital anomalies. It is interesting that with these varied and "softer" indications the rate of chromosomally abnormal fetuses was 1.7%.

It is important to stress that although the figures given above and in Table 5.2 appear straightforward, there are many pitfalls in the prenatal detection of chromosomal abnormalities. One of these pitfalls is the occurrence of de novo clones of cytogenetically aberrant cells that do not represent the true karyotype of the fetus. These clones can be induced in amniotic fluid cells by the presence of mycoplasma in the culture medium,[75] but there is also evidence that aberrant clones can arise in the absence of contamination.[76, 77]

Polyploidy is a normal variant in cultured amniotic fluid cells. Tetraploidy is found in a majority of amniotic fluid cell cultures, usually in only a small percentage of cells, but occasionally in 80–100% of the cells.[78, 79] The incidence of tetraploidy varies with the concentration of colcemid used before harvesting and with the cell type, being higher in fibroblast-like than in epithelial-like cells.[80] Prior to the recognition that tetraploidy is a normal variant in this type of cell culture, one normal fetus was aborted because of this finding.[81]

Another pitfall is the diagnosis of mosaicism, the existence of two different cell lines, in the fetus. One aspect of the problem is finding mosaicism in the cultured cells when none exists in the fetus, secondary to an aberrant clone arising in culture.[82] The concept of mosaicism has also been used to explain situations in which the amniotic fluid cell karyotype differed from that of the fetus,[82, 83] but it is more likely that such cases represent culture or processing errors. To obviate such errors, any abnormal findings should be verified by harvesting a second parallel culture. The second aspect of this problem is whether a true fetal mosaicism would be recognized by amniotic fluid cell karyotyping. One case of 46,XX/47,XX,13+ mosaicism has been prenatally diagnosed and verified at the time of therapeutic abortion.[84] In this particular case the two cell lines were present in approximately equal quantities, and it is unknown whether mosaicism for 10 or 20% of the cells would be recognizable.

A fourth type of pitfall is related to the fact that even if the karyotype is correct we may not know its clinical significance for the fetus. The classic examples are 47,XYY and 47,XXX. These karyotypes are not "normal" but they are not associated with malformations or marked mental retardation. No measure of the risk of a 47,XYY male's being socially deviant or of a 47,XXX female's having gamete nondisjunction exists. Our approach is to present parents of such a fetus, in as neutral a fashion as possible, with all of the relevant information. It may help to give the data in the form of a historic review and to place their risk in the context of the 2 to 3% risk of having a malformed infant that exists in every pregnancy.

During the last 5 years there have been rapid advances in cytogenetics occasioned by the development of staining techniques which allow the identification of each individual chromosome. Prior to this it was possible only to separate the chromosomes into groups. These new staining methods and their applications have been well summarized by Miller et al.[85] Relatively small deletions, translocations, and inversions can be recognized using banding techniques, and we believe all amniotic fluid lines should be studied using one of these methods. Using chromosome polymorphic variations elucidated by these stains it may be possible, for example, to prove that a 46,XX line must be fetal and not maternal, or to conduct prenatal paternity investigations.[60] However, the new techniques demonstrate many new polymorphisms of the chromosomes, and this raises new problems. Higher frequencies of these variants have been reported to occur among children with various defects.[86] Currently it is difficult to evaluate the significance of these variants in the individual case, and it will require a substantial cumulative experience of many centers to define the risks, if any, associated with these polymorphisms. Until such data are available, it is our policy to karyotype the parents when a fetal chromosomal variant is found. If the variant is present in one of the parental karyotypes we interpret it as being familial, and if it is not present we explain that we do not know what additional risk this indicates for the fetus but that we believe it to be quite small. Followup of these pregnancies will aid in determining the significance of such polymorphisms.

X-linked Disorders

Attempts to predict the sex of an unborn child are as old as recorded history. As early as 1350 B.C. the pregnant Egyptian woman was told to place barley and wheat in separate bags moistened with her urine. If the wheat germinated she would given birth to a boy; if the barley, a girl; and if neither, she was not pregnant.[87] Today, fetal sex is determined by demonstration of the Barr body (sex chromatin mass), by Y chromosome fluorescence, and by fetal karyotyping. Amniotic fluid cells can be stained directly for the sex chromatin mass or Y body, but the accuracy of these methods is only about 95%, as reported on 327 samples examined in five different laboratories.[88] Therefore, we feel that preparing a full karyotype is the only acceptable method of prenatal sex determination. Note that among the pregnancies monitored for sex one fetus with trisomy 21 was discovered (Table 5.2).

Women who are carriers of X-linked disorders can have the fetal sex ascertained and abort male fetuses. At present only in Fabry disease, the Hunter syndrome, and the Lesch-Nyhan syndrome, all of which are enzymatically defined, can an affected male be distinguished from an unaffected male. In all other situations, such as hemophilia or Duchenne muscular dystrophy, the parent should understand that 50% of the male abortuses would not have had the disease.

For X-linked disorders in which the affected males do not reproduce, the disease incidence is three times the mutation rate for that trait. This means that one-third of the males with such a disorder represent new mutations and that the trait is not carried by the mother. Therefore, she is not at an increased risk for future sons having the disorder. In some instances the mother's carrier status is demonstrable by pedigree analysis, e.g. if her father is affected, if she has two affected sons, if she has an affected son and an affected brother or maternal uncle. When the pedigree is not a help, an attempt should be made to clarify whether or not the mother is a carrier of the trait if suitable methods are available. Since pregnancy may alter the assayed factor e.g. factor VIII is raised, making the pregnant carrier of hemophilia "appear normal", it is desirable to investigate the carrier status prior to conception. Statistical methods to aid carrier detection for hemophilia A and Duchenne muscular dystrophy have been described.[89, 90]

The results in Table 5.2 indicate that close to the expected 50% of pregnancies monitored for X-linked diseases were male. One error in fetal sex prediction was reported in this group, and that involved using chromatin mass determination for sexing.[53] A significant difference from the pregnancies monitored for a chromosomal indication or to determine an inborn error of metabolism was noted in that a number of families elected not to terminate the pregnancy even though a male offspring was predicted. A number of the disorders for which fetal sex determination was performed have milder effects than the chromosomal aneuploidies or metabolic errors. This and the fact that 50% of the predicted males would be unaffected appear to be the two major factors contributing to the decision not to terminate the pregnancy.

Sex Selection

In many areas of the world there is a decided preference for male offspring. In India, for example, the desire for a son is very strong and sex preselection would ensure that son and decrease the number of daughters. The overall effect would be to lower the birth rate. Recent surveys[91, 92] have shown that if Americans had only one child most would prefer a son. There is also a slight tendency to prefer males in families with equal numbers of male and female children already born, but a strong preference for equalizing the number of males and females in families with a preponderance of one sex. The long range effect of sex preselection on the sex ratio would be minimal.[91, 92] Our experience has been that there is an increasing number of families that would like to use prenatal sex determination and selective abortion to control the sex and number of children they bear. Currently, most prenatal detection centers (ours included) will not determine fetal sex unless a specific genetic indication exists. However, in a country where one million elective abortions are performed annually, it is difficult to support this as a logically consistent position regarding acceptable and unacceptable indications for prenatal diagnosis. One practical problem is that to accept such cases would make it logistically impossible to perform prenatal diagnosis for families in which a genetic indication exists.

A simpler and perhaps more socially acceptable method of sex selection would be sex predetermination at the time of conception. This would allow women carriers of X-linked disorders selectively to conceive females. The most promising approach is separation of the X-bearing and the Y-bearing sperm, followed by artificial insemination. Physical methods for the separation of sperm have included centrifugation and electrophoresis.[93, 94] The centrifugal techniques assume that Y-bearing sperm have a mass slightly less than that of X-bearing sperm. The electrophoretic separation depends upon the sperm having different isoelectric points on their surfaces. Neither technique has met with much success. A recent report[95] purporting to separate the Y-bearing sperm has not been substantiated.[96] Moreover, this is not the desired end point from a geneticist's viewpoint, since it would be of more value to recover the X-bearing sperm and enhance the conception of daughters who would not manifest X-linked disorders. A preliminary report employing Sephadex column separation claims to allow selective recovery of the X-bearing sperm.[97] When such techniques are followed by artificial insemination it will be necessary to monitor these pregnancies by amniocentesis to verify the fetal sex.

Inborn Errors of Metabolism

The demonstration that a disease state could be due to the absence of a functionally normal enzymatic or structural protein was a key step in molecular genetics. Since this discovery, in 1952, there has been a virtually logarithmic growth in the number of conditions found to be secondary to a single molecular defect. Most of these diseases are inherited in an autosomal recessive or X-linked manner. Of the over 2,000 presently defined human genetic traits,[98] almost one-half are transmitted in one of these two modes, and inherited biochemical disorders of metabolism are known to occur in 0.8% of liveborns.[99] These conditions have a 25% occurrence rate when both parents are heterozygous for the deleterious autosomal gene or when the mother carries an abnormal X-linked gene. The presence of the abnormal gene(s) in the parent(s) is usually established by the birth of an affected child.

There has been a fundamental observation that cultured skin fibroblasts normally possess the enzyme activity that is deficient in many of these conditions and retain this enzymatic machinery through successive generations in culture. Cultured amniotic fluid cells are usually fibroblastic in their growth characteristics and express a biochemical phenotype similar to skin fibroblasts. It is important to note, however, that quantitative enzyme activities in cultured amniotic fluid and skin fibroblasts may be considerably different.[100] Therefore, enzyme studies on amniotic fluid cells must be controlled using normal amniotic fluid cells grown at the same time and under identical conditions. The medium used, the confluency of the cells, how often the medium was changed, the gestational age at which the cells were obtained, the length of time in culture, and the cellular morphology have all been shown to influence the enzymatic activity of the cells.[101-104] This last variable can be used to advantage in that, although histidase activity (the deficient enzyme, in histidinemia) is normally not manifest in amniotic fluid fibroblastic cells, it is present in epithelial-like cells. By cloning and selecting the latter for analysis the prenatal diagnosis of this condition becomes feasible.[104]

The prenatal diagnosis of the inborn errors of metabolism is generally by enzyme activity assays of cultured amniotic fluid cells. However, diagnoses have been made using amniotic fluid, per se, or uncultured amniotic fluid cells. Amniotic fluid may be used for defects in transport or metabolism of amino acids,[41] for defects such as the mucopolysaccharidoses where abnormal fetal urinary products accumulate,[105] for defects such as Tay-Sachs where the deficient enzyme is normally present in the fluid,[106] or for defects such as adrenogenital syndrome where the enzyme deficiency is not demonstrable in cultured fibroblasts.[107] However, the use of amniotic fluid analysis for prenatal diagnosis is fraught with danger. Maternal blood contamination may alter results, the changing protein content of the fluid makes interpretation difficult, and the unknown qualitative and quantitative contribution of fetal urine to the fluid further obscures analysis results. Uncultured amniotic fluid cells have detectable levels of most enzymes found in cultured amniotic fluid cells,[108] and have been used for prenatal diagnosis. In fact, ornithine carbamyltransferase, the enzyme deficient in hyperammonemia Type II, appears to be absent in cultured cells but present in uncultured cells. This example aside, the variation in amniotic fluid cell number and viability makes the use of uncultured cells unreliable and has led to the abortion of a normal fetus with the misdiagnosis of Tay-Sachs disease.[109] The major stimulus to avoid using cultured cells is the 4- to 6-week time period required to grow enough cells for enzyme analysis. Another approach to the problem is the development of sensitive assays that can be carried out on small numbers of cells, and this has been done in a few instances.[110-112]

Table 5.3 lists the hereditary biochemical disorders which have been detected in utero. It also details several other deficiency diseases in which the deficient enzyme has been demonstrated in normal skin or amniotic fluid fibroblasts, although the prenatal diagnosis of the disease has not yet been made. From the combined data of Table 5.2 and Milunsky[41] there have been 239 pregnancies monitored for an inborn error of metabolism, of which 44 (18.4%) have been affected. Tay-Sachs disease, Pompe disease, and the mucopolysaccharidoses have been the commonest indications for prenatal biochemical studies thus far.

Congenital Malformations

Most congenital malformations occur without demonstrable chromosomal or biochemical abnormalities and are produced by a combination of environmental and genetic factors. Prenatal diagnosis of such malformations has been attempted by fetal visualization and by detection of substances quantitatively or qualitatively abnormal as a result of the defect.

Indirect fetal visualization has been by sonography or contrast radiography. Ultrasound measurements of the biparietal diameter of the fetal head can be used to diagnose anencephaly.[171] We have had the experience of serendipitously discovering anencephaly when a fetal sonogram was obtained as a baseline because the mother had had a previous intra-uterine growth-retarded infant. With the introduction of "gray scale" and "real time" sonography more subtle anomalies such as myelomeningocele, omphalocele, or gastroschesis should become diagnosable. Serial measurements of fetal biparietal diameter to evaluate hydrocephalus

TABLE 5.3

Potentially Detectable Inborn Errors of Metabolism

Disease	Enzyme defect	Prenatal diagnosis[a]	Reference
Acatalasia	Catalase	Possible	113
Adenosine deaminase deficiency	Adenosine deaminase	Yes	114
Adrenogenital syndrome	C-11 or C-21 steroid hydroxylase	Yes (term)	115
Arginosuccinicaciduria	Arginosuccinase	Yes	116
Chediak-Higashi syndrome	Unknown (intracellular inclusion body)	Possible	117
Citrullinemia	Arginosuccinic acid synthetase	Yes	118
Cystathionuria	Cystathionase	Probable	119
Cystinosis	Unknown (cystine accumulation)	Yes	120
Ehlers-Danlos Syndrome Type IV	Unknown (lack of Type III collagen)	Possible	121
Fabry's disease[b]	Ceramidetrihexoside galactosidase	Yes	122
Farber's disease	Ceramidase	Possible	123
Fucosidosis	α-Fucosidase	Probable	41
Galactokinase deficiency	Galactokinase	Yes	124
Galactosemia	Galactose-1-P uridyl transferase	Yes	125
Generalized gangliosidosis (G_{M1} gangliosidosis, Type I)	β-Galactosidase	Yes	126
Juvenile gangliosidosis (G_{M1} gangliosidosis, Type II)	β-Galactosidase	Yes	127
Juvenile G_{M2} gangliosidosis	Partial deficiency of hexosaminidase A	Possible	128
Gaucher's disease	Glucocerebrosidase	Yes	129
Glycogen storage, Type II (Pompe's disease)	α-1,4-Glucosidase	Yes	130
Glycogen storage, Type III	Amylo-1,6-glucosidase	Probable	131
Glycogen storage, Type IV	Branching enzyme	Probable	132
Hemoglobinopathies	Synthesis of abnormal hemoglobin	Yes	133
Histidinemia	Histidase	Probable	134
Homocystinuria	Cystathionine synthetase	Probable	135
Hunter's syndrome[b]	α-L-Iduronic acid-2 sulfatase	Yes	136
Hurler's syndrome	α-L-Iduronidase	Yes	136
Hyperammonemia, Type II	Ornithine carbamyltransferase	Probable	108
Hyperlysinemia	Lysine-ketoglutarase reductase	Possible	137
Hypervalinemia	Valine transaminase	Possible	138
Hypophosphatasia	Alkaline phosphatase	Yes	139
I-cell disease	Nonspecific lysosomal enzymes	Yes	140
Ketotic hyperglycinemia	Propionyl-CoA carboxylase	Yes (late gestation)	141
Krabbe's disease	Galactocerebroside β-galactosidase	Yes	142
Lesch-Nyhan syndrome[b]	Hypoxanthine-guanine phosphoribosyltransferase	Yes	143
Lysosomal acid phosphotase deficiency	Lysosomal acid phosphatase	Yes	144
Mannosidosis	α-Mannosidase	Probable	41
Maple syrup urine disease	Branched chain ketoacid decarboxylase	Yes	145
Maroteaux-Lamy syndrome	Arylsulfatase B	Possible	146
Metachromatic leukodystrophy	Arylsulfatase A	Yes	147
Methylmalonicaciduria	Methylmalonic-CoA isomerase	Yes	148
Methyltetrahydrofolate methyltransferase deficiency	Methyltetrahydrosulfate methyltransferase	Possible	149
Methyltetrahydrofolate reductase deficiency	Methyltetrahydrofolate reductase	Possible	150
Morquio's syndrome	Chondroitin sulfate-*N*-acetylhexo-samine sulfate sulfatase	Possible Possible	151 151
Niemann-Pick disease	Sphingomyelinase	Yes	152
Ornithine-α-ketoacid transaminase deficiency	Ornithine-α-ketoacid transaminase	Probable	153
Oroticaciduria	Orotidylic pyrophosphorylase and decarboxylase	Possible	154
Osteogenesis imperfecta[c]	Unknown (sulfate incorporation)	Probable	155
Phosphohexose isomerase deficiency	Phosphohexose isomerase	Possible	156
Placental sulfatase deficiency[b]	Placental sulfatase	Yes	157

TABLE 5.3—*Continued*

Disease	Enzyme defect	Prenatal diagnosis[a]	Reference
Porphyria, congenital erythropoietic type	Cosynthetase	Possible	158
Pyruvate decarboxylase deficiency	Pyruvate decarboxylase	Possible	159
Refsum's disease	Phytanic acid α-hydroxylase	Probable	160
Sandhoff's disease	Hexosaminadase A and B	Yes	161
Sanfilippo syndrome, Type A	Heparin sulfatase	Yes	162
Sanfilippo syndrome, Type B	N-acetyl-α-D-glucosaminidase	Possible	163
Scheie's syndrome	α-L-Iduronidase	Possible	164
Tay-Sachs disease	Hexosaminidase A	Yes	165
α-Thalassemia	Decreased synthesis of α chain hemoglobin	**Yes**	166
β-Thalassemia	Decreased synthesis of β chain hemoglobin	Yes	167
Vitamin B_{12} metabolic defect	Vitamin B_{12} coenzyme	Possible	168
Wolman's disease	Acid lipase	Yes	169
Xeroderma pigmentosum	UV endonuclease	Yes	170

[a] Yes, prenatal diagnosis accomplished; Probable, enzyme activity present in normal amniotic fluid cells; Possible, enzyme activity present in normal skin fibroblasts.

[b] X-linked.

[c] Autosomal dominant.

or microcephaly probably will not be of value because these defects are not demonstrable until later in the pregnancy.[172]

Direct radiography has been used to demonstrate the absence of an autosomal recessively inherited syndrome in which radial aplasia is one of the components.[173] The fatal infantile form of osteopetrosis has been radiologically diagnosed in the second trimester of pregnancy,[174] but an attempt to make the prenatal diagnosis of achondroplasia was unsuccessful.[175] Contrast radiography may use a water-soluble dye such as hypaque to demonstrate fetal swallowing and the presence of esophageal or duodeneal atresia and/or may use a fat-soluble dye such as lipiodol to outline the fetal silhouette and the presence of a myelomeningocele or omphalocele.[176] The use of direct radiography for prenatal diagnosis appears to be quite limited, and the use of contrast radiography will probably be largely susperseded by the development of better sonographic techniques.

Direct fetal visualization is performed using a small bore fiberoptic endoscope. The original impetus for the development of such an instrument was for visualization of neural tube defects, e.g. anencephaly and spina bifida, but in the interim a better method for the prenatal diagnosis of such defects has been developed (see below). Our personal experience with the currently available 2-mm diameter endoscope (Dyonics, Inc.) has been such that we feel it will not be useful for the prenatal identification of congenital malformations. In fact, a fetus with a spina bifida and meningomyelocele was examined in utero with a fetoscope and the defect was missed![177] The fetoscope could be of great value, however, in facilitating the obtaining of fetal red cells or fetal serum.

The discovery that increased quantities of α-fetoprotein were present in the amniotic fluid and maternal sera of pregnancies in which the fetus had a neural tube defect has led to the prenatal diagnosis of a number of such fetuses (see Table 5.2). α-Fetoprotein is a normal fetal serum protein synthesized by the fetal liver and yolk sac.[178] The fetal serum and amniotic fluid concentrations of α-fetoprotein are highest during the 12th to 14th gestational weeks.[179] Brock and Sutcliffe[180] first drew attention to the fact that the amniotic fluid α-fetoprotein concentration was abnormally high in the presence of a fetal neural tube defect. The increase in α-fetoprotein is presumably due to transudation from exposed fetal capillaries or meninges, and a closed neural tube defect probably will not be recognized by this method. Since individuals with a neural tube defect are at a 4 to 5% risk of having first degree relatives (siblings or children) with such a defect, these have been the families referred for prenatal diagnosis. Table 5.2 lists 221 such "at risk" pregnancies monitored, with 20 "affected" fetuses having been found. That this is higher than the 4 to 5% "expected positives" reflects the tendency to report single positive cases. An increased amniotic fluid α-fetoprotein level appears to be nonspecific and has been found in conjunction with a number of other congenital defects such as the Turner syndrome,[181] sacrococcygeal teratoma,[182] nephrosis,[183] omphalocele[184, 185] and esophageal atresia.[186]

Of the children born with a neural tube defect, 90% are the first affected individual in the family, so that even if amniocentesis were employed in all families with a previous child with a neural tube defect the disease incidence would only be lowered by 10%. Thus there is great interest in a usable diagnostic test that might be based on raised α-fetoprotein levels in maternal serum. The prenatal diagnosis of a neural tube defect has been made using the maternal serum α-fetoprotein concentration with confirmation by ultrasonic and x-ray scan.[187] In a collation of data from a number of centers,[188] it was found that 12 of 15 anencephalic and 10 of 17 open spina bifida fetuses were associated with maternal serum α-fetoprotein levels above the highest value for normal pregnancies. The overall detection rate of 68% suggests that the number of infants born with neural tube defects could be more than halved with widespread application of maternal serum screening. If, as a practical point, the 98th percentile of the normal range of our values is used as an indication for a confirmatory amniocentesis, then 20 amniocenteses would be needed per thousand pregnancies. With an incidence rate of 1.7 per thousand liveborns in the United States[189] and a detection rate of 68%, there would be positive confirmation in 5.8% of these amniocenteses. This compares very well with the current results for amniocentesis for prenatal diagnosis of chromosomal disorders.

Recently a second marker, the cerebrospinal fluid β-trace protein, was found to be elevated in the amniotic fluid of pregnancies in which the fetus had a neural tube defect.[190] A retrospective study[191] has suggested this marker would also be useful for prenatal diagnosis, but β-trace protein is probably no more specific than the α-fetoprotein.[185] There is no evidence this protein could be used in a maternal serum screening test, and there is now some question just what is being measured.

Fetal Tissue Biopsy

Many genetic defects are not reflected in amniotic fluid constituents but are demonstrable using other fetal tissues or cells. The ability to obtain these cells or tissues would allow prenatal diagnosis of such disorders. One example is the use of fetal red cells to determine the normality or abnormality of the hemoglobin chains being synthesized. As little as 10 μl of fetal blood obtained in the second trimester makes possible the prenatal diagnosis of aberrant chains, as in sickle cell anemia, or abnormal rates of hemoglobin synthesis (thalassemia).[192] The prenatal exclusion of β-thalassemia has already been reported.[193] The major need is for a safe, reliable method of obtaining the fetal red cells. The fetal blood may be obtained using a 27-gauge needle under direct visualization (fetoscopy)[194, 195] or by sonographic directed aspiration from the placenta with a 20-gauge needle.[196, 197] Which of these methods will prove to be the safer and more reliable is not yet known. The prenatal diagnosis of hemoglobinopathies is currently available at only two centers in the United States.

The fetal red blood cells needed for hemoglobin chain synthesis may be contaminated with maternal blood or amniotic fluid without influencing the results. Obtaining uncontaminated fetal blood would make possible the prenatal diagnosis of (1) defects of lymphocytes, polymorphonuclearleukocytes, and platelets, (2) red cell structural abnormalities or enzyme defects that cause hemolytic anemias, and (3) defects of serum proteins such as immunoglobulins, fibrinogen, ceruloplasmin, or clotting factors. In each of these cases it will be necessary to first demonstrate that the fetal serum concentration accurately reflects the status of the fetus. Although most amniotic fluid proteins are of maternal origin,[198] this is unlikely to be true of fetal serum constituents in view of the placental endothelial barrier between the two circulations. Obtaining uncontaminated fetal blood will be very difficult and will probably require cannulization of a fetal vessel with a 30-gauge catheter under fetoscopic visualization.

The other fetal tissue that has been biopsied thus far is skin.[199] Although it may be possible to obtain enough fibroblasts for karyotype analysis or biochemical studies somewhat more rapidly from skin explants, I do not feel the time saved is worth the risk to the fetus. Very few metabolic disorders are demonstrable in skin fibroblasts that are not demonstrable in amniotic fluid cells, so there probably will be little practical value of fetal skin biopsies. Muscle biopsies, however, might be of considerable aid in the prenatal diagnosis of myopathies.

Complications

Although no matched-control studies are yet available, the cumulative experience of prenatal detection centers has been that early amniocentesis is associated with minimal risks and complications. Parents must be informed of the possibility of failure to obtain amniotic fluid or to grow amniotic fluid cells. Among the 3,452 monitored pregnancies in Table 5.2 there were 88 (2.6%) failures to obtain a result. This certainly reflects under-reporting, as some series never discussed failures or complications. In our first 600 monitored pregnancies we had 15 failures to obtain a result.

The cumulative experience with spontaneous abortion following early amniocentesis included 51 abortions occurring 1 day to 12 weeks after the procedure. This also reflects serious under-reporting. The relationship of the abortion to the preceding amniocentesis is difficult to establish. There is a spontaneous abortion rate of 3% between the 14th and 18th gestational weeks in large surveys of pregnant women.[200] Among our first 600 patients there were four abortions that occurred within the first week following amniocentesis and seven that occurred 18 to 50 days after the procedure. We are making the unsubstantiated assumption that the four early losses may be related to the procedure and the seven late losses reflect the "expected" losses at this time of gestation. We, therefore, tell patients there is a ½ to 1% risk of miscarrying related to having an early amniocentesis. The issue is further clouded by the fact that more than 20 of our patients have aborted in the week prior to their appointment!

Families also should be counseled that prenatal diagnosis is not infallible and that the results obtained may not reflect the fetal status. Three nonconsequential errors due to culturing maternal cells have been reported,[54, 60] but one misdiagnosis leading to a therapeutic abortion was made when sex chromatin masses were used to determine the sex of fetuses at risk for X-linked diseases.[53] In addition, a normal fetus was aborted because of tetraploid amniotic fluid cells before the true meaning of such cells was recognized,[57] a prenatally diagnosed XXY fetus was found to have a normal karyotype postabortion,[42] a normal fetus was aborted with the prenatal diagnosis of a neural tube defect when samples became interchanged,[202] and an incorrect diagnosis of Tay-Sachs disease was made because of unrecognized technological problems and a normal fetus aborted.[109] Four errors of the reverse nature have been reported where a fetus was prenatally diagnosed as being unaffected but after delivery was found to be affected. These include fetuses at risk for the Hurler syndrome,[203] galactosemia,[41] Tay-Sachs disease,[204] and the Down syndrome.[82] Couples who choose to have prenatal diagnosis must understand its limitation. Most of the above errors occurred very early in the cumulative experience and are avoidable with current methodology.

Perhaps the greatest "risk" of the procedure is that it might have a positive result. The family must consider this in order to evaluate their options, and this possibility should be discussed during the counseling session. We recently conducted psychometric testing and psychiatric interviews on 13 families who upon receiving positive results elected to have a therapeutic abortion.[205] The incidence of depression following selective abortion may be as high as 92% among the women and as high as 82% among the men studied, and was greater than that usually associated with elective abortion for psychosocial indications or with delivery of a stillborn. Four families experienced separation during the pregnancy-abortion period. Despite the emotional trauma of the procedure, most of the families studied would repeat their course of action and consider abortion preferable to the birth of a defective child.

Cost-Effectiveness

In the United States there has been little legislative aid to the prenatal detection centers. One argument for such aid is the cost-benefit analysis demonstrating the economic gains to society of such programs. The reduction in emotional cost for the involved families is, of course, immeasurable.

Genetic counseling, amniocentesis, cell culture, and the appropriate genetic studies cost about $300 in our center. Of the approximately three million infants born in this country annually, some 7% (210,000) are born to mothers 35–39 years of age and some 3% (90,000) are born to mothers aged forty or more.[41] If we assume a utilization rate of 50%, then 150,000 amniocenteses would be done annually at a cost of $45 million.

If the risk of bearing a chromosomally abnormal child is 1% for the 35- to 39-year-old mother and 2% for the mother 40 or over (between the reported liveborn rate and the cumulative experience rate in Table 5.2), then a total of 1,950 chromosomally defective fetuses will be found among those women opting for prenatal diagnosis. Our institution charges $300 for a second trimester therapeutic abortion, so the cost of terminating the 1,950 pregnancies would be $565,000, assuming all couples requested such action. Thus the total cost of prenatal diagnosis and therapeutic abortion when necessary would be just over $45.5 million.

The cost of caring for the 1,950 chromosomally abnormal offspring that would otherwise be born is difficult to compute. For many of these defects institutionalization or subsidized care would eventually result. If we use a conservative figure of 10 years of such care per individual and the Massachusetts annual care cost of $6,100,[41] then the care of these abnormal offspring would cost society almost $116 million, or two and one-half times the cost of prevention through prenatal diagnosis and selective abortion.

Ethical Questions

The purpose of the prenatal detection center is to assure families that they can selectively have unaffected offspring when the risk for having genetically defective children becomes unacceptably high. Currently, "unacceptably high" is defined at most centers as greater than 1%, on the philosophy that the procedural risk seems to be under that figure. If the risk is less than 1/2% and the overall frequency of chromosomal aneuploidy is 1:200, the question arises as to whether all pregnant women should be offered this diagnostic test. This is not economically justifiable since many of the sex chromosome disorders would not require institutional care, but the cost in human terms is significant. The definition of "genetically defective" also requires clarification. Should this include only lethal defects or only nonlethal defects? Should a metabolic error such as galactosemia which is at least partially treatable be considered a valid indication for prenatal diagnosis? Should *any* defect, regardless how minor, that causes consternation to the parents be an acceptable indication? Today, the genetic counselors at prenatal detection centers are providing the explicit or implicit guidelines—not always consistently. Since these questions are of basic importance to society, it seems more reasonable that society as a whole should consider these questions and define guidelines of "ethical acceptability."

The decision for amniocentesis and intervention for an affected fetus must be made by the parents. Many families in a high risk category would not desire prenatal diagnosis. A request for an amniocentesis should not be construed as a commitment for therapeutic abortion of an affected fetus, and such a commitment should never be a prerequisite for the study. We do discuss this problem with parents and if they feel that they would not have an abortion of an affected fetus, we ask them to be sure they wish to place the fetus at even the small risk of amniocentesis. If their decision is an informed one we abide by their wishes. The suggestion that parents who knowingly give birth to an abnormal child do not have the right to society's help in caring for their child is mentioned only to be deplored.

The question of patient privacy *vs.* the relatives' right to information that may influence their lives and those of their offspring remains unresolved. If a woman is found to be a carrier of a serious deleterious X-linked allele, whose responsibility will it be to inform her sisters of their risks? The physician obviously breaches the patient's right of privacy if he informs the sisters. Yet many patients are reticent about informing relatives about genetic defects. In the near future the principle of the greatest good for the greatest number may have to supersede the principle of patient-physician privileged communication. Eventually it is hoped that public education about genetics and genetic diseases will allow unstigmatized sharing of genetic information among family members.

The fear has been voiced that selective abortion of affected fetuses and reproductive compensation with offspring likely to be carriers of the deleterious gene would have long term implications for the gene pool. Motulsky et al.[206] showed that for autosomal recessive diseases the case reduction would be 12.5 to 34% if prenatal diagnosis was initiated after the birth of an affected child. Reproductive compensation with normal children, two-thirds of whom would be heterozygotes for the mutant gene, would have a definite but minimal effect on the gene frequency.[206, 207] For the X-linked diseases it is more likely that the gene carrier would be identified prior to childbearing, and selective abortion of all-male fetuses would result in a two-thirds reduction in the disease incidence. The remaining one-third would represent new mutations. Reproductive compensation by these known carriers would increase the prevalence of female heterozygotes by 50% each generation.[207] This rapid rise in gene frequency would be manageable provided that prenatal diagnosis became routine for these individuals.

Future Prospects

As noted above, our current method of identifying heterozygotes for the autosomal recessive disorders is by the birth of the index case. Even widespread application of prenatal diagnosis will provide only a small reduction in disease incidence. We are now entering an era of mass screening for heterozygote detection. The criteria for such a program are: (1) a defined population group at risk, (2) an accurate, reliable, inexpensive method of carrier detection, and (3) the ability to provide prenatal diagnosis of the entity in question. Tay-Sachs disease is the first disorder to meet these criteria, and the Baltimore-Washington screening established the practicality of such an approach.[208] Since then a number of cities have embarked upon Tay-Sachs heterozygote detection programs, and California has established the first statewide legislatively supported program. In California alone there are 33,000 carriers of the Tay-Sachs gene and 350 "at risk" couples in which both are carriers with a 25% risk of Tay-Sachs disease for each offspring. Identification of these couples will allow the use of prenatal diagnosis without the index case being born. The recent prenatal diagnosis of a hemoglobinopathy[193] indicates that this class of disorders may be tackled with similar mass screening efforts.

Artificial insemination using a sperm donor (AID) is an approach to the control of autosomally inherited diseases that has been biologically feasible since the end of the eighteenth century but is only now becoming socially acceptable. Prior to utilization of this technique for a family with one child with an autosomal recessive inherited entity, it is advisable to demonstrate that the husband is a heterozygote and that the planned donor is not. Various authors have demonstrated in different communities that up to 30% of the husbands could not have been the fathers of their children.[209, 210] We are informing couples whom we counsel regarding autosomally inherited diseases about AID as one option they could choose. Muller[211] suggested an effort should be made to improve the quality of our species using AID, but Medawar[212] concluded that positive eugenics could not be achieved since our genetic system would not improve with selective inbreeding. Our genetic diversity contributes to our species' well-being. We would do better to expend our efforts on educational and cultural measures for self-improvement.

It is likely that many of the autosomal dominant diseases will not be identifiable by an abnormal gene product. These entities and the X-linked diseases (in males) which manifest themselves in the presence of one abnormal gene may be detected in the fetus by the use of closely linked genetic markers. The approach is to determine whether the marker gene, known to be closely linked to the mutant disease-causing gene, is present on the same or different chromosome as is the defective gene. The fetal cells are analyzed for the presence of the marker gene, and its presence or absence indicates whether or not the fetus is affected.

The first application of the linkage technique was for the autosomal dominant disorder myotonic dystrophy.[213] The gene for this disease is closely linked to the gene for ABH-secretor status.[214] Since amniotic fluid reflects the secretor status of the fetus,[215] this linkage can be used, with the understanding that the 8% crossover rate between these two loci will give erroneous results in that percentage of fetuses. A significant drawback to this technique is that a favorable combination of marker and disease genes will occur in only about one-third of the families.[213]

The linkage technique could be applied to hemophilia A, since the gene for factor VIII production and the gene for glucose 6-phosphate dehydrogenase (G6PD) are close to one another on the X chromosome.[216] Amniotic fluid cells do express G6PD variants,[217] and so could be used for the prenatal diagnosis. Easily detectable G6PD variants are most common in the black population, where this approach would therefore be most helpful. As somatic cell hybridization techniques assign more and more human genes to specific chromosomes, it is likely that numerous other marker gene-disease gene linkages will be discovered.

A number of recognized inherited enzyme defects occur only in one or two tissues which are not represented in amniotic fluid cells or by other fetal cells liable to biopsy. Since the entire genome is present in each fetal cell, the question is one of activating unexpressed genes in that cell. The approach envisioned is to fuse easily obtainable fetal cells with "activator" cell lines. That this is a feasible concept has been demonstrated by obtaining mouse albumin from mouse fibroblasts fused with rat hepatoma cells.[218] The gene for albumin synthesis is normally only "on" in liver cells but it is activated in the fibroblasts by the hepatoma cells.

Another new approach to prenatal diagnosis is suggested by the recent discovery that α-thalassemia is due to absence of the structural gene (DNA) for the alpha chain of hemoglobin.[166, 219] Since it can be demonstrated that cultured amniotic cells do have the gene,[220] the prenatal diagnosis of α-thalassemia can be made by finding the absence of this specific DNA in an "at risk" couple. A number of disorders probably will be shown to be secondary to absent structural genes, and this technique may be applicable for their prenatal diagnosis if the specific mRNA can be isolated.

It has been suggested that an alternate goal of prenatal diagnosis should be treatment of the affected fetus and correction of the defect. For those disorders involving physical abnormalities such as congenital malformations or chromosomal aneuploidy it is very unlikely that effective preventive therapy will be developed. Publicity regarding the successful induction of galactose-1-P-uridyl transferase activity in galactosemic skin fibroblasts has led to premature conclusions that alteration of the basic genome is now possible. There is concern that in some enzyme deficiencies irreversible fetal damage may have occurred by the time the prenatal diagnosis is made.[126, 127, 221, 222] A recent editorial has appraised the potential and liabilities of gene therapy, with emphasis on its limitations and hazards.[223]

The future of prenatal diagnosis holds great promise for exciting advances. The number of disorders diagnosable in utero will undoubtedly steadily increase, and amniocentesis will become routine for women at increased risk of producing defective offspring. This will probably develop in tandem with computerized metaphase chromosome scanning and microanalysis of biochemical defects. The education of the obstetrician-gynecologists to take a central role in the genetic history taking and initial counseling of prenatal (and pre-pregnant) patients is taking its place as a significant part of specialty training.

REFERENCES

1. Fuchs, F, Amniocentesis: Techniques and Complications, in Harris, M, ed., *Early Diagnosis of Human Genetic Defects*, Fogerty Proc 6:11, 1970.

2. Hahnemann, N, Possibility of Culturing Foetal Cells at Early Stages of Pregnancy, Clin Genet 3:286, 1972.

3. Wahlstrom, J, The Quantity of Viable Cells at Various Stages of Gestation, Humangenetik 22:335, 1974.

4. Fuchs, F, Volume of Amniotic Fluid at Various Stages of Pregnancy, Clin Obstet Gynecol 9:449, 1966.

5. Golbus, MS, Conte, FA, Schneider, EL, and Epstein, CJ, Intrauterine Diagnosis of Genetic Defects: Results, Problems, and Follow-up of 100 Cases in a Prenatal Genetic Detection Center, Am J Obstet Gynecol 118:897, 1974.

6. Bibring, GL, Dwyer, TF, Huntington, DS, and Valenstein, AF, A Study of the Psychological Processes in Pregnancy and of the Earliest Mother-Child Relationship. I. Some Propositions and Comments, Psychoanal Stud Child 16:9, 1961.

7. Raphael, B, Psychosocial Aspects of Induced Abortion: Its Implication for the Woman, Her Family and Her Doctor, Med J Aust 2:98, 1972.

8. Burnett, RG, and Anderson, WR, The Hazards of Amniocentesis, J Iowa Med Soc 58:130, 1968.

9. Creasman, WT, Lawrence, RA, and Thiede, HA, Fetal Complications of Amniocentesis, JAMA 204:91, 1968.

10. Aickin, DR, The Significance of Rises in Rhesus Antibody Titre Following Amniocentesis, J Obstet Gynecol Brit Comm 78:149, 1971.

11. Scrimgeour, JB, The Diagnostic Use of Amniocentesis: Techniques and Complications, Proc Roy Soc Med 64:29, 1971.

12. Bartsch, FK, Lundberg, J, and Wahlstrom, J, Amniocentesis and Cytogenetic Study of Amniotic Fluid Cells: Technique, Risks and Results in 180 Cases (Abstract), 4th International Conference on Birth Defects, Vienna, 1973, Excerpta Medica 297:77, 1973.

13. Morris, JA, Hustead, RF, Robinson, RG, and Haswell, GL, Measurement of Feto-

placental Blood Volume in the Human Previable Fetus, Am J Obstet Gynecol *118:*927, 1974.

14. Zipursky, Alvin, The Universal Prevention of Rh Immunization, Clin Obstet Gynecol *14:*869, 1971.

15. Abbo, G, and Zellweger, H, Prenatal Determination of Fetal Sex and Chromosomal Complement, Lancet *1:*216, 1970.

16. Gray, C, Davidson, RG, and Cohen, MM, A Simplified Technique for the Culture of Amniotic Fluid Cells, J Ped *79:*119, 1971.

17. Knorr-Gartner, H, and Harle, I, A Modified Method of Culturing Human Amniotic Fluid Cells for Prenatal Detection of Genetic Disorders, Humangenetik *14:*333, 1972.

18. Cederqvist, WL, Wennerstrom, C, Senterfit, LB, Baldridge, PB, and Rothe, DJ, Simplified Method for the Accelerated Growth of Amniotic Fluid Cell Cultures, Am J Obstet Gynecol *116:*871, 1973.

19. Sutherland, GR, and Bain, AD, Antenatal Diagnosis of Inborn Errors of Metabolism: Tissue Culture Aspects, Humangenetik *20:*251, 1973.

20. Hoehn, H, Bryant, EM, Karp, LE, and Martin, GM, Cultured Cells from Diagnostic Amniocentesis in Second Trimester Pregnancies. I. Clonal Morphology and Growth Potential, Pediat Res *8:*746, 1974.

21. Golbus, MS, and Erickson, RP, Midtrimester Abortion Induced by Intraamniotic Prostaglandin $F_{2\alpha}$: Fetal Tissue Viability, Am J Obstet Gynecol *119:*268, 1974.

22. Sergovich, F, Valentine, G, Chen, A, Kinch, R, and Stout, M, Chromosome Aberrations in 2159 Consecutive Newborn Babies, New Engl J Med *280:*851, 1969.

23. Lubs, H, and Ruddle, F, in Jacobs, P, Price, W, and Law, P, eds., *Human Population Cytogenetics*, Williams & Wilkins, Baltimore, 1970, p. 119.

24. Gerald, P, and Walzer, S, *ibid*, p. 143.

25. Turner, J, and Wald, N, *ibid*, p. 153.

26. Smith, P, and Jacobs, P, *ibid*, p. 159.

27. Hamerton, J, Manoranjan, R, Abbott, J, Williamson, C, and Ducasse, G, Chromosome Studies in a Neonatal Population, Canad Med Assoc J *106:*776, 1972.

28. Friedrich, U, and Nielsen, J, Chromosome Studies in 5,049 Consecutive Newborn Children, Clin Genet *4:*333, 1973.

29. Chen, A, and Falek, A, Chromosome Aberrations in Full-term Low Birth Weight Neonates, Humangenetik *21:*13, 1974.

30. Machin, G, Chromosome Abnormality and Perinatal Death, Lancet *1:*549, 1974.

31. Sutherland, G, Bauld, R, and Bain, A,

32. Mulcahy, M, and Jenkyn, J, Results of 538 Chromosome Studies on Patients Referred for Cytogenetic Analysis. Med J Aust *2:*1333, 1972.

33. Mitchell, A, J Ment Sci *98:*174, 1876, quoted in Richards, BW, Mongols and Their Mothers, Brit J Psych *122:*1, 1973.

34. Jenkins, R, Etiology of Mongolism, Am J Dis Child *45:*506, 1933.

35. Penrose, LS, The Relative Effects of Paternal and Maternal Age in Mongolism, J Genet *27:*219, 1933.

36. Ratcliffe, SG, personal communication.

37. Collmann, RD, and Stoller, A, A Survey of Mongoloid Births in Victoria, Australia, 1942–1957, Am J Pub Health Nat Health *52:*813, 1962.

38. Smith, DW, Patau, K, and Therman, E, Autosomal Trisomy Syndromes, Lancet *2:*211, 1961.

39. Smith, D, Autosomal Abnormalities, Am J Obstet Gynecol *90:*1055, 1964.

40. Mikkelson, M, and Stene, J, Genetic Counselling in Down's Syndrome, Hum Hered *20:*457, 1970.

41. Milunsky, A, *The Prenatal Diagnosis of Hereditary Diseases*, Charles C Thomas, Springfield, Il, 1973.

42. Milunsky, A, and Atkins, L, Prenatal Diagnosis of Genetic Disorders, JAMA *230:*232, 1974.

43. Polani, PE, Prenatal Cytological Recognition of Sex-linked and Chromosomal Abnormalities, J Obstet Gynecol Brit Common *78:*1024, 1974.

44. Ebbin, AJ, Wilson, MG, Towner, JW, and Slaughter, JP, Prenatal Diagnosis of an Inherited Translocation Between Chromosomes No. 9 and 18, J Med Genet *10:*65, 1973.

45. Aula, P, and Karjalainen, O, Prenatal Karyotype Analysis in High Risk Families, Ann Clin Res *5:*142, 1973.

46. Tayski, K, Bobrow, M, Balci, S, Madan, K, Atasu, M, and Say, B, Duplication Deficiency Product of a Pericentric Inversion in Man: A Cause of D_1 Trisomy Syndrome, J Pediat *82:*263, 1973.

47. Aarskog, D, Down's Syndrome Transmitted through Maternal Mosaicism, Acta Pediat Scand *58:*609, 1969.

48. Hsu, LY, Gertner, M, Leiter, E, and Hirschhorn, K, Paternal Trisomy 21 Mosaicism and Down's Syndrome, Am J Hum Genet *23:*592, 1971.

49. Hauschka, TS, Hasson, JE, Goldstein, MN, Koepf, GH, and Sandberg, AA, An XXY Man with Progeny Indicating Familial Tendency to Non-Disjunction.

Am J Hum Genet *14:*22, 1962.

50. Penrose, LS, and Smith, GF, *Down's Anomaly*, J & A Churchill, London, 1966.

51. Court-Brown, WM, *Human Population Cytogenetics*, North-Holland, Amsterdam, 1967.

52. Hamerton, JL, Robertsonian Translocation: Evidence on Segregation from Family Studies, in Jacobs, P, Price, WH, and Law, P, eds., *Human Population Cytogenetics*, Williams & Wilkins, Baltimore, 1970, p. 143.

53. Fuchs, F, Genetic Information from Amniotic Fluid Constituents, Clin Obstet Gynecol *9:*565, 1966.

54. Gerbie, AB, Nadler, HL, and Gerbie, MY, Amniocentesis in Genetic Counseling, Am J Obstet Gynecol *109:*765, 1971.

55. Barakat, BY, Heller, RH, and Jones, HW, Fetal Quality Control in Pregnancies with High Risk for Genetic Disorders, Fertil Steril *22:*409, 1971.

56. Ferguson-Smith, ME, Ferguson-Smith, MA, Nevin, NC, and Stone M, Chromosome Analysis Before Birth and its Value in Genetic Counseling, Brit Med J *4:*69, 1971.

57. Robinson, A, Bowes, W, Droegemuller, W, Puck, M, Goodman, S, Shikes, R, and Greenshur, A, Intrauterine Diagnosis: Potential Complications, Am J Obstet Gynecol *116:*937, 1973.

58. Prescott, GN, Pernoll, ML, Hecht, F, and Nicholas, A, A Prenatal Diagnosis Clinic: An Initial Report, Am J Obstet Gynecol *116:*942, 1973.

59. Doran, TA, Rudd, NL, Gardner, HA, Lowden, JA, Benzie, RJ, and Liedgreen, SI, The Antenatal Diagnosis of Genetic Disease, Am J Obstet Gynecol *118:*314, 1974.

60. Linsten, J, Therkelsen, AJ, Friedrich, U, Jonasson, J, Steenstrup, OR, and Wiquist, N, Prenatal Cytogenetic Diagnosis, Int J Gynecol Obstet *12:*101, 1974.

61. Hsu, LYF, Serutkin, AV, Kim, HJ, and Hirschhorn, K, 415 Cases of Prenatal Cytogenetic Diagnosis: Experience and Prospects, Amer Soc Hum Genet Abst, 1974 p. 42a.

62. Allen, HH, Sergovich, F, Stuart, EM, Pozsonyi, J, and Murray, B, Infants Undergoing Antenatal Genetic Diagnosis: A Preliminary Report, Am J Obstet Gynecol *118:*310, 1974.

63. Philip, J, Bang, J, Hahnemann, N, Mikkelsen, M, Niebuhr, E, Rebbe, H, and Weber, J, Chromosome Analysis of Fetuses in Risk Pregnancies, Acta Obstet Gynecol Scand *53:*9, 1974.

64. Laurence, KM, Fetal Malformations and Abnormalities, Lancet *2:*939, 1974.

65. Bartsch, FK, Lundberg, J, and Wahlstrom, J, The Technique, Results and Risks of Amniocentesis for Genetic Reasons, J Obstet Gynecol Brit Comm, *81:*991, 1974.

66. Larget-Piet, L, Le Lirzin, R, Berthelot, J, Larget-Piet, A, and Rouchy, R, Diagnostic Prenatal des Affections Genetiques, Sem Hosp Paris *51:*1151, 1975.

67. Niermeijer, MF, Sachs, ES, Jahodova, M, Tichelaar-Klepper, C, Kleiter, WJ, and Galjaard, H, Prenatal Diagnosis of Genetic Disorders in 350 Pregnancies, J Med Genet, 1975, in press.

68. Brock, DJH, and Sutcliffe, JB, Early Prenatal Diagnosis of Anencephaly, Lancet *2:*1252, 1972.

69. Lorber, J, Stewart, CR, and Ward, AM, Alpha-Fetoprotein in Antenatal Diagnosis of Anencephaly and Spina Bifida, Lancet *1:*1187, 1973.

70. Seller, MJ, Campbell, S, Coltart, TM, and Singer, JD, Early Termination of Anencephalic Pregnancy after Detection by Raised Alpha-Fetoprotein Levels, Lancet *2:*73, 1973.

71. Allen, LD, Ferguson-Smith, MA, Donald, I, Sweet, EM, and Gibson, AAM, Amniotic Fluid Alpha-Fetoprotein in the Antenatal Diagnosis of Spina Bifida, Lancet *2:*522, 1973.

72. Field, B, Mitchell, G, Garrett, W, and Kerr, C, Prenatal Diagnosis and Selected Abortion for Anencephaly and Spina Bifida, Med J Aust *1:*608, 1974.

73. Leek, AE, Leighton, PC, Kitau, MJ, and Chard, T, Prospective Diagnosis of Spina Bifida, Lancet *2:*1511, 1974.

74. Campbell, S, Pryse-Davies, J, Coltart, TM, Seller, MJ, and Singer, JD, Ultrasound in the Diagnosis of Spina Bifida, Lancet *1:*1065, 1975.

75. Schneider, EL, Stanbridge, EJ, Epstein, CJ, Golbus, MS, Abbo-Halsbach, G, and Rodgers, G, Mycoplasma Contamination of Cultured Amniotic Fluid Cells: Potential Hazard to Prenatal Chromosomal Diagnosis, Science *184:*477, 1974.

76. Cox, DM, Niewczas-Late, V, Riffell, MI, and Hamerton, JL, Chromosomal Mosaicism in Diagnostic Amniotic Fluid Cell Cultures, Pediat Res *8:*679, 1974.

77. Sutherland, GR, Bowser-Riley, SM, and Bain, AD, Chromosome Mosaicism in Amniotic Fluid Cell Cultures, Clin Genet *7:*400, 1975.

78. Walker, S, Lee, CLY, and Gregson, NM, Polyploidy in Cells Cultured from Amniotic Fluid, Lancet *2:*1137, 1970.

79. Milunsky, A, Atkins, L, and Littlefield, JW, Polyploidy in Prenatal Genetic Diagnosis,

J Ped *79:*303, 1971.

80. Tegenkamp, JR, and Hux, CH, Incidence of Tetraploidy as Related to Amniotic Fluid Cell Types, Am J Obstet Gynecol *120:*1066, 1974.

81. Kohn, G, and Robinson, A, Tetraploidy in Cells Cultured from Amniotic Fluid, Lancet *2:*778, 1970.

82. Katayama, KP, Park, IJ, Heller, RN, Barakat, BY, Preston, E, and Jones, HW, Errors of Prenatal Cytogenetic Diagnosis, Obstet Gynecol *44:*693, 1974.

83. Kardon, NB, Chernay, PR, Hsu, LYF, Martin, JL, and Hirschhorn, K, Problems in Prenatal Diagnosis Resulting from Chromosomal Mosaicism, Clin Genet *3:*83, 1972.

84. Bloom, AD, Schmickel, R, Barr, M, and Burdi, AR, Prenatal Detection of Autosomal Mosaicism, J Ped *84:*732, 1974.

85. Miller, O, Miller, D, and Warburton, D, Applications of New Staining Techniques to the Study of Human Genetics, Prog Med Genet *9:*1, 1973.

86. Lubs, N, Neonatal Cytogenetic Surveys, in *Perspectives in Cytogenetics: The Next Decade*, Charles C Thomas, Springfield, Il, 1972, p. 297.

87. Blakely, SB, Diagnosis of the Human Fetus in Utero, Am J Obstet Gynecol *34:*322, 1937.

88. Nadler, HL, Indications for Amniocentesis in the Early Prenatal Detection of Genetic Disorders, Birth Defects, Original Article Series *7:*5, 1971.

89. Bennett, B, and Ratnoff, OD, Detection of the Carrier Status for Classical Hemophilia, New Eng J Med *288:*342, 1973.

90. Emery, AEH, and Morton, R, Genetic Counseling in Lethal X-linked Disorders, Acta Genet *18:*534, 1968.

91. Markle, GE, and Nam, CB, Sex Predetermination: Its Impact on Fertility, Soc Biol *18:*73, 1971.

92. Westoff, CF, and Rindfuss, RR, Sex Preselection in the United States: Some Implications, Science *184:*633, 1974.

93. Jones, RJ, Sex Predetermination and the Sex Ratio at Birth, Soc Biol *20:*203, 1973.

94. Gordon, MJ, The Control of Sex, Sci Am *199:*87, 1958.

95. Ericsson, RJ, Langevin, CN, and Nishino, M, Isolation of Fractions Rich in Human Y Sperm, Nature (Lond) *246:*421, 1973.

96. Ross, A, Robinson, JA, and Evans, HJ, Failure to Confirm Separation of X and Y Bearing Human Sperm using BSA Gradients, Nature (Lond) *253:*354, 1975.

97. Steeno, O, Adimoelja, A, and Steeno, J, Separation of X and Y Bearing Human Spermatozoa with the Sephadex Gel-Filtration Method, Andrologia *7:*95, 1975.

98. McKusick, VA, *Mendelian Inheritance in Man*, 4th ed, Johns Hopkins Press, Baltimore, 1975.

99. Polani, PE, Incidence of Developmental and Other Genetic Abnormalities, Proc Roy Soc Med *66:*1118, 1973.

100. Kaback, MM, Leonard, CO, and Parmley, TH, Intrauterine Diagnosis: Comparative Enzymology of Cells Cultivated from Maternal Skin, Fetal Skin, and Amniotic Fluid Cells, Ped Res *5:*366, 1971.

101. Ryan, CA, Lee, SY, and Nadler, HC, Effect of Culture Conditions on Enzyme Activities in Cultivated Human Fibroblasts, Exp Cell Res *71:*388, 1972.

102. Butterworth, J, Broadhead, DM, Sutherland, GR, and Bain, AD, Lysosomal Enzymes of Amniotic Fluid in Relation to Gestational Age, Am J Obstet Gynecol *119:*821, 1974.

103. Sutherland, GR, Butterworth, J, Broadhead, DM, and Bain, AD, Lysosomal Enzyme Levels in Human Amniotic Fluid Cells in Tissue Culture, Clin Genet *5:*351 and 356, 1974.

104. Gerbie, AB, Melancon, SB, Ryan, C, and Nadler, HL, Cultivated Epithelial-like Cells and Fibroblasts from Amniotic Fluid: Their Relationship to Enzymatic and Cytologic Analysis, Am J Obstet Gynecol *114:*314, 1972.

105. Matalon, R, Dorfman, A, Nadler, HL, and Jacobson, CB, A Chemical Method for the Antenatal Diagnosis of Mucopolysaccharidosis, Lancet *1:*83, 1970.

106. Friedland, J, Perle, G, Saifer, A, Schneck, L, and Volk, BW, Screening for Tay-Sachs Disease in Utero using Amniotic Fluid, Proc Soc Exp Biol Med *136:*1297, 1971.

107. Golbus, MS, Siiteri, PK, and Conte, FA, unpublished results.

108. Nadler, HL, and Gerbie, AB, Enzymes in Noncultured Amniotic Fluid Cells, Am J Obstet Gynecol *103:*710, 1969.

109. Rattazzi, MC, and Davidson, RG, Limitations of Amniocentesis for the Antenatal Diagnosis of Tay-Sachs Disease, Abstract, Am Soc Hum Genet, 1970.

110. Richardson, BJ, and Cox, DM, Rapid Tissue Culture and Microbiochemical Methods for Analyzing Colonially Grown Fibroblasts from Normal, Lesch-Nyhan and Tay-Sachs Patients and Amniotic Fluid Cells, Clin Genet *4:*376, 1973.

111. Galjaard, H, Mekes, M, De Josselin De Jong, JE, and Niermeijer, MF, A Method for Rapid Prenatal Diagnosis of Glycogenosis II (Pompe's Disease). Clin Chim Acta *49:*361, 1973.

112. Galjaard, H, Niermeijer, MF, Hahnemann, N, Mohr, J, and Sorenson, SA, An Exam-

ple of Rapid Prenatal Diagnosis of Fabrey's Disease Using Microtechniques, Clin Genet 5:368, 1974.

113. Krooth, RS, Howell, RR, and Hamilton, HB, Properties of Acatalasic Cells Growing in Vitro, J Exp Med 115:313, 1962.

114. Hirschhorn, R, Beratis, N, Rosen, FS, Parkman, R, Stern, R, and Polmar, S, Adenosine-deaminase Deficiency in a Child Diagnosed Prenatally, Lancet 1:73, 1975.

115. Jeffcoate, TNA, Fliegner, JRH, Russell, SH, Davis, JC, and Wade, AP, Diagnosis of Adrenogenital Syndrome before Birth, Lancet 2:553, 1965.

116. Goodman, SI, Mace, JW, Turner, B, and Garrett, WJ, Antenatal Diagnosis of Arginosuccinic Aciduria, Clin Genet 4:236, 1973.

117. Danes, BS, and Bearn, AG, Cell Culture and the Chediak-Higashi Syndrome, Lancet 2:65, 1967.

118. Roerdink, FH, Gouw, WLM, Okken, A, van der Bilj, JF, Luit-de Haan, G, Hommes, FA, and Huistes, HJ, Citrullinemia, Report of a Case, with Studies on Antenatal Diagnosis, Ped Res 7:863, 1973.

119. Scott, CR, Dasjell, SW, Clark, SH, Chiang-Teng, C, and Swroberg, KR, Cystathioninemia: A Benign Genetic Condition, J Ped 76:571, 1970.

120. Schneider, JA, Verroust, FM, Kroll, WA, Garvin, AJ, Horger, EO, Wong, VG, Spear, GS, Jacobson, CB, Pellett, OL, and Becker, FLA, Prenatal Diagnosis of Cystinosis, New Eng J Med 290:878, 1974.

121. Pope, FM, Martin, GR, Lichtenstein, JR, Penttinen, R, Gerson, B, Rowe, DW, and McKusick, VA, Patients with Ehlers-Danlos Syndrome Type IV Lack Type III Collagen, Proc Nat Acad Sci 72:1314, 1975.

122. Brady, RO, Uhlendorf, BW, and Jacobson, CB, Fabry's Disease: Antenatal Detection, Science 172:174, 1971.

123. Sugita, M, Dulaney, JT, and Moser, HW, Ceramidase Deficiency in Farber's Disease (Lipogranulomatosis), Science 178:1100, 1972.

124. Donnell, G, personal communication.

125. Fensom, AH, Benson, PF, and Blunt, S, Prenatal Diagnosis of Galactosemia, Brit Med J 4:386, 1974.

126. Lowden, JA, Cutz, E, Conen, PE, Rudd, N, and Doran, TA, Prenatal Diagnosis of G_{M1}-Gangliosidosis, New Eng J Med 288:225, 1973.

127. Booth, CW, Gerbie, AB, and Nadler, HL, Intrauterine Detection of G_{M1} Gangliosidosis, Type 2, Pediatrics 52:521, 1973.

128. Menkes, JH, O'Brien, JS, Okada, S, Grippo, J, Andrews, JM, and Cancilla, PA, Juvenile G_{M2} Gangliosidosis, Arch Neurol 25:14, 1971.

129. Schneider, EL, Ellis, WG, Brady RO, McCullach, JR, and Epstein, CJ, Infantile Gaucher's Disease: In Utero Diagnosis and Fetal Pathology, J Ped 81:1134, 1972.

130. Nadler, HL, and Messina, AM, In Utero Detection of Type II Glycogenosis (Pompe's Disease), Lancet 2:1277, 1969.

131. Justice, P, Tyan, C, and Hsia, DYY, Amylo-1,6-Glucosidase in Human Fibroblasts: Studies in Type III Glycogen Storage Disease, Biochem Biophys Res Commun 39:301, 1970.

132. Howell, RR, Kaback, MM, and Brown, BI, Glycogen Storage Disease Type IV. Branching Enzyme Deficiency in Skin Fibroblasts and Possible Heterozygote Detection, J Ped 78:638, 1971.

133. Kan, YW, Dozy, AM, Alter, BP, Frigoletto, FD, and Nathan, DG, Detection of the Sickle Gene in the Human Fetus, New Eng J Med 287:1, 1972.

134. Melancon, SB, Lee, SY, and Nadler, HL, Histidase Activity in Cultivated Human Amniotic Fluid Cells, Science 173:627, 1971.

135. Fleisher, LD, Longhi, RC, Tallan, HH, Beratis, NG, Hirschhorn, K, and Gaull, GE, Homocystinuria: Investigations of Cystathionine Synthetase in Cultured Fetal Cells and the Prenatal Determination of Genetic Status, J Ped 85:677, 1974.

136. Fratantoni, JC, Neufeld, EF, Uhlendorf, BW, and Jacobson, CB, Intrauterine Diagnosis of the Hurler and Hunter Syndrome, New Eng J Med 280:686, 1969.

137. Levy, HL, Shih, VE, and MacReady, RA, Inborn Errors of Metabolism and Transport: Prenatal and Neonatal Diagnosis, Abstract, Genetics 5:1, 1971.

138. Dancis, J, Hutzler, J, Tada, K, Wada, Y, Morikawa, T, and Arakawa, T, Hypervalinemia: A Defect in Valine Transamination, Pediatrics, 39:813, 1967.

139. Rattenbury, JM, Blau, K, Sandler, M, Pryse-Davies, J, and Clark, PJ, Prenatal Diagnosis of Hypophosphatasia, Lancet 1:306, 1976.

140. Warren, RJ, Condron, CJ, Hollister, D, Huijing, F, Neufeld, EF, Hall, CW, McLeod, AGW, and Lorinez, AE, Antenatal Diagnosis of Mucolipidosis II (I-Cell Disease), Abstract, Pediat Res 7:343, 1973.

141. Gomperts, D, Goodey, PA, Thom, H, Russell, G, MacLean, MW, Ferguson-Smith, ME, and Ferguson-Smith, MA, Antenatal Diagnosis of Propionicacidaemia,

Lancet *1:*1009, 1973.

142. Suzuki, K, Schneider, EL, and Epstein, CJ, In Utero Diagnosis of Globoid Cell Leukodystrophy (Krabbe's Disease), Biochem Biophys Res Commun *45:*1363, 1971.

143. Boyle, JA, Raivio, KO, Astrin, KH, Schulman, JD, Graf, ML, Seegmiller, JE, and Jacobson, CB, Lesch-Nyhan Syndrome: Preventive Control by Prenatal Diagnosis, Science *169:*688, 1970.

144. Nadler, HL, and Egan, TJ, Deficiency and Lysosomal Acid Phosphatase: A New Familial Metabolic Disorder, New Eng J Med *282:*302, 1970.

145. Wendel, CL, Rudiger, HW, Passarge, E, and Mikkelsen, M, Maple Syrup Urine Disease: Rapid Prenatal Diagnosis by Enzyme Assay, Humangenetik *19:*127, 1973.

146. Kihara, H, Fluharty, AL, and Steven, RL, Arylsulfatase B Deficiency in Marteaux-Lamy Fibroblasts, Abstract, Am Soc Human Genet 1974, p. 48a.

147. Leroy, JG, Van Elsen, AF, Martin, JJ, Dumon, JE, Hulet, AE, Okada, S, and Navarro, C, Infantile Metachromatic Leukodystrophy: Confirmation of a Prenatal Diagnosis, New Eng J Med *288:*1365, 1973.

148. Morrow, G, Schwartz, RH, and Hallock, JA, Prenatal Detection of Methylmalonic Acidemia, J Ped *77:*120, 1970.

149. Goodman, SI, Moe, PG, Hammond, KB, Mudd, SH, and Uhlendorf, BW, Homocystinuria with Methylmalonic Aciduria: Two Cases in a Sibship, Biochem Med *4:*500, 1970.

150. Mudd, SH, Uhlendorf, BW, Freeman, JM, Finkelstein, JD, and Shin, VE, Homocystinuria Associated with Decreased Methylenetetrahydrofolate Reductase Activity, Biochem Biophys Res Commun *46:*905, 1972.

151. Matalon, R, and Dorfman, A, Marquio's Syndrome: A Deficiency of Chondroitin Sulfate *N*-Acetylhexamine Sulfate Sulfatase, Abstract, Res *8:*436, 1974.

152. Epstein, CJ, Grady, RO, Schneider, EL, Bradley, D, and Shapiro, D, In Vitro Diagnosis of Niemann-Pick Disease, Am J Hum Genet *23:*533, 1971.

153. Shin, VE, and Schulman, JD, Ornithine-Ketoacid Transaminase Activity in Human Skin and Amniotic Fluid Cell Culture, Clin Chim Acta *27:*73, 1970.

154. Krooth, RS, Properties of Diploid Cell Strains Developed from Patients with an Inherited Abnormality of Uridine Biosynthesis, Symp Quant Biol *29:*189, 1964.

155. Solomons, C, Armstrong, D, Van Wormer, D, Roberts, J, Golbus, M, and Pettet, G, Prenatal Diagnosis of Osteogenesis Imperfecta, Abstract, 9th Int Cong Clin Chem, 1975.

156. Krone, W, Schneider, G, and Schulz, D, Detection of Phosphohexose Isomerase Deficiency in Human Fibroblast Cultures, Humangenetik *10:*224, 1970.

157. Tabei, T, and Heinrichs, WL, Prenatal Diagnosis of a Sex-Specific Placental Sulfatase Deficiency, Abstract, Gynecol Invest *6:*27, 1975.

158. Romeo, G, Kaback, MM, and Levin, EY, Uroporphyrinogen. III. Cosynthetase Activity in Fibroblasts from Patients with Congenital Erythropoietic Porphyria, Biochem Genet *4:*659, 1970.

159. Blass, JP, Avigan, J, and Uhlendorf, BW, A Defect in Pyruvate Decarboxylase in a Child with an Intermittent Movement Disorder, J Clin Invest *49:*423, 1970.

160. Herndon, JH, Steinberg, D, Uhlendorf, BW, and Fales, HM, Refsum's Disease: Characterization of the Enzyme Defect in Cell Culture, J Clin Invest *48:*1017, 1969.

161. Desnick, RJ, Krivit, W, and Sharp, HL, In Utero Diagnosis of Sandhoff's Disease, Biochem Biophys Res Commun *51:*20, 1973.

162. Harper, PS, Laurence, KM, Parkes, A, Wusteman, FS, Kresse, H, Von Figura, K, Ferguson-Smith, MA, Duncan, DM, Logan, W, Hall, F, and Whiteman, P, Sanfillippo Disease in the Fetus, J Med Genet *11:*123, 1974.

163. O'Brien, JS, Sanfilipo Syndrome: Profound Deficiency of α-Acetylglucosaminidase Activity in Organs and Skin Fibroblasts from Type-B Patients, Proc Nat Acad Sci *69:*1720, 1972.

164. Bach, G, Friedman, R, Weissmann, B, and Neufeld, EF, The Defect in the Hurler and Scheie Syndromes: Deficiency of α-L-Iduronidase, Proc Nat Acad Sci *69:*2048, 1972.

165. Schneck, L, Friedland, J, Valenti, C, Adachi, M, Amsterdam, D, and Volk, BW, Prenatal Diagnosis of Tay-Sachs Disease, Lancet *1:*582, 1970.

166. Kan, YW, Golbus, MS, and Dozy, AM, Application of Molecular Hybridization to Prenatal Diagnosis of α-Thalassemia (abstract), Clin Res, in press.

167. Kan, YW, Golbus, MS, Klein, P, and Dozy, AM, Successful Application of Prenatal Diagnosis in a Pregnancy at Risk for Homozygous β-Thalassemia, New Eng J Med *292:*1096, 1975.

168. Mudd, SH, Levy, NL, and Abeles, RH, A Derangement in the Metabolism of B_{12} Leading to Homocystinemia, Cystathioninemia, and Methylmalonic Aciduria, Biochem Biophys Res Commun *35:*121, 1969.

169. Cortner, JA, and Swoboda, E, Wolman's Disease: Prenatal Diagnosis: Electrophoretic Identification of the Missing Lysosomal Acid Lipase, Abstract, Am Soc Human Genet Meeting, 1974, p. 23a.

170. Ramsay, CA, Coltart, TM, Blunt, S, Pawsey, SA, and Giannelli, F, Prenatal Diagnosis of Xeroderma Pigmentosum, Lancet 2:1109, 1974.

171. Campbell, S, Johnston, FD, Holt, EM, and May, P, Anencephaly: Early Ultrasonic Diagnosis and Active Management, Lancet 2:1226, 1972.

172. Campbell, S, Pryse-Davies, J, Coltart, TM, Seller, MJ, and Singer, JD, Ultrasound in the Diagnosis of Spina Bifida, Lancet 1:1065, 1975.

173. Omenn, GS, Figley, MM, Graham, CB, and Heinrichs, WL, Prospects for Radiographic Intrauterine Diagnosis—The Syndrome of Thrombocytopenia with Absent Radii, New Eng J Med 288:777, 1973.

174. Jenkinson, EL, Pfisterer, WN, Latteier, KK, and Martin, A, A Prenatal Diagnosis of Osteopetrosis, Am J Roentgenol 49:455, 1943.

175. Golbus, MS, and Hall, BD, Failure to Diagnose Achondroplasia in Utero, Lancet 1:629, 1974.

176. Queenan, JT, and Gadoin, EC, Amniography for Detection of Congenital Malformations, Obstet Gynecol 35:648, 1970.

177. Scrimgeour, JB, personal communication.

178. Gitlin, D, and Boesman, M, Sites of Serum α-Fetoprotein Synthesis in The Human and in the Rat, J Clin Invest, 46:1010, 1967.

179. Gitlin, D, and Boesman, M, Serum α-Fetoprotein, Albumin, and Gamma-Globulin in the Human Conceptus, J Clin Invest 45:1826, 1966.

180. Brock, DJH, and Sutcliffe, RG, Alpha-Fetoprotein in the Antenatal Diagnosis of Anencephaly and Spina Bifida, Lancet 2:197, 1972.

181. Seller, MJ, Creasy, MR, and Alberman, ED, Alpha-Fetoprotein Levels in Amniotic Fluids from Spontaneous Abortions, Brit Med J 2:524, 1974.

182. Schmid, W, and Muhlethaler, JP, High Amniotic Fluid Alpha-1-Fetoprotein in a Case of Fetal Sacrococcygeal Teratoma, Humangenetik 26:353, 1975.

183. Kjessler, B, Johansson, SGO, Sherman, M, Gustavson, KH, and Hultquist, G, Alpha-Fetoprotein in Antenatal Diagnosis of Congenital Nephrosis, Lancet 1:432, 1975.

184. De Bruijn, HWA, and Huisjes, HJ, Omphalocele and Raised Alpha-Fetoprotein in Amniotic Fluid, Lancet 1:525, 1975.

185. Golbus, MS, Hall, BD, and Creasy, RK, Prenatal Diagnosis of Congenital Anomalies in an Intra-Uterine Growth Retarded Fetus, Hum Genet, in press.

186. Seppala, MS, Increased Alpha Fetoprotein in Amniotic Fluid Associated with a Congenital Esophageal Atresia of the Fetus, Obstet Gynecol 42:613, 1973.

187. Brock, DJH, Bolton, AE, and Monaghan, JM, Prenatal Diagnosis of Anencephaly through Maternal Serum Alpha-Fetoprotein Measurement, Lancet 2:923, 1973.

188. Laurence, KM, Clinical and Ethical Considerations on Alpha-Fetoprotein Estimation for Early Prenatal Diagnosis of Neural Tube Malformations, Dev Med Child Neurol 16(6 Suppl 32):117, 1974.

189. Janerich, DT, Epidemic Waves in the Prevalence of Anencephaly and Spina Bifida in New York State, Teratology 8:253, 1973.

190. Macri, JN, Weiss, RR, Joshi, MS, and Evans, MI, Antenatal Diagnosis of Neural-Tube Defects Using Cerebrospinal-Fluid Proteins, Lancet 1:14, 1974.

191. Macri, JN, Weiss, RR, and Joshi, MS, Beta-Trace Protein and Neural-Tube Defects, Lancet 1:1109, 1974.

192. Hollenberg, MD, Kaback, MM, and Kazazian, HH, Jr, Adult Hemoglobin Synthesis by Reticulocytes from the Human Fetus at Midtrimester, Science 174:698, 1971.

193. Kan, YW, Golbus, MS, Klein, P, and Dozy, MT, Successful Application of Prenatal Diagnosis in a Pregnancy at Risk for Homozygous β-Thalassemia, New Eng J Med 292:1096, 1975.

194. Hobbins, JC, and Mahoney, MJ, Progress Toward In Utero Diagnosis of Hemoglobinopathies. I. Technique for Obtaining Fetal Blood, New Eng J Med 290:1065, 1974.

195. Valenti, C, Antenatal Detection of Hemoglobinopathies, Am J Obstet Gynecol 115:851, 1973.

196. Kan, YW, Valenti, C, Carnazza, V, Guidotti, R, and Rieder, RF, Foetal Blood Sampling In Utero, Lancet 1:79, 1974.

197. Golbus, MS, Kan, YW, and Naglich-Craig, M, Fetal Blood Sampling in Midtrimester Pregnancies, Am J Obstet Gynecol, in press.

198. Johnson, AM, Umansky, I, Alper, CA, Everett, C, and Greenspan, G, Amniotic Fluid Proteins: Maternal and Fetal Contributions, J Ped 84:588, 1974.

199. Valenti, C, Endoamnioscopy and Fetal Biopsy: A New Technique, Am J Obstet Gynecol 114:561, 1972.

200. Carr, DH, Chromosome Studies in Spontaneous Abortions, Obstet Gynecol 26:308, 1965.

201. Shapiro, S, Levine, HS, and Abramowicz, M, Factors Associated with Early and Late Fetal Loss, Excerpta Med Int Congr Ser *224:*45, 1970.
202. Golbus, MS, and Milunsky. A, unpublished data.
203. Brock, DJH, Gordon, H, Seligman, S, and Lobo, E de H, Antenatal Detection of Hurler's Syndrome, Lancet *2:*1324, 1971.
204. Michael, CA, Hahnel, R, Hockey, A, and Wysocki, S, Pitfalls in the Prenatal Diagnosis of Tay-Sachs Disease. Aust Paediat J *10:*23, 1974.
205. Blumberg, BD, Golbus, MS, and Hanson, KH, The Psychological Sequelae of Abortion Performed for a Genetic Indication, Am J Obstet Gynecol *122:*799, 1975.
206. Motulsky, AG, Fraser, GR, and Felsenstein, J, Public Health and Long-Term Genetic Implications of Intrauterine Diagnosis and Selective Abortion, Birth Defects, Original Article Series *7:*22, 1971.
207. Fraser, GR, Genetical Implications of Ante-Natal Diagnosis, Ann Genet *16:*5, 1973.
208. Kabach, MM, Zeiger, RS, Reynold, LW, and Sonneburn, M, Approaches to the Control and Prevention of Tay-Sachs Disease, Prog Med Genet *10:*103, 1974.
209. Philipp, EE, in *Law and Ethics of A.I.D. and Embryo Transfer*, Excerpta Medica, New York, Ciba Found Symp *17:*63, 1973.
210. Edwards, JH, A Critical Examination of the Reputed Primary Influence of ABO Phenotype on Fertility and Sex Ratio, Brit J Prev Med Soc *11:*79, 1957.
211. Muller, HJ, Genetical Progress by Voluntarily Conducting Germinal Choice, in Wolstenholme, G, ed., *Man and His Future*, Churchill, London, 1963.
212. Medawar, PB, The Genetic Improvement of Man, Austral Ann Med *4:*317, 1969.
213. Schrott, HG, Karp, L, and Omenn, GS, Prenatal Prediction in Myotonic Dystrophy: Guidelines for Genetic Counseling, Clin Genet *4:*38, 1973.
214. Renwick, JN, Bundy, SE, Ferguson-Smith, MA, and Izatt, MM, Confirmation of Linkage of the Loci for Myotonic Dystrophy and ABH Secretion, J Med Genet *8:*407, 1971.
215. Harper, P, Bias, WB, Hutchinson, JR, and McKusick, VA, ABH Secretor Status of the Fetus: A Genetic Marker Identifiable by Amniocentesis, J Med Genet *8:*438, 1971.
216. Boyer, SH, and Graham, JB, Linkage Between the X Chromosome Loci for Glucose-6-Phosphate Dehydrogenase Electrophoretic Variation and Hemophilia A, Am J Hum Genet *17:*320, 1965.
217. Nadler, HL, Patterns of Enzyme Development Utilizing Cultivated Human Fetal Cells Derived from Amniotic Fluid, Biochem Genet *2:*119, 1968.
218. Peterson, JA, and Weiss, MC, Expression of Differentiated Functions in Hepatoma Cell Hybrids: Induction of Mouse Albumin Production in Rat Hematoma-Mouse Fibroblast Hybrids, Proc Nat Acad Sci *69:*571, 1972.
219. Taylor, JM, Dozy, A, Kan, YW, Varmus, HE, Lee-Injo, LE, Gannesan, J, and Todd, D, Genetic Lesion in Homozygous α-Thalassemia, Nature, *251:*392, 1974.
220. Kan, YW, and Golbus, MS, unpublished data.
221. Schneider, EL, Ellis, WG, Brady, RO, McCulloch, JR, and Epstein, CJ, Prenatal Niemann-Pick Disease: Biochemical and Histologic Examination of a 19-Gestational Week Fetus, Pediat Res *6:*720, 1972.
222. Ellis, WG, Schneider, EL, McCulloch, JR, Suzuki, K, and Epstein, CJ, Fetal Globoid Cell Leukodystrophy (Krabbe's Disease), Arch Neurol *29:*253, 1973.
223. Fox, MS, and Littlefield, JW, Reservations Concerning Gene Therapy, Science *173:*195, 1971.

6

THE ABNORMAL PAP SMEAR

JOHN McL. MORRIS, M.D.

The diagnosis of gynecologic cancer belongs in the hands of any physician, surgeon, or gynecologist who sees women. The use of cytologic smears has been a major advance in the earlier detection of cervical cancer, especially in the recognition of the disease in the preinvasive stages. It is of some value in other forms of pelvic carcinoma, but with a much lesser degree of accuracy.

The smear is only an indicator. False negatives are not uncommon and, on occasion, false positives may be reported. The final diagnosis must be made on pathologic sections, which may also be in error because the biopsies were taken from the wrong area, were inadequately sectioned, or were improperly interpreted.

INDICATIONS FOR CYTOLOGIC SMEARS

Annual smears in patients over 25 are generally considered desirable, but the cytologic smear is only one of many tests for diagnosing pelvic cancer. Screening programs without concomitant pelvic examination may provide false assurance for the patient. Suspicious areas of the vulva, vagina, or cervix should be biopsied regardless of cytologic findings.

Cost and yield must be considered in planning cytologic screening programs. For example, the age-specific incidence of cancer of the cervix in the 15- to 19-year-old girl in Connecticut is 1.5 per million. Routine screening at $5 in this group would therefore cost $3,333,333 per case. In terms of maximum utilization of medical and scientific manpower, smears in the young nulliparous patient should be limited to those who have suspicious areas on the cervix or who have additional cause for concern, such as maternal estrogen medication during pregnancy. The age-specific incidence of cervical carcinoma rises to 1 per 100,000 at 20–24 years of age and over 50 per 100,000 in the 45 to 65 age group.[1] The disease is almost nonexistent in virginal patients.

Even the repeat annual screening in normal patients has been questioned. Most screening programs yield roughly 5 abnormal smears per 1,000 on the initial visit, which rapidly falls off to a tenth or less of this figure in succeeding years.[2] If 10% false negatives are encountered, 0.05% of these women might receive false assurance, but after the second or third negative smear the incidence of carcinoma is negligible.

While vaginal recurrence is not uncommon in patients treated by hysterectomy for pelvic cancer or in situ disease, and semiannual evaluation of such patients is warranted, the yield of cytology in the patient who has had hysterectomy for benign disease is very nearly zero. In some instances, however, smears may be demanded by the patient and may be necessary to calm a cancerophobia.

TECHNIQUE AND REPORTS

Smears are usually taken with a spatula or pipette from the posterior fornix of the vagina. In addition direct scraping from the squamocolumnar junction of the cervix or from any suspicious area of vagina or vulva is desirable. The fixative (usually an alcohol-ether mixture) should be applied promptly before drying occurs.

Recently endometrial cytology (brushings or washings) has come into vogue, but most pathologists prefer suction biopsies if endometrial carcinoma is suspected because of difficulty in interpretation of smears.

Cytologic laboratories may report findings unrelated to cancer, including degree of cornification (estrogen effect), presence of endometrial cells, infection, trichomonads, yeasts, hyphae, or starch granules and poor fixation.

Basal cells are small round or oval cells with large rounded nuclei. A smear consisting predominantly of basal cells indicates vaginal atrophy and low estrogen because the superficial cornified layer of cells is decreased or absent. This may be abnormal in patients in the reproductive age group. Precornified cells from just above the transitional layer of the squamous epithelium are usually large cells with basophilic cytoplasm and small vesicular nuclei. The completely cornified cell has irregular angulated borders, eosinophilic cytoplasm, and a pyknotic nucleus without visible structural detail. Predominance of cornified cells indicates a high estrogen effect. Thus the smear may serve as an inexpensive biologic assay for estrogen. This may be of clinical significance, especially in the postmenopausal patient.

Cells from the glandular epithelium of endocervix and endometrium are also frequently seen in the vaginal smear and sometimes result in false positive reports. They are usually of no clinical significance except that in the postmenopausal woman the occurrence of endometrial cells is sometimes reported as "suspicious" because desquamation of endometrium after the menopause may be a cause for concern.

The presence of leukocytes, red blood cells, histiocytes, or trichomonads may be noted, as well as foreign body giant cells. In the presence of severe infection, degeneration of cells may lead to misinterpretation as false positives. After radiotherapy, radiation changes in cells with bizarre forms may also be very difficult to interpret.

Smears may be reported as negative, suspicious, or positive. If reported by "classes," local practices may vary. In general,

> Class I = negative
> Class II = abnormal, not suggestive of malignancy
> Class III = suspicious
> Class IV or V = consistent with carcinoma

The Class II smear should not cause the clinician to overreact, as is sometimes the case. It may only show the presence of endometrial cells or may be an indication of vaginitis. It does not indicate cancer. The cytologist may point out the problem or suggest that vaginitis is present. The source of abnormal cells in suspicious or positive smears should always be investigated.

COURSE OF ACTION

The decision as to what course to take in the event of a suspicious or positive smear does not lend itself to a single answer. Unfortunately there is sometimes a tendency to push too many panic buttons. The smear should be regarded as a red signal on the railroad track, not a train wreck.

Time is usually on the side of the patient. Figures from the Connecticut State Tumor Registry show that cervical cancer may have an extremely long life history, with a median of 7.9 years between development of carcinoma in situ and development of invasive carcinoma, and a median of 8.5 years between local invasive carcinoma and distant metastases.[3] As it is generally recognized that cervical dysplasia may precede carcinoma in situ, the total period of development of the disease may be even longer.

When an unsuspected suspicious or positive smear is reported, a repeat smear should be routine. Because of the unnecessary anguish caused by borderline smears or false positives, it is probably wiser not to announce to the patient that she has a positive smear for cancer, but merely inform her that the smear must be repeated. The surface of the cervix can be stained with Lugol's solution and nonstaining areas biopsied. Toluidine blue, Schiller's solution, colposcopy, or other techniques may be employed.

Colposcopy, favored for many years in certain European clinics, has (with support from manufacturers of optical devices) become the "in" thing recently in many clinics in the United States. While a cervical dysplasia clinic with a colposcope may be a desirable thing for a community to have, a colposcope is unnecessary in the average gynecologist's office, and the expense of purchase will ultimately have to be borne by the patient.

The experienced gynecologist may do equally well with punch biopsies of suspicious areas of the exocervix which do not stain with Lugol's iodine. Significant exocervical growth is usually recognizable. The danger is unrecognized endocervical tumor. For this purpose a small endocervical curette is of great value. Endometrial cancers can be similarly diagnosed with one of several available suction endometrial biopsy curettes. The majority of gynecologic cancer cases, including those of the vulva, vagina, cervix, and corpus, may be diagnosed by an office procedure. To admit a patient to a hospital for an operation without first attempting outpatient directed biopsy, endocervical curettage, or endometrial aspiration biopsy is to involve the patient in unnecessary risk and expense.[4]

Routine cervical conization as an initial procedure in the event of a positive cytologic smear has, in addition to the disadvantages of the expense of hospitalization and the risk of anesthesia, a traumatic psychologic effect on the patient. The operation is not simple and without complications. Hemorrhage or infection not only relate to the procedure itself, but also to any subsequent therapy which may be undertaken.[5-7] There is a marked increase in abortion if subsequent pregnancy occurs. The morbidity in hysterectomy postcone is significantly increased. It may delay treatment if invasive tumor is found. Furthermore, unless a cone is carefully cut, fragments of unoriented tissue, particularly if cauterized or inadequately sectioned, may prove of less value than carefully chosen punch biopsies.

Conization should be limited to:

1. Cases with repeated positive cytology in which office biopsies have failed to demonstrate the source of the cells.

2. Cases with carcinoma in situ on biopsy in which it may be necessary to rule out significant undetected invasive tumor.

3. An occasional therapeutic procedure in cases of dysplasia or localized carinoma in situ in instances where the patient wishes to preserve child bearing. The margins of the cone should be free of disease.

The proper handling of all malignant or premalignant disease requires as an initial step a review of the pathologic material available. It must be determined whether it is representative and adequate. Many times lesions are borderline and opinions of pathologists vary. It is not correct to assume all cases are black or white, cancer or benign. Severe dysplasias should at times be treated as premalignant lesions. Microinvasive tumors do not necessarily require as rigorous treatment as Stage I cancer. Lymphatic involvement or anaplastic disease may require more extensive therapy.

Should the pathology report show severe dysplasia or carcinoma in situ, some programs have proposed cryosurgical treatment, others have advocated conization or cauterization, and one series was merely observed. Long term followup in such groups (10 years or more) usually will reveal a 10 to 20% incidence of invasive carcinoma. While conservative measures may be permissible as a temporizing procedure in young patients who want to have more children, most authorities favor hysterectomy for severe dysplasia, carcinoma in situ, or microinvasive carcinoma. Invasive cancer is best handled in an organized cancer program.

SUMMARY

In the event of a suspicious or positive smear:

1. A repeat smear should be taken.

2. Outpatient diagnosis by cervical biopsy and endocervical curette should be routine in most cases. This is facilitated by "directed biopsy," applying Lugol's solution (Schiller test) with attention to nonstaining areas, or using colposcopic techniques.

3. In cases where biopsies show severe dysplasia, carcinoma in situ, or microinvasion, cervical conization may sometimes be necessary to rule out undetected invasive tumor. At the time of conization, immediate cryostat sections should be taken in the operating room, and appropriate treatment may be instituted under the same anesthesia.

REFERENCES

1. Morris, JMcL, Carcinoma of the Cervix, Conn Med 30:477, 1966.
2. Christopherson, WM, and Parker, JE, Control of Cervix Cancer in Women of Low Income in a Community, Cancer 24:64, 1969.
3. Bailar, JC, III, Uterine Cancer in Connecticut: Late Deaths among 5-Year Survivors, J Nat Can Inst 27:239, 1961.
4. Holley, MR, Management of the Patient with an Abnormal Papanicolaou Smear, Am J Obstet Gynec 110:979, 1971.
5. Doran, TA, and Shier, CB, Conization of the Cervix, Am J Obstet Gynecol 88:367, 1964.
6. Ferguson, JH, and Brown, GC, Cervical Conization during Pregnancy, Surg Gyn Obstet 111:603, 1960.
7. Laubach, JB, and McGanity, WJ, Hysterectomy post Conization of the Cervix, Am J Obstet Gynecol 91:437, 1965.

7

COLPOSCOPY

DUANE E. TOWNSEND, M.D.

The first studies on the use of the colposcope in critically evaluating the visible portion of the female genital tract were reported by Hans Hinselmann,[1] of Hamburg, Germany, in 1925. His initial publications were the result of several years of effort to develop a method for the early detection of cervical cancer. The stimulus for Hinselmann to develop the colposcope evolved from an assignment to rewrite a textbook chapter on the cervix. During his labors to upgrade the knowledge of cervical disease, Hinselmann was struck by the fact that cervical cancer often presented as advanced disease with poor patient salvage. He logically deduced that magnification should be able to detect this disease at an early stage. Although the original instrument, when compared to modern colposcopes, may appear crude, the basic design has changed little. The colposcope is essentially a dissecting microscope on a stand with excellent illumination.

Despite this apparent breakthrough in early cancer detection, virtually all English-speaking countries rejected the technique. The major problem appeared to be related to Hinselmann's interpretation of colposcopic patterns which resulted in a terminology that many English and American physicians found cumbersome, lengthy, occasionally contradictory, and practically impossible for English translation. Despite these handicaps, efforts were made to stimulate interest in this technique in North America. Ries[2] in 1931 reviewed the concepts upon which the technique was based and concluded that colposcopy provided an avenue for the reduction of deaths from cervical cancer. Martlzloff[3] studied the technique for a decade, but his results in 1940 reinforced many doubts that North American physicians had about the method. He concluded that the colposcope offered little advantage over a carefully performed pelvic examination with the unaided eye.

The introduction of cytology in the later 1940's[4] further dampened North American interest in colposcopy.

Efforts were made to reintroduce the technique in the United States during the 1950's and 60's. Invariably, it was placed in competition with cytology and invariably cytology was found to be more economical, easier to learn, with a lower false negative rate.[5-8] As a result of this consistent competitiveness, critics of the technique became quite vocal and at one time colposcopy was called the greatest "gynecologic hoax" in this or any century. In a prominent author's book on the management of early cervical neoplasia, the colposcope is indexed as "the uselessness of."[9]

With such an inauspicious background, it is somewhat surprising to note the recent burgeoning interest in the technique in North America. However, several major developments probably account for this change in attitude.

1. A logical, scientifically based, simplified English terminology was introduced.[10]

2. Improved reference materials, teaching aids, and instructional techniques were developed.

3. Articles began to appear in the English literature pointing out the value of colposcopy in avoiding the hazards and complications of diagnostic conization in the patient with the abnormal Papanicolaou test, i.e. Pap test suggestive of dysplasia or worse.[11-26]

4. Colposcopy is recommended primarily as a technique to assist the physician in the examination of the visible portion of the female genital tract, i.e. vulva, vagina, and cervix, therefore not placing it in competition with, but rather complementing, cytology. In the patient with neoplasia of the visible portion of the female genital tract, cytology will suggest the presence of the neoplastic process, while colposcopy can usually determine its location and extent.

The colposcope is different from the colpomicroscope, another tool for examining the cervix. The colpomicroscope employs a magnification between 150 and 200x in contrast to colposcopy, which ranges from 6 to 20x. Colpomicroscopy is much more difficult to master, requires an expert knowledge of cytology, and takes a considerably longer period of time to perform.

THE COLPOSCOPIC EXAMINATION

The examination of the visible portion of the female genital tract by colposcopy usually takes no more than a few minutes. If the patient happens to have an abnormality, then the examination will be longer: 15 to 20 minutes in experienced hands. Initially the vulva is inspected in a systematic fashion. If abnormal tissue is present, it is sampled. A nonlubricated speculum is then slipped into the vagina and the cervix is exposed. Should excess mucus and cellular debris obscure the cervix, dry cotton balls are gently used to improve the view. A cytologic sample is first taken from the endocervical canal either with a saline-moistened cotton tip applicator or with an endocervical canal aspirator. The canal sample is followed by a scrape of the ectocervix. The vaginal pool should be avoided because of its high false negative rate.[27, 28]

Next, acetic acid (2 to 4%) delivered by soaked cotton balls is used to thoroughly cleanse the cervix and the anterior and posterior vaginal fornices. The colposcope is then swung into view and focused on the cervix. The transformation zone and the squamocolumnar junction are viewed. The color tone and vascular architecture are carefully noted. It is recommended by some authors that the vascular architecture be viewed before application of acetic acid, using saline to keep the tissue moist. However, should acetic acid be applied initially, the vascular changes will reappear once the acetic acid effect has lessened in 3 to 4 minutes. After the squamocolumnar junction and the transformation zone have been thoroughly inspected, any abnormal or suspect areas are biopsied. If the patient has an abnormal Papanicolaou test and the entire limits of the squamocolumnar junction are not visible, then the patient must undergo some type of canal sampling, preferably with an endocervical curette. After the cervix has been examined the vagina can be viewed in its entirety by gradually withdrawing and rotating the speculum. The vaginal epithelium will fold down over the end of the speculum, permitting an end-on view of this tissue. A bimanual completes the examination.

Bleeding is seldom a problem after biopsies since they are taken with special instruments, i.e. Kevorkian, which remove only a small piece of epithelium and stroma.[29] However, excess bleeding is easily controlled with Monsel's solution (ferric subsulfate) and cotton balls. Depending upon the results of the Pap test and tissue sampling, a logical and appropriate management may be initiated. Details of management will be covered in the latter part of this chapter.

THE TRANSFORMATION ZONE

One of the major concepts upon which contemporary colposcopy is based is the transformation zone. An understanding of this area is vital not only to colposcopy but also in comprehending the origin and development of cervical neoplasia. The transformation zone is defined as the area of the cervix or cervix and vagina which was initially covered by columnar epithelium and which, through a process called metaplasia, has been replaced all or in part by squamous epithelium.

It had been believed for many years that the cervix is normally covered by squamous epithelium and that the presence of columnar tissue on the ectocervix is abnormal. Studies in Australia,[30] complemented by work in the United States, have shown conclusively that columnar tissue normally exists on the ectocervix in at least 70% of females and extends onto the vagina in an additional 4 to 5% of subjects. Moreover, the location of columnar epithelium on the ectocervix is determined during embryologic development.

The replacement of columnar by squamous epithelium occurs both as a peripheral ingrowth from the original squamous tissue laid down early in fetal life and from multipotential cells that are adjacent to columnar epithelium. In instances where the peripheral ingrowth appears to be the major contribution, an irregular border of the metaplastic squamous epithelium will be found at the periphery of the grapelike columnar epithelium. In cases where there is an equal or greater contribution from the multipotential cells, islands of squamous metaplasia will be found within the area covered by columnar tissue.

The initial phase of transformation from metaplastic derived islands is a fusion of the grapelike columnar tissue, forming ridges. On the surface of the ridges the glandular epithelium is lost and is replaced by immature metaplastic squamous epithelium. Accompanying this process is an infiltrate of inflammatory-like cells. The multiple foci of metaplastic epithelium broaden, coalesce, and eventually join the peripheral contribution from the original squamous epithelium. Gland openings become prominent and appear as white spots or rings from which mucus may be expressed. The openings permit the egress of mucus from the deeper secreting columnar cells which are afforded protection from the acid environment by the buffering effect of the mucus. Whenever the gland openings become occluded and buried, columnar epithelium continues to secrete mucus and Nabothian cysts form. The complete transformation from columnar to squamous epithelium requires many years. Patients who are on oral contraceptives seem to have a slower transformation, probably because of the buffering effect of increased mucus production, a response to the high concentration of steroids in the pills. As a patient ages, the transformation zone matures, the Nabothian cysts and gland openings disappear, and the squamocolumnar junction is usually found at or just within the external os. The junction then gradually moves up the canal. The upward migration is extremely slow because of the neutral pH of the environment.

In the teenage years, the transformation zone is characterized by areas of columnar epithelium intermingling with metaplastic squamous epithelium. As an individual matures the sheets of metaplastic squamous epithelium enlarge, and gland openings and Nabothian cysts are prominent. With advancing age the transformation zone becomes less apparent and only its very fine vascular structure will reveal its location. In some cases the metaplastic squamous epithelium appears slightly whiter than the original squamous epithelium. This is due to the increased number of relatively large nuclei in the intermediate and parabasal cell layers. It is of interest that when these immature cells exfoliate and are picked up on a Pap smear, they are occasionally misinterpreted as mild dysplasia or atypia. Moreover, in some instances, this immature metaplastic squamous epithelium lacks sufficient glycogen and only partially stains with iodine.

In most women a normal transformation zone develops and the cytology will be normal. However, in a few instances, because of an as yet unknown cause or causes, a change in DNA occurs in the immature metaplastic squamous epithelium and potentially malignant cells develop; an atypical transformation zone evolves. It is within the atypical transformation zone that the abnormal patterns that characterize the earliest forms of cervical neoplasia reside.

ATYPICAL TRANSFORMATION ZONE

A transformation zone is classified as atypical when one or more of the following patterns are seen: white epithelium, mosaic structure, punctation, leukoplakia, or abnormal vascular patterns. Although each pattern may exist as a separate and distinct entity, in most cases several patterns exist simultaneously. In fact, the atypical vascular pattern associated with neoplasia is never found alone and always exists with either white epithelium, punctation, mosaic, or leukoplakia. Although each pattern of the atypical transformation zone is a separate entity, they are all primarily white epithelium which, when having certain vascular structures, takes on specific appearances, i.e. punctation, mosaic, and atypical vessels. The term leukoplakia is generally reserved for the raised white plaque that is due to hyperkeratosis. Leukoplakia is recognized with the naked eye before the application of acetic acid, while white epithelium, mosaic, and punctation become apparent *after* the application of acetic acid. The abnormal patterns that make up the atypical transformation zone are invariably sharply demarcated from the surrounding areas. They will be found within the boundaries of the original squamocolumnar junction, the junction that developed around the fifth month of fetal life, and the physiologic junction, that junction which is observed at the time the patient is examined. Except for leukoplakia and atypical vessels, one edge of the lesion will invariably be located at the physiologic squamocolumnar junction.

White epithelium is due to an increased number of nuclei which also have an increase in DNA. When light from the colposcope illuminates an area with increased nuclear concentrations the light does not completely penetrate the tissue and is reflected back to the instrument. As a consequence, these areas appear white. The optical density and therefore the degree of whiteness will vary directly with the nuclear concentration. Normal epithelium, which has small pyknotic nuclei, is pinkish-white. Dysplasia and carcinoma in situ which have varying degrees of nuclear density vary in degrees of whiteness. White epithelium due to neoplastic tissue is usually unifocal, slightly raised, and sharply demarcated from surrounding normal tissue. Examples of white epithelium are presented in Figures 7.1 and 7.2.

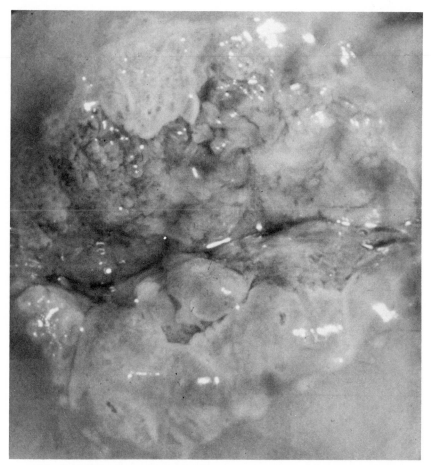

FIG. 7.1 Colpophotograph (x12) of cervix in a 19-year-old female whose Pap test was consistent with mild dysplasia: transverse os in center of photo. Atypical transformation zone present on anterior and posterior cervical lip. The small anterior lip pattern at 11 o'clock is characterized by white epithelium and faint punctation. The posterior lip pattern from 9 o'clock is white epithelium. Directed biopsies of the two lesions revealed moderate dysplasia. Treatment was outpatient cryosurgery.

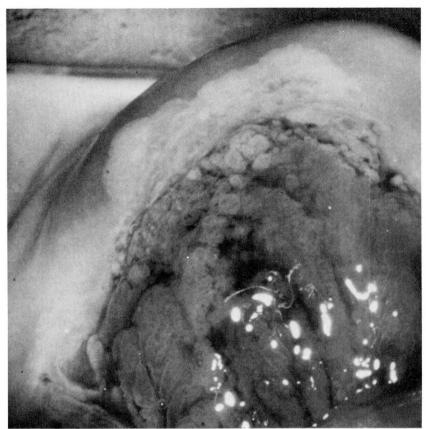

FIG. 7.2. Colpophotograph (x12) of anterior lip of cervix from 25-year-old gravida 3, para 3 whose Pap test was consistent with moderate dysplasia. Cervical os at posterior border. Vertical furrows and ridges of columnar epithelium are in the center of the photo. White epithelium is present at anterior rim of the transformation zone. Directed biopsy showed mild dysplasia. Treatment was by excision biopsy of this small lesion.

In cases where the individual villus capillaries are retained, completely or partially, punctation and mosaic structures predominate. Punctation is the result of the retention of each individual villus capillary during the metaplastic process. Instead of fusing, the villi persist and the abnormal nuclei multiply around the villi. As the abnormal epithelium expands, the villi are compressed so that only the individual capillary remains. When viewed on end the capillaries appear as red dots (Figs. 7.3 and 7.4).

Mosaic structure is likewise due to preservation of many of the villus capillaries, but in this case some villus capillaries are lost and the remaining capillaries link to one another to form a mosaic pattern (Fig. 7.5). Mosaic and punctation can be considered exact opposites of one another. Neither, however, carries any greater or lesser degree of significance. Mosaic and punctation often coexist (Fig. 7.6).

Infrequently, the abnormal epithelium will produce an excess amount of keratin resulting in leukoplakia. Leukoplakia alone is usually not significant; however, each keratinized plaque must be thoroughly sampled since it is impossible to recognize any significant vascular pattern beneath the keratin crust (Fig. 7.7).

The last abnormal pattern seen in the atypical transformation zone is atypical vessels. This is the most important entity, since it may herald the site of early invasive carcinoma. It is an infrequent finding. An atypical vascular structure rarely, if ever, exists alone; occurring with it will be either white epithelium, punctation, mosaic, or leukoplakia. The vascular patterns that are considered atypical are usually termed commas, spaghetti, corkscrews, or earthworms. They are to be differentiated from the regular branching normal vessels often present over Nabothian cysts. Examples of atypical vessels are shown in Figure 7.8, which should be contrasted with the regular branching vessels over Nabothian cysts in Figure 7.9.

COLPOSCOPICALLY OVERT CARCINOMA

There are instances when to the naked eye there is no evidence of invasive carcinoma but, when the patients are examined colposcopically, features consistent

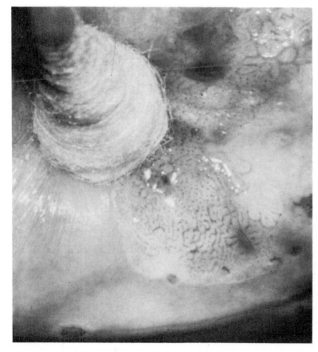

FIG. 7.3. Colpophotograph of the posterior cervix in a 32-year-old gravida 3, para 3 whose Pap test was consistent with carcinoma in situ. A highly atypical transformation zone characterized by punctation and mosaic is present. In this photograph the cotton-tipped applicator is lifting the posterior lip of the cervix to demonstrate punctation. The borders of the lesion are quite sharp and the area was quite white; it was graded as a carcinoma in situ, which it proved to be on biopsy. The lesion did extend into the canal for some distance and the patient therefore required a conization since curettage of the canal was positive. Conization showed only carcinoma in situ. Since the conization cleared the lesion, it was unnecessary to perform a hysterectomy.

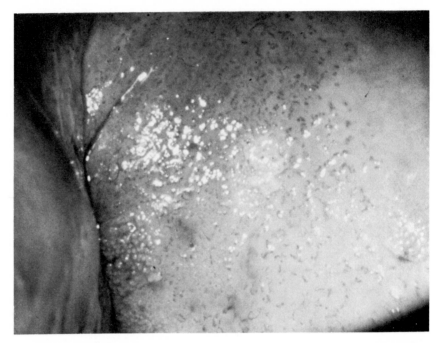

FIG. 7.4. Colpophotograph of vagina in 63-year-old female who had had a hysterectomy for carcinoma in situ 10 years previous. There are areas of coarse punctation with surface branching of vessels. The pattern was consistent with microinvasion, confirmed by directed biopsy. Because of the patient's age, treatment was by irradiation.

with invasive disease are apparent, i.e. raised, irregular surface contour and markedly atypical vascular pattern. In these cases the colposcope is particularly valuable in pinpointing the exact area for sampling for early diagnosis and prompt initiation of therapy. An example of colposcopic overt carcinoma is shown in Figures 7.10 and 7.11.

SATISFACTORY OR UNSATISFACTORY EXAMINATION

Critical to every colposcopic evaluation, in the patient with the abnormal Papanicolaou test or in routine colposcopic screening, is the ability to view the entire limits of the active or physiologic squamocolumnar junction. If the entire limits of this important landmark cannot be seen, then the examination must be judged unsatisfactory and exclusion of invasive cancer in the patient with the abnormal Papanicolaou test cannot be made. However, if invasive cancer has been recognized and confirmed by biopsy, then the patient has had appropriate evaluation. In those cases where preinvasive cervical neoplasia is present or suspected and the entire junction cannot be seen, the examination must be followed by endocervical curettage. Depending upon the results of the curettings, further evaluation may be necessary, i.e. diagnostic conization.

OTHER COLPOSCOPIC FINDINGS

The largest subdivision of colposcopic findings is comprised of those which usually have minor significance but at times are associated with an abnormal Pap test. Those most frequently encountered include condyloma, papilloma, cervical polyps, true erosions (which are usually traumatic due to speculum insertion), vaginocervicitis, and atrophic epithelium.

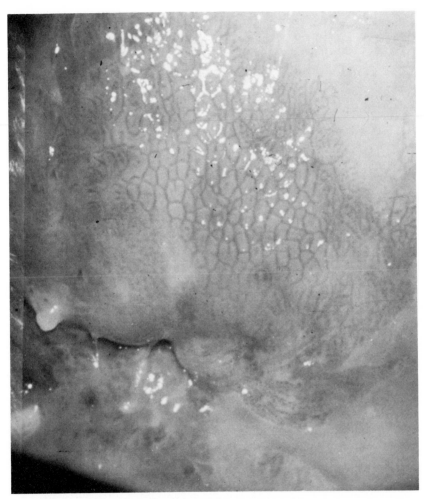

FIG. 7.5. Colpophotograph of cervix in 23-year-old female whose Pap test was consistent with carcinoma in situ. There is a large atypical transformation zone characterized by mosaic structure and punctation. Directed biopsy of the abnormality showed carcinoma in situ. The lesion extended well into the endocervical canal. Endocervical curettage showed neoplastic tissue. The upper limits of the lesion could not be seen; conization showed only carcinoma in situ. Hysterectomy was not performed since patient was nulliparous and cone had cleared the lesion.

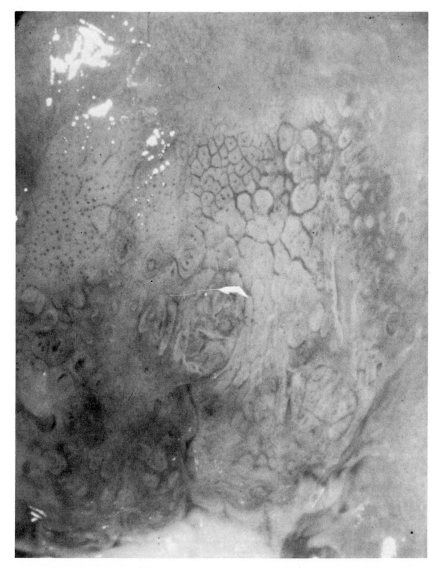

FIG. 7.6. Colpophotograph of anterior lip of cervix in a 26-year-old
pregnant woman whose Pap test was consistent with carcinoma in situ.
The cervical os is on the lower border of the photograph. A large atypical
transformation zone characterized by heavy mosaic and punctation is
present. Directed biopsy showed carcinoma in situ. The patient was
permitted to continue through pregnancy, delivered vaginally, and was
treated by shallow conization, which showed only carcinoma in situ.

The most important of the miscellaneous patterns are condyloma and papilloma
(Figs. 7.12 and 7.13) since they often give rise to slightly abnormal Papanicolaou
tests, particularly in pregnancy where they are most frequently encountered. They
are recognized by their striking surface contour and vascular pattern. Most are

associated with vulvar and vaginal condyloma and are usually multifocal. They should always be biopsied because there have been instances where an inexperienced colposcopist mistook a keratinizing invasive cancer for condyloma.

With the recognition of the above colposcopic patterns it is possible to divide these changes into a simplified and logical terminology (Table 7.1).

GRADING OF ABNORMAL PATTERNS

With experience, it is possible to grade the abnormal transformation zone and to make an extremely accurate prediction as to the histologic diagnosis. Factors

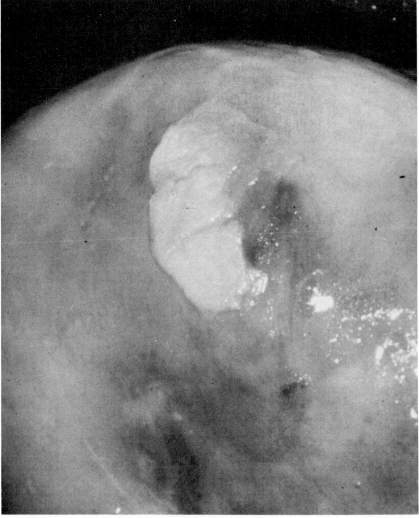

FIG. 7.7. Colpophotograph (x12) of anterior lip of cervix in a 31-year-old gravida 4, para 4. Patient had grossly visible white lesion on anterior cervical lip. Pap test was normal. Directed biopsy showed hyperkeratosis, no nuclear atypia. Since the lesion could be seen with naked eye and before the application of acetic acid, it is called leukoplakia.

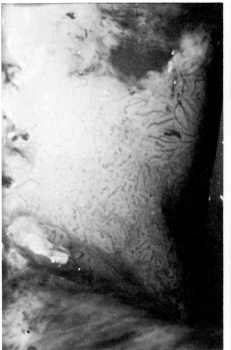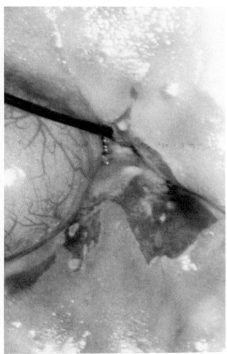

FIG. 7.8. (*Left*). Colpophotograph of the vagina of an early invasive carcinoma showing a highly atypical blood vessel pattern. Note the irregular branching of vessels, corkscrews, and spaghetti-like configuration. It is important to contrast these abnormal vessels with those seen in the Nabothian cyst in Figure 7.9.

FIG. 7.9. (*right*). Colpophotograph of the cervix in a 35-year-old female showing a large Nabothian cyst along the left-hand border of the photo. The cervical os is in the center; an IUD string is passing anteriorly. Note the regular branching vessels overlying the Nabothian cyst. Normal vessels have a regular direction. It is important to recognize and appreciate the normal blood vessel pattern in order to contrast normal with abnormal vessels, with the latter being associated with carcinoma.

considered in grading include the vascular structure, regular or irregular; the surface contour, flat, depressed, smooth, or irregular; the color and opacity or degree of whiteness and line of demarcation of apparently normal epithelium. A green filter enhances the color tone differences and the vascular changes. The latter are perhaps best viewed before acetic acid application. The most important factor in grading is the degree of whiteness, which is directly related to nuclear density. The earlier forms of dysplasia are less white than carcinoma in situ and early invasive carcinoma. Immature metaplastic squamous epithelium may appear white owing to the increased number of immature nuclei. However, it is possible to differentiate it from dysplastic epithelium in that the border between the metaplastic and normal epithelium is usually irregular whereas the border between normal and potentially neoplastic tissue is invariably sharp.

Most of the abnormal patterns will be unifocal, although in some instances multifocal appearances are seen. Multifocal cervical lesions will lie within the transformation zone. Cases of neoplastic disease high in the canal and low on the ectocervix without an intervening bridge of tissue have not been found in the nontraumatized cervix.

APPLICATION OF COLPOSCOPY

Abnormal Papanicolaou Test

The single greatest value of colposcopy is in the patient whose Pap test is abnormal, i.e. suggestive of dysplasia or worse, or Class III or worse. With colposcopy it is usually possible to determine the site of the abnormal smear, thereby eliminating the need for diagnostic conization. In addition, selection of therapy with colposcopy is based more upon the extent of the neoplastic epithelium than the histologic diagnosis. In some cases the lesser forms of dysplasia are quite vast and are of greater challenge than small focal areas of carcinoma in situ. Invariably the preinvasive lesion will be found within the transformation zone and with one border at the physiologic squamocolumnar junction (PSC). The lesions stay superficial for many years, but some will eventually develop into invasive

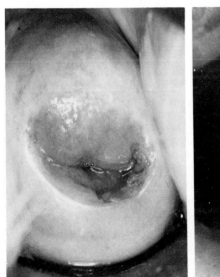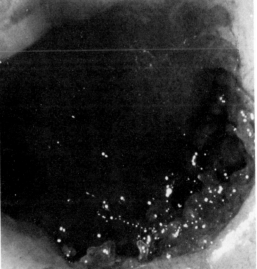

FIGS. 7.10. and 7.11. Gross (Fig. 7.10) (*left*) and colposcopic (Fig. 7.11, *right*) appearance of cervix in a 42-year-old female who had a Pap test suggestive of carcinoma in situ. Four quadrant biopsies, *i.e.* 12, 3, 6, and 9, showed carcinoma in situ. Directed biopsy from irregular lesion within the endocervical canal at 5 o'clock showed invasive carcinoma. The abnormal pattern was one of a highly irregular surface contour apparent in Figure 7.11. Patient did not require diagnostic cone biopsy and was given prompt and effective treatment for her disease, i.e., radical hysterectomy and bilateral pelvic lymphadenectomy.

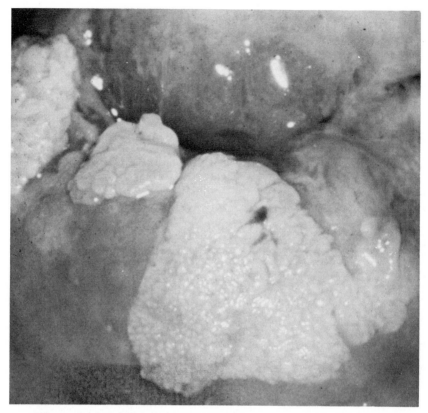

FIG. 7.12. Colpophotograph of posterior lip of cervix in a 21-year-old woman, 26 weeks pregnant. Several grossly visible raised white lesions were seen on the posterior lip. Colposcopically, these lesions showed irregular surface contour with an occasional double-branching vessel. Impression was condyloma acuminata confirmed by directed biopsy. These lesions disappeared spontaneously following vaginal delivery. Pap test on this patient was Class II.

cancer.[31-34] In over 90% of women with abnormal Papanicolaou tests, colposcopy, coupled with appropriate biopsies, can either confirm or exclude the presence of invasive cancer. When invasive cancer can be excluded without the need for conization, the patient can be treated in the manner most appropriate for her age, desire for childbearing, size of lesion and histologic diagnosis.[9]

Depending upon the ability to view the limits of the PSC, patients are separated into several treatment categories (Table 7.2).

Entire Limits of PSC Seen

If the entire limits of the PSC and the lesion are viewed, it is only necessary to take 1 to 3 biopsies of the most colposcopically abnormal appearing areas. Endocervical curettage (ECC) is probably not necessary in these patients since they will not have disease beyond the upper limits of the lesion. However, ECC has been performed routinely in our program for several reasons. First, it permits an expeditious grouping of patients into two major categories based upon the presence or absence of neoplastic disease in the curettings. Second, the multifocal concept of cervical neoplasia is an unproven entity and needs to be substantiated or refuted by experience. Third, the early asymptomatic, cytologically negative adenocarcinoma may be revealed by routine curettage. Last, patients with a negative curettage have rarely been found to have invasive cancer.

In those patients in whom noninvasive disease is present, several treatment techniques can be employed. Outpatient methods include excision biopsy, cryosurgery,

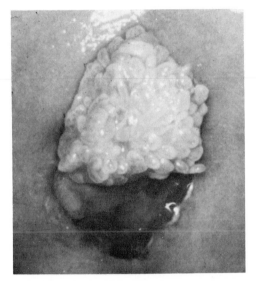

FIG. 7.13. Colpophotograph of cervix in a 19-year-old female referred for possible carcinoma. Close inspection of the cervix in this patient revealed a raised, irregular mass which colposcopically showed double-branching vessels and a contour consistent with condyloma acuminata. Biopsies were necessary in this patient, since the appearance of some condyloma is very similar to that of early invasive cancer.

TABLE 7.1
Colposcopic Terminology

Normal colposcopic findings
   1. Original squamous epithelium
   2. Columnar epithelium
   3. Transformation zone
Abnormal colposcopic findings
   1. Atypical transformation zone
      White epithelium
      Punctation
      Mosaic structure
      Leukoplakia
      Abnormal blood vessels
   2. Suspect frank invasive cancer
Unsatisfactory colposcopic findings
Other colposcopic findings
  Vagino-cervicitis
  True erosion
  Atrophic epithelium
  Condyloma, papilloma

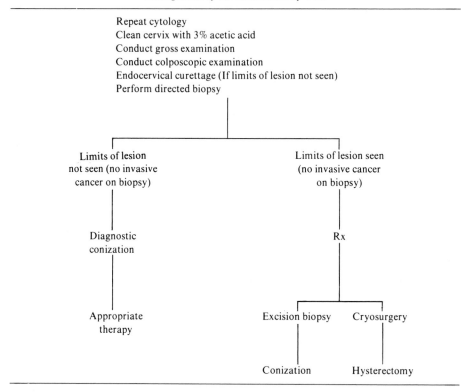

and hot cautery. Excision biopsies are used when lesions are 1 cm or less in size. Once the lesion has been treated, patients are seen every 3 months for 1 year and then every 6 months thereafter with cytology and colposcopy.

Surgery is recommended in the minority of patients with preinvasive cervical neoplasia. Therapeutic conization is used in those patients who refuse outpatient therapy or in individuals who are considered poor followup risks. Hysterectomy is restricted to patients who desire sterilization by hysterectomy or who have some other gynecologic problem such as pelvic relaxation, uterine myoma, chronic salpingitis, adenomyosis, etc. A simple vaginal or abdominal hysterectomy is sufficient. A vaginal cuff excision is necessary only when neoplastic tissue extends onto the vagina (under 5% of the time).

Entire Limits of the Lesion Not Seen

In about 10% of the patients with an abnormal Pap test the lesion will extend well into the endocervical canal or will be present solely within the canal. In these patients a firm and vigorous ECC should be carried out since invasive cancer may be diagnosed by canal sampling. Those patients in whom there is only evidence of dysplasia or carcinoma in situ must undergo diagnostic conization. Depending upon the results of the conization, further treatment may be necessary.

If invasive cancer is found then radical surgery or irradiation is undertaken. When microinvasive cancer is present a simple hysterectomy is sufficient.

If only preinvasive disease is present and the conization has cleared the lesion, treatment has been completed. On the other hand, if the cone biopsy has not cleared the lesion then either repeat conization or hysterectomy must be employed. If conization is properly performed, this should occur in no more than 5% of instances.

Routine Endocervical Curettage

An often raised question is the routine use of the endocervical curettage in the patient with the abnormal smear. In our earlier studies with colposcopy the ECC was routinely used. However, as experience was gained it became apparent that in the patient in whom the limits of the lesion, as well as the squamocolumnar junction, could be easily viewed, the ECC would not contain any neoplastic epithelium. As a consequence, the routine use of the ECC was dropped.

However, recent review of this policy was prompted by several physicians who reported invasive cervical disease high in the canal when in the opinion of the physician the squamocolumnar junction and the limits of the ectocervical lesions (which were noninvasive) could be seen. If the ECC had been performed in these patients, then the disease in the canal would have been detected. The patients then would have been subjected to conization and proper therapy for their disease. Therefore, it is recommended that for the less experienced colposcopist, the ECC be performed routinely on all patients and that conization be used in those patients in whom abnormal epithelium is found in the endocervical curetting.

In the nonpregnant patient colposcopy has significantly reduced the need for diagnostic conization. In most cases in the reproductive years the entire limits of the lesion can be viewed. In those cases where the lesion does extend into the canal, its upper limits can often be viewed with an endocervical speculum. Colposcopy in pregnant patients is more difficult because the colposcopic patterns are exaggerated, owing to the increased vascularity of the organ. An additional problem in these patients is an inflammatory component. When redundant vaginal folds prevent adequate visualization, the blades of the speculum must be fully extended. Cervical mucus in pregnancy is quite tenacious and requires gentle teasing to avoid bleeding. Enzymatic powders containing papaya derivatives may be helpful in lysing the mucus. Those patients who have a diffuse punctation due to inflammation should have local therapy for at least 2 to 3 weeks before a final decision is made regarding the most atypical area for sampling. Biopsies in pregnancy are often associated with brisk bleeding, and for this reason we now restrict our biopsies to those patients in whom only carcinoma in situ or early invasive cancer is suspected. When biopsies are taken a thick Monsel's solution is close at hand, along with a generous supply of cotton balls. Biopsy sites are immediately cauterized followed promptly by packing for 15 to 20 minutes.

Following radiotherapy the Papanicolaou test is occasionally abnormal. With colposcopy it is possible to locate the areas of white epithelium due to radiation dysplasia. These areas may be subtle, and the intravaginal application of estrogen cream will enhance the contrast between normal and abnormal tissue. Since minimal therapy is required for radiation dysplasia, the patients are spared the need for hospitalization and possible traumatic radical surgery. In other cases an early recurrence may be picked up, thereby permitting a more expedient route for further therapy.

Benign Changes

Physicians are often faced with a patient who has a red, "angry"-appearing cervix. Colposcopic evaluation in these instances permits an accurate assessment of the red epithelium, assuring both the physician and the patient that a more serious problem is not present. The red hypertrophied granular appearance is invariably due to the single cell columnar epithelium overlying the highly vascular stroma. This appearance is exaggerated in the patient taking birth control pills and may be accentuated when the patient has some type of vaginal infection.

Patients with cervical polyps can be assessed by colposcopy. In most cases the base of the polyp can be viewed.

The vaginocervicitis of trichomonas often has a classic appearance and can be diagnosed readily with colposcopy. Herpes infections of the cervix have no characteristic appearance, although small vesicles may be seen. The later stages of ulceration may be small, although in some cases it may be so extensive that the cervix is totally involved, resulting in a picture not too dissimilar to invasive carcinoma.

Vulva

Vulvar diseases amenable to colposcopic evaluation include those that are inflammatory and benign, as well as premalignant and malignant. Papillomas and condylomas are characteristic and usually do not require biopsy. However, several young patients referred to our clinic who were diagnosed clinically as having condyloma and not biopsied, when viewed colposcopically had abnormal epithelial foci. On biopsy, these proved to be Bowen's disease.

Vulvar neoplasia is frequently multifocal, and with the colposcope it is possible to locate all foci. In cases where only a single focus is present local therapy is used thereby avoiding disfiguring surgery. The most frequent pattern encountered is white epithelium which may have a keratin crust. Whenever the lesions are keratinized total excision is necessary. Mosaic and punctation are infrequent, since the vulva lacks columnar epithelium. Although herpes genitalis has no specific characteristics, evaluation may disclose vesicles, permitting an early initiation of therapy and possibly aborting the full blown disease.

Vagina

The predominant patterns of the vagina are white epithelium and punctation. Where there has been columnar tissue in the vagina, particularly at the apex, or in patients exposed before birth to diethylstilbestrol (DES), then all the features seen in the transformation zone, such as mosaic, punctation, leukoplakia, and atypical vessels, may be present. It is important in evaluating vaginal intraepithelial lesions that Lugol's solution be used to assist in the location of small foci which may be hidden in vaginal folds.

DES-exposed Offspring

The recent finding of clear cell adenocarcinoma and other abnormalities in DES-exposed offspring has sparked a debate as to the best means to evaluate and follow these individuals. Clear cell adenocarcinoma is still rare in DES-exposed offspring, and the squamous cell lesions have not "exploded" in frequency as initially expected.

Although a thorough colposcopic examination by an experienced colposcopist would be ideal for all DES-exposed offspring, it is not practical. Moreover, all of the clear cell adenocarcinomas to date have been detected by careful palpation, inspection, and cytologic sampling of the cervix and vagina. The colposcopic examination has not proven useful for early detection of these malignancies.

In addition, the colposcopic examination in the DES-exposed individual can be very confusing. Invariably a large transformation zone is present, usually covering the entire ectocervix and often extending onto the vagina, occasionally to the introitus. Vast areas of mosaic structure, punctation, and white epithelium are encountered in almost all patients. However, biopsies of these "abnormal" areas are almost always interpreted as squamous metaplasia. As a consequence, the interpretation of abnormal changes in the DES-exposed patient is much more difficult and should be attempted only by the more experienced colposcopist. However, when these individuals have an abnormal Pap test, colposcopy is mandatory. Examples of the changes in the DES-exposed individual are shown in Figures 7.14 to 7.16.

Research and Education

With the aid of the colposcope, it is now possible to demonstrate in a logical manner the development of both benign and malignant disease of the cervix, vulva, and vagina. It is particularly satisfying to point out those areas where cervical neoplasia is most likely to occur so that Papanicolaou sampling is more accurate, thereby lowering the false negative rate. When specific tissue sampling is needed for research, one can precisely locate the area and take a small sample without significantly disturbing the cervical architecture or surface epithelium.

Infertility

In selected cases colposcopic inspection of the infertile patient is of assistance in determining the cause of postcoital bleeding and has been of assistance in collecting cervical mucus. Whether the use of the instrument has been of significant value in enhancing the possibility of fertility is doubtful, although it does provide a more thorough assessment of the cervix in the infertile woman.

COMMENT

Currently, the availability of colposcopy is limited. Certainly, every major teaching hospital and university should be employing this technique for patient care as well as providing a consultation service for the community. The Medical College of Wisconsin has developed an innovative program to make colposcopy available on a consultation basis for the entire state by organizing hospital-based colposcopy

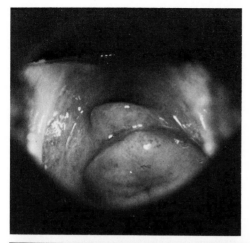

FIG. 7.14. Gross photograph of the cervix and upper vagina in a 23-year-old nulliparous female whose mother had taken diethylstilbestrol throughout pregnancy. This low power examination shows an anterior cervical ridge.

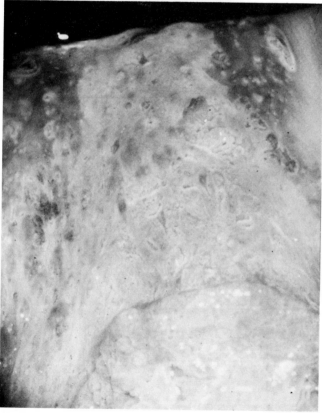

FIG. 7.15. Colpophotography of anterior vagina and cervical ridge shown in Figure 7.14. There is an irregular surface contour, and grape-like clusters of columnar tissue in the anterior vagina (adenosis); the numerous white dots are gland openings. This is a finding one sees in about 30% of females who were exposed to DES, that is, columnar tissue in the vagina. The vast majority of the adenosis has disappeared and is in the process of being transformed to metaplastic squamous epithelium.

clinics in major communities. A similar program has been developed in Southern California at several major community hospitals.

Colposcopy is eminently suited to office gynecology, and its utilization is particularly applicable to group practice. However, the interested solo practitioner may also find the instrument useful with sufficient frequency to warrant its acquisition.

It is anticipated that the current interest in colposcopy will lead to its widespread use and that it will finally take its place as an indispensable addition to the diagnostic armamentarium of the gynecologist.

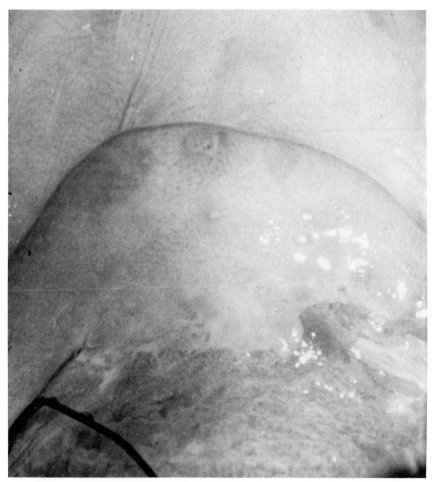

FIG. 7.16. Colpophotograph of anterior cervix and upper one-third of vagina in a 17-year-old DES-exposed offspring. The cervix has a slight peaking deformity suggestive of a cock's comb. A portion of the IUD string is present in the lower left-hand portion of the photograph. Grape-like columnar tissue is present in the lower portion of the photograph. The grape-like columnar tissue blends into a large area of metaplastic squamous epithelium characterized by punctation. This punctation pattern continues onto the anterior vaginal wall, down to the upper one-third of the vagina. In the center of the photograph a vaginal Nabothian cyst is faintly visible.

REFERENCES

1. Hinselmann, H, Verbesserung de Inspektionsmoglichkeiten von Vulva, Vagina and Portio, Munch Med Wschr 77:1733, 1925.

2. Ries, E, Erosion, Leukoplakia, and the Colposcope in Relation to Carcinoma of the Cervix, Am J Obstet Gynecol 23:393, 1932.

3. Scheffey, LC, Lang WR, and Tataria, G, Experimental Program with Colposcopy (Discussion by Martlzloff), Am J Obstet Gynecol 70:886, 1955.

4. Papanicolaou, GN, and Traut, HF, Diagnosis of Uterine Cancer by the Vaginal Smear, New York Commonwealth Fund, 1943.

5. Wilds, PL, Is Colposcopy Practical? Obstet Gynecol 20:645, 1962.

6. Scheffey, LC, Bolten, KA, and Lang, WR, Colposcopy: Aid in Diagnosis of Cervical Cancer, Obstet Gynecol 5:294, 1955.

7. Limburg, H, Comparison between Cytology and Colposcopy in the Diagnosis of Early Cervical Carcinoma, Am J Obstet Gynecol 75:1298, 1958.

8. Hill, E, Preclinical Cervical Carcinoma, Colposcopy, and the "Negative" Smear, Am J Obstet Gynecol 95:308, 1966.

9. Way, S, *The Diagnosis of Early Carcinoma of the Cervix*, Little, Brown, Boston, 1963.

10. Coppleson, M, Pixley, E, and Reid, B, *Colposcopy*, Charles C Thomas, Springfield, Ill, 1971.

11. Creasman, WT, Weed, JC, Curry, SL, Johnston, WM, and Parker, RT, Efficacy of Cryosurgical Treatment of Severe Intraepithelial Neoplasia, Obstet Gynecol 41:501, 1973.

12. Donohue, L, Meriwether, D, Colposcopy as a Diagnostic Tool in the Investigation of Cervical Neoplasias, Am J Obstet Gynecol 113:107, 1972.

13. Gondos, B, Townsend, DE, and Ostergard, DR, Cytologic Diagnosis of Squamous Dysplasia and Carcinoma of the Cervix, Am J Obstet Gynecol 110:107, 1971.

14. Hollyock, VE, and Chanen, W, The Use of the Colposcope in the Selection of Patients for Cervical Cone Biopsy, Am J Obstet Gynecol 114:185, 1972.

15. Kolstad, P, Carcinoma of the Cervix, Stage 0, Am J Obstet Gynecol 96:1098, 1966.

16. Kolstad, P, and Stafl, A, *Atlas of Colposcopy*, University Park Press, Baltimore, 1972.

17. Krumholz, BA, and Knapp, RC, Colposcopic Selection of Biopsy Sites, Obstet Gynecol 39:22, 1972.

18. Ortiz, R, and Newton, M, Colposcopy in the Management of Abnormal Cervical Smear in Pregnancy, JAMA 109:44, 1971.

19. Ortiz, R, Newton, M, and Langlois, PL, Colposcopic Biopsy in the Diagnosis of Carcinoma of the Cervix, Obstet Gynecol 34:303, 1969.

20. Ortiz, R, and Odell, L, Observations on the Use of the Colposcope for Cervical Neoplasia, J Reprod Med 4:97, 1970.

21. Ostergard, D, and Gondos, B, Outpatient Therapy of Preinvasive Cervical Neoplasia: Selection of Patients with the Use of Colposcopy, Am J Obstet Gynecol 115:783, 1973.

22. Stafl, A, and Mattingly, RF, Colposcopic Diagnosis of Cervical Neoplasia, Obstet Gynecol 41:168, 1973.

23. Thompson, BH, Woodruff, JD, Julian, CG, and Silva, FG, Cytopathology, Histopathology, and Colposcopy in the Management of Cervical Neoplasia, Am J Obstet Gynecol 114:329, 1972.

24. Townsend, DE, and Ostergard, DR, Cryocauterization for Preinvasive Cervical Neoplasia, J Reprod Med 6:55, 1971.

25. Townsend, DE, Ostergard, DR, Mishell, DR, Jr, and Hirose, FM, Abnormal Papanicolaou Smears: Evaluation by Colposcopy, Biopsies, and Endocervical Curettage, Am J Obstet Gynecol 108:429, 1970.

26. Tredway, DR, Townsend, DE, Hovland, DN, and Upton, RT, Colposcopy and Cryosurgery in Cervical Intra-Epithelial Neoplasia, Am J Obstet Gynecol 114:1020, 1972.

27. Graham, RM, *The Cytologic Diagnosis of Cancer*, W. B. Saunders, Philadelphia, 1964.

28. Richart, RM, and Vaillant, HW, Influence of Cell Collection Techniques upon Cytological Diagnosis, Cancer 18:1474, 1969.

29. Richart, RM, The Handling of Small Tissue Samples for Pathologic Examination, Bull Sloane Hosp 9:113, 1963.

30. Fox, CH, Biologic Behavior of Dysplasia and Carcinoma in Situ, Am J Obstet Gynecol 99:960, 1967.

31. Fox, CH, Time Necessary for Conversion of Normal to Dysplastic Cervical Epithelium, Obstet Gynecol 31:749, 1968.

32. Koss, LG, Significance of Dysplasia, Clin Obstet Gynecol 13:873, 1970.

33. Koss, LG, Stewart, FW, Foote, FW, Jordan, MJ, Bader, GM, and Day, E, Some Histological Aspects of Behavior of Epidermoid Carcinoma in Situ and Related Lesions of the Uterine Cervix—Long Term Prospective Study, Cancer 16:1160, 1963.

34. Richart, RM, Natural History of Cervical Intraepithelial Neoplasia, Clin Obstet Gynecol 10:748, 1967.

8

DIETHYLSTILBESTROL-EXPOSED FEMALES

ARTHUR L. HERBST, M.D.

ROBERT E. SCULLY, M.D.

STANLEY J. ROBBOY, M.D.

INTRODUCTION

In 1971 the unusual occurrence of clear-cell adenocarcinoma of the vagina in seven females 14 to 22 years of age was associated in a carefully controlled epidemiologic study with their mothers' ingestion of diethylstilbestrol (DES) during the pregnancies of which they had been products.[1] Only two or three of these cancers in patients in this age group had been recorded in the world literature prior to the usage of this drug for high risk pregnancies.[2]

DES was synthesized by Dodds and his associates in 1938. Soon it became readily available as an inexpensive, potent, orally active estrogen that had many medical uses. In the 1940's it was first used to treat high risk pregnancies on the basis of data available at that time, which suggested that its administration improved fetal salvage. Subsequently DES treatment during pregnancy became widespread. In the early 1950's the efficacy of this approach was questioned, and thereafter its popularity gradually diminished. In November, 1971, the Food and Drug Administration issued a bulletin proscribing the use of DES during pregnancy because of its documented association with the development of malignancy in the exposed female offspring.

The precise number of females in the United States who have been exposed to DES *in utero* is unknown, but the estimate is one-half to two million. In this population clear-cell adenocarcinomas have fortunately been very rare, with fewer than 200 involving the vagina or cervix having been related unequivocally to prenatal DES exposure.[3] In contrast, several striking non-neoplastic alterations of the lower genital tract have been found with great frequency.[4, 5] The most common of these has been the ectopic presence of benign glandular epithelium in the vagina or on the exocervix. Depending on its location, this has been termed vaginal adenosis (the presence of columnar epithelium or its mucinous products in the vagina) or cervical erosion or ectropion (the presence of columnar epithelium or its mucinous products on the exocervix or portio vaginalis). In addition, congenital transverse fibrous bands or ridges have been observed less frequently in the vagina, often close to its junction with the cervix (Fig. 8.1).

This chapter will present guidelines for the gynecologist in his or her approach to

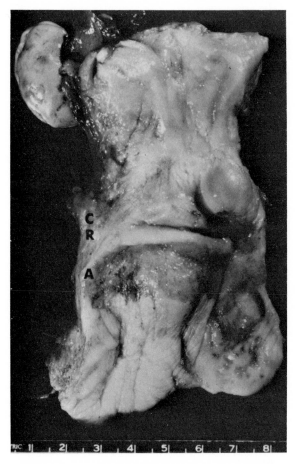

Fig. 8.1. Open uterus and vagina with attached adnexa. Note transverse ridge (R), cervix (C), and zone of adenosis (A). A nabothian cyst of the cervix is visible along the right margin of the specimen. (Used with permission of New Eng J Med, Herbst et al. *287:*1261, 1972.)

the large DES-exposed population. First, some observations from the Registry of Clear-cell Adenocarcinoma of the Genital Tract in Young Females will be presented, insofar as the data accumulated therein bear on the assessment of those without known carcinoma. Second, the methods and results of the clinical examination of DES-exposed females will be discussed, with consideration of their appropriate management.

RELEVANT FINDINGS FROM THE REGISTRY OF CLEAR-CELL ADENOCARCINOMA

The startling association of ingestion of DES during pregnancy with vaginal and cervical cancer in offspring led to the establishment in 1971 of the Registry of Clear-cell Adenocarcinoma of the Genital Tract in Young Females. This Registry gathers clinical, pathologic, and epidemiologic data on all cases of clear-cell cancer occurring in females born after 1940, whether or not a history of maternal hormone ingestion has been obtained. The earliest reported cases of carcinoma associated with a history of maternal DES ingestion occurred in patients in New England, but these tumors are now known to have occurred throughout the United States and in many foreign countries, including Australia, Belgium, Canada, France, and

Mexico. The maternal histories are not yet available in all the cases reported to the Registry, but among the completely investigated cases, histories of maternal ingestion of DES, dienestrol, or hexestrol (all chemically related nonsteroidal synthetic estrogens) have been obtained in approximately two-thirds. In an additional 10% of the cases the mothers were treated for high risk pregnancy but the drug administered could not be identified, and in the remaining 20 to 25% of the cases no history of maternal therapy was uncovered. It should be emphasized that in many of these cases the medical records were incomplete and the mothers, who had been treated 15 to 20 years previously, did not recall the details of the pregnancies. Thus there is a high correlation between the occurrence of these cancers and maternal ingestion of DES-type drugs, but very few carcinomas have developed among the exposed. Furthermore, the known rare occurrence of these carcinomas in the pre-DES era, coupled with the identification of cases with negative maternal hormone histories, indicates that factors other than prenatal exposure to DES are also involved in the genesis of these cancers. So far, intrauterine exposure to steroidal estrogens has not been linked to the subsequent development of vaginal and cervical clear-cell adenocarcinoma in the offspring.

Analysis of the maternal therapy data from the Registry cases has revealed a wide variation in both dosages and patterns of administration of DES (Table 8.1). In six cases the daily dosage never exceeded 5 mg, while in two, only 1.5 mg per day were prescribed. The duration of treatment varied from as short as 1 week to many months. The timing of the therapy, however, has proved to be important. In all the cases where precise information was available, therapy began prior to the 18th week of pregnancy, and no cases of cancer have yet been recorded when therapy commenced in the second half of the pregnancy. The minimal dosage that can be

TABLE 8.1
Details of Dosage of Stilbestrol Therapy

Total DES dosage	Daughters with clear-cell adenocarcinoma	
	Vaginal	Cervical
mg		
<500	3	3
501–1,000	0	3
1,001–5,000	3	4
5,001–10,000	11	3
10,001–15,000	5	4
>15,000	2	2
Total	24	19
Time during pregnancy stilbestrol started		
Week 8 or before	33	15
Weeks 9–13	37	18
Weeks 14–17	5	4
Week 18 or greater	0	0
Total	75	37

associated with the development of carcinoma in the offspring is still unknown. At present any intrauterine exposure to these compounds must be considered potentially dangerous, necessitating appropriate examination and follow-up.

The age of the cancer patients with histories of exposure has varied from 7 to 27 years, with an average of 17.5 years; 90% have been 14 years of age or older. As shown in Table 8.2, most of the patients presented with bleeding or discharge, as might be expected in cases of lower genital tract carcinoma. The symptomatic lesions varied greatly in size and involved the cervix or vagina or both. All were readily detectable on pelvic examination. Asymptomatic patients, however, often had smaller tumors which were less readily detected on visual examination. A few tumors were submucosal and were found only after careful palpation of the vaginal wall. Of 37 asymptomatic patients, 35 are free of disease after treatment, emphasizing the importance of screening examinations to detect early lesions. Table 8.2 also reveals that cytologic smears were abnormal in 71% of the 122 cancer cases, and in 11 of these cases an abnormal cytologic report was the initial finding that led to a more intensive investigation and detection of the carcinoma. Nonetheless, the smear was negative in 27% of the cases, indicating that cytology cannot be relied upon to exclude the diagnosis.[6] From these data we have concluded that DES-exposed females deserve a screening evaluation once they have begun to menstruate or, if they have not begun, by the age of 14 years. The very rare occurrence of these cancers before puberty, combined with the difficulties of repeated examination of the prepubertal group, makes screening examinations of these very young individuals unwarranted unless abnormal symptoms such as bleeding or persistent discharge develop.

METHOD OF EXAMINATION OF DES-EXPOSED FEMALES

An adequate screening examination includes cytologic sampling of the vagina and cervix and careful gross inspection and palpation of the vaginal and cervical mucosa, followed by colposcopy, iodine staining, or both, to delineate abnormal areas that should be biopsied. A careful digital examination should not only reveal any nodularity or tumor but should also indicate the size of the speculum that can be introduced into the vagina. After the cervix is exposed, excess mucus should be wiped away and a spatula used to obtain a direct scrape of the cervix and a separate sample from the vagina.[7] An endocervical specimen should also be obtained, either with a saline-soaked cotton-tipped applicator or by aspiration with a pipette. The

TABLE 8.2
Presenting Symptoms and Cytology of Registry Patients

Presenting symptoms	Number of cases	Cytology report	Number of cases
Bleeding or discharge	152 (73%)	Positive (IV or V)	65 (53%)
None	37 (18%)	Doubtful (IIR or III)	22 (18%)
Pain	6 (3%)	Negative (I or II)	33 (27%)
Other or unknown	13 (6%)	Unsatisfactory	2
Total	208		122

endocervical sample is then usually placed on the same slide as the cervical scrape, and the vaginal and cervical slides are submitted separately for cytologic evaluation. Following careful inspection and palpation, a colposcopic examination may be performed after the application of 3% acetic acid. The details of colposcopic evaluation of the vagina and cervix are presented in Chapter 7. A Schiller (iodine) test can then be performed after excess acetic acid is removed. Half-strength Lugol's solution provides greater contrast than Schiller's solution between the staining and nonstaining areas, and is preferable to full strength Lugol's which frequently causes drying of the mucosal surface and an annoying irritation to the patient. Biopsies are taken of areas that appear red or nodular on naked-eye examination or that are most abnormal on colposcopic examination. If colposcopy is not performed, multiple biopsies should be taken from the areas that appear abnormal or that fail to stain with iodine solution (Fig. 8.2). As a rule a small Eppendorfer* or Kevorkian punch can remove millimeter-sized samples from the vagina or cervix without undue discomfort to the patient. Excessive bleeding is rare and, if it occurs, it can usually be controlled by chemical cauterization. The examination is facilitated if the speculum is as large as possible without causing discomfort. For girls with intact hymens, narrow specula are available that allow examination of the vagina and cervix (Fig. 8.3). If the initial evaluation is unsatisfactory, the subsequent use of vaginal tampons often makes a second office evaluation easier. Rarely, hospitalization and anesthesia may be necessary to permit an adequate evaluation.

RESULTS OF EXAMINATION OF DES-EXPOSED FEMALES

Recently we have completed a prospective case-controlled study comparing the findings in DES-exposed females to those in unexposed controls.[5] The exposed group was made up of female offspring whose mothers were treated at the stilbestrol clinic of the Boston Lying-in Hospital between 1947 and 1958. The control group consisted of unexposed females born at the same hospital closest in time and always within five days of the birth of the exposed. The health histories of the mothers after the study pregnancies, as well as the health and reproductive histories of the daughters, were similar in both groups, as were the general physical and pelvic examinations. Additional gynecologic evaluation consisted of vaginal cytology, careful inspection and palpation of the vagina and cervix, iodine staining, and biopsies of areas that appeared red or failed to stain with iodine solution. At the time the subject was seen, the examiner did not know whether she had been exposed.

The results of the pelvic examinations showed highly significant differences between the two groups (Table 8.3). The types of alterations observed in the exposed were typical of those seen in DES-exposed females.[8] Mucosa that failed to stain with iodine solution were found in at least part of the vagina in 56% of the exposed but in only 1% of the unexposed subjects. A similar finding on the exocervix was observed in 95% of the exposed subjects in contrast to only 49% of the controls. Biopsy specimens from the abnormal areas of the vagina revealed

---

*Gynemed, Inc., Palo Alto, California.

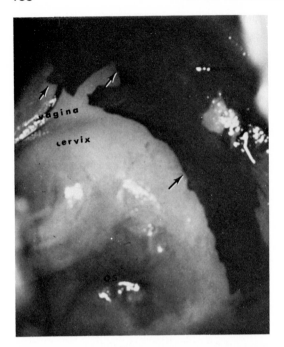

Fig. 8.2. Abnormal Schiller stain in which aglycogenated (nonstaining) areas in both the vagina and the cervix appear white in the photograph. The glycogenated epithelium (staining area) appears black. Arrows indicate the demarcation between staining and nonstaining areas. (Used with permission of J Reprod Med, Robboy et al. *15:*13, 1975.)

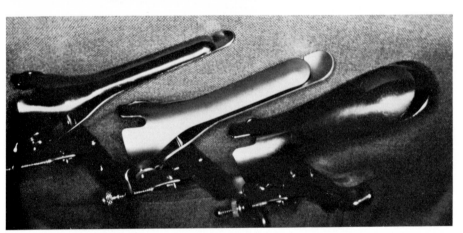

Fig. 8.3. Narrow (geriatric type) specula (Milex Company, Chicago) that can be used for examination of the patient with intact hymen are shown on the left, with a normal-sized Graves' speculum on the right.

adenosis in 35% of the exposed subjects but in only 1% of the controls, and biopsy of the cervix revealed erosion in 85% of the exposed subjects in contrast to only 38% of the controls. Those biopsy specimens in which no glandular epithelium was identified in the vagina or cervix usually were found to be lined by glycogen-free metaplastic squamous epithelium, which resulted in the failure of the surface to stain with iodine solution and which is thought to represent a healing phase of adenosis and erosion. Approximately 20% of the exposed had transverse ridges in the vagina and cervix (Figures 8.1 and 8.4 to 8.6). No evidence of malignancy was found in either group.

Additional DES-exposed subjects who were not part of the controlled portion of the study were also examined. These included 18 Caucasians aged 13 to 17 years and 5 non-Caucasians aged 19 to 24 years. An analysis of these 23 subjects in addition to the 110 exposed in the controlled study revealed a striking correlation between the incidence of adenosis and the time of initiation of DES exposure

TABLE 8.3
Results of Pelvic Examinations[a]

Examination results	Exposed (110 examined)	Control (82 examined)	P values
	%	%	
Failure of part of the vagina to stain with iodine	56%	1%	0.0001
Vaginal adenosis identified in biopsy specimens	35%	1%	0.0001
Failure of part of cervix to stain with iodine	95%	49%	0.0001
Cervical erosion identified in biopsy specimens	85%	38%	0.0001
Vaginal or cervical fibrous ridges	22%	0%	0.0001

[a] Used with permission of *New Eng J Med*, Herbst et al. *292:*336, 1975.

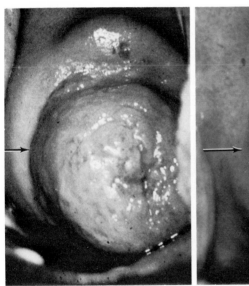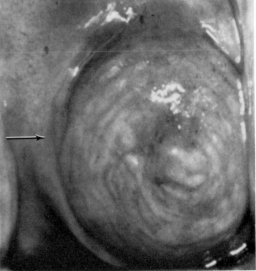

Fig. 8.4. (*left*). Concentric ridge (arrow) in the cervix creating the appearance of a "pseudopolyp," in the center of which is the external os. A circular fold gives the appearance of a hood covering the cervix. (Used with permission of J Reprod Med, Robboy et al. *15:*13, 1975.)

Fig. 8.5. (*right*). Transverse ridge at the junction of the vagina and the cervix, giving the appearance of a cervical collar (arrow). An erosion covers the entire outer cervix, and vaginal adenosis was detected on microscopic examination. (Used with permission of Obstet Gynecol, Herbst et al. *40:*293, 1972.)

(Table 8.4). No cases of vaginal adenosis were detected in the 11 offspring whose mothers began treatment after the 18th week of gestation.

A wide variation in the incidence of vaginal adenosis in DES-exposed females has been reported in the literature,[9, 10] with higher frequencies noted following colposcopic examination than after direct inspection and iodine staining. However, a number of factors other than the method of examination are probably primarily responsible for these wide discrepancies.[11] They include: (1) the use of the term "adenosis" by some investigators to denote the presence of columnar (glandular) epithelium on the cervix as well as in the vagina, (2) the categorization of biopsy specimens of ridges and rims near the cervix as vaginal by some investigators and

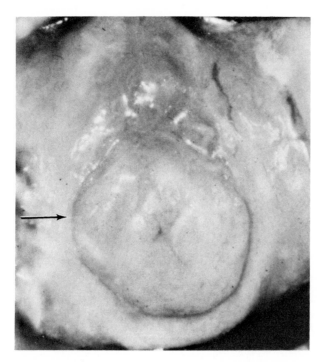

Fig. 8.6. Concentric ridge (arrow) in the cervix giving a "pseudopolyp" appearance. The cervical os is located in the center of the pseudopolyp. (Used with permission of Obstet Gynecol, Herbst et al. *40:*294, 1972.)

TABLE 8.4

Frequency of Abnormalities in 133 Exposed Subjects Related to Week of Initiation of DES Therapy during Pregnancy[a]

Week	Total number	Percentage with		
		Vaginal adenosis	Cervical erosion	Ridge
		%	%	%
≤8	22	73	100	23
9–12	39	49	92	28
13–16	42	29	81	19
≥17	30	7	70	13

[a] Used with permission of *New Eng. J Med*, Herbst et al. *292:*337, 1975.

as cervical by others, and (3) the time in pregnancy during which DES therapy was begun. Thus the examination of patients exposed earlier during pregnancy, the inclusion of a ridge near the cervix as part of the vagina, and the designation of all columnar epithelium found on any biopsies as "adenosis" all contribute to an increase in the reported incidence of adenosis. Comparison between series is not possible unless these variables are standardized. It is conceivable that other factors such as age or contraceptive practices may also alter the results of these examinations, but their influence, if any, is unknown at present.[9]

We have recently compared our reported findings based on iodine staining and multiple random biopsies of the vagina with those of Townsend et al., who performed colposcopic examinations on 500 exposed females and who used the same definitions of vaginal adenosis we have employed in the Boston Lying-in DES study. These investigators identified adenosis in 30% of the subjects and a metaplastic transformation zone in the vagina (corresponding to the non-iodine-staining squamous mucosa) in an additional 30%. Somewhat surprisingly, the results of their series and ours are almost identical, in spite of the different methods of examination.[12]

CURRENT MANAGEMENT OF DES-EXPOSED FEMALES

It is important that DES-exposed females receive thorough screening examinations, including colposcopy if the examiner is trained in its use. The colposcope provides a magnified view of the vaginal and cervical mucosa and enables the gynecologist to take directed and usually fewer biopsies. It should be emphasized, however, that in a few cases a clear-cell adenocarcinoma has not been visualized by the colposcope because of its location either behind an obstructing ridge or in the submucosa unaccompanied by an abnormal surface colposcopic pattern. In addition, a few words of caution are needed in regard to the interpretation of colposcopic findings in DES-exposed subjects. On the basis of our experience and that of others, it has become evident that many colposcopic abnormalities, such as marked mosaic and punctation, which would be suspicious of intraepithelial carcinoma in an unexposed individual are common in DES-exposed subjects. Biopsy specimens of these areas almost always show squamous metaplasia or other non-neoplastic changes in DES-exposed subjects. In other words, squamous metaplasia (Fig. 8.7) in the vagina and cervix of the DES-exposed female may be confused colposcopically with dysplastic or other premalignant processes. Great care must be taken before initiating any therapy in these young patients, because of the danger of undertaking treatment that might not be necessary.

Vaginal adenosis, cervical erosion, and areas of squamous metaplasia are common histologic findings in DES-exposed females. Moreover, in spite of the fact that adenosis has been found in almost all patients with vaginal carcinoma, a direct transition from adenosis to cancer has not been histologically identified, adding further support to the contention that adenosis is primarily non-neoplastic, with a very small premalignant potential. It has been suggested that squamous cell carcinomas may eventually prove to be more common than clear-cell adenocarcinoma in the exposed population in view of the large areas of metaplastic squamous epithelium in the vagina and cervix at risk for malignant change and the

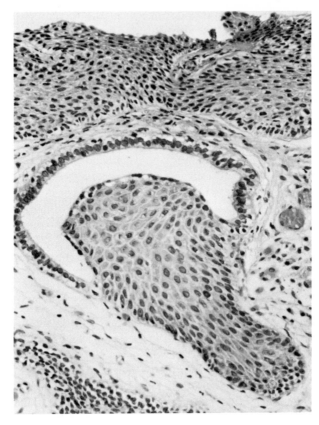

Fig. 8.7. Vaginal biopsy. The gland shows focal squamous metaplasia. Hemotoxylin and eosin, ×250. (Used with permission of Am J Obstet Gynecol, Herbst et al. *118:*611, 1974.)

occasional finding of squamous dysplasia in the cervix and vagina of exposed individuals.[13] Although evidence for an increase in squamous cell carcinoma in DES-exposed females does not exist at the present time, this possibility is an additional reason for close followup.

The question has frequently arisen as to what contraceptive advice should be given to DES-exposed females. In the study performed on the Boston Lying-in DES-exposed group, there was a slight decrease in the incidence of vaginal adenosis among those who used oral contraceptives. However, we have refrained from advocating the use of the pill in these subjects because it introduces an additional unknown variable into an already complicated situation, even though there is no evidence as yet that the pill is harmful. It has been suggested by some that acidification of the vagina promotes squamous metaplasia, leading to healing of adenosis and erosion, but there are no statistically valid studies at present to verify this hypothesis.

Many DES-exposed females have successfully achieved pregnancy and delivery, and there is no evidence at present to suggest that infertility is more common among them than in the unexposed population. However, most of the DES-exposed subjects are just beginning to attempt pregnancy. The reproductive histories of the exposed subjects from the small Boston Lying-in Hospital series were comparable to those of the controls.

Excision of areas of vaginal adenosis has been advocated by some who have assumed that such therapy is justified by the risk of development of cancer. In our opinion current evidence does not support such active radical therapeutic intervention. The universal adoption of such treatment would result in extensive therapy of 90 to 95% of DES-exposed subjects, and much of this may be unnecessary. In view of the multifocal distribution of the lesions, two or three procedures might be required in a single patient. Hemorrhage, stenosis, and scarring can result. We recommend that local destruction by cautery, cryosurgery, or excision be reserved for those patients in whom premalignant changes are histologically identified.

For the few exposed subjects whose initial pelvic examination is normal, yearly checkups are recommended. For those in whom adenosis or extensive erosion is found, examination two or three times a year seems reasonable. Direct cytologic sampling of the abnormal areas may provide a nontraumatic adjunct to the followup.

Clearly a great deal more needs to be learned about the natural history of the various changes noted in the DES-exposed female. Careful followup of this population in the future should provide many of the answers as well as afford early diagnosis for the occasional exposed subjects in whom clear-cell adenocarcinoma may develop.†

REFERENCES

1. Herbst, AL, Ulfelder, H, and Poskanzer DC, Adenocarcinoma of the Vagina: Association of Maternal Stilbestrol Therapy with Tumor Appearance in Young women, New Eng J Med 284:878, 1971.
2. Herbst, AL, and Scully, RE, Adenocarcinoma of the Vagina in Adolescence, Cancer 25:745, 1970.
3. Herbst, AL, Robboy, SJ, Scully, RE, and Poskanzer, DC, Clear-cell Adenocarcinoma of the Vagina and Cervix in Girls: Analysis of 170 Registry Cases, Am J Obstet Gynecol 119:713, 1974.
4. Herbst, AL, Kurman, RJ, and Scully, RE, Vaginal and Cervical Abnormalities after Exposure to Stilbestrol in Utero, Obstet Gynecol 40:287, 1972.
5. Herbst, AL, Poskanzer, DC, Robboy, SJ, Friedlander, L, and Scully, RE, Prenatal Exposure to Stilbestrol: A Prospective Comparison of Exposed Female Offspring with Unexposed Controls, New Eng J Med 292:334, 1975.
6. Taft, PD, Robboy, SJ, Herbst, AL, and Scully, RE: Cytology of Clear-cell Adenocarcinoma of the Genital Tract in Young Females: Review of 95 Cases from the Registry, Acta Cytol 18:279, 1974.
7. Ng, AB, Reagan, JW, Hawliczek, S, and Wentz, WB, Cellular Detection of Vaginal Adenosis, Obstet Gynecol 46:323, 1975.
8. Scully, RE, Robboy, SJ, and Herbst, AL, Vaginal and Cervical Abnormalities including Clear-cell Adenocarcinoma Related to Prenatal Exposure to Stilbestrol, Ann Clin Lab Sci 4:222, 1974.
9. Sherman, AI, Goldrath, M, Berlin, A, Vakhariva, V, Banooni, F, Michaels, W, Goodman, P, and Brown, S, Cervical-Vaginal Adenosis after in Utero Exposure to Synthetic Estrogens, Obstet Gynecol 44:531, 1974.
10. Stafl, A, Mattingly, RF, Foley, DV, and Fetherston, WC, Clinical Diagnosis of Vaginal Adenosis, Obstet Gynecol 43:118, 1974.
11. Herbst, AL, Scully, RE, Robboy, SJ, Problems in the Examination of the DES-exposed Female, Obstet Gynecol 46:353, 1975.
12. Townsend, DE, Personal Communication.
13. Stafl, A, and Mattingly, RF, Vaginal Adenosis: A Precancerous Lesion? Am J Obstet Gynecol 120:666, 1974.

† Supported in part by Grant RO1 CA 13139-04 from the National Cancer Institute.

9

OFFICE SEX COUNSELING

ANN K. SPENCE, M.D.

JAY MANN, PH.D.

You are just completing an annual checkup on Mrs. Smith. The time is 4:30 in the afternoon. Still waiting in your office are three prenatal patients, two postoperative checks, and another annual examination. This is the night you have promised your spouse you are going to be home at a decent hour to go out for dinner. As you prepare to leave the examining room, Mrs. Smith quietly says, "Doctor, I think I have a sexual problem."

You ask yourself, "Should I do sex counseling in office practice?" The information provided in the following chapter may help you to decide.

INTRODUCTION

Every physician can do some sexual counseling. How much any given individual can do, will depend on how comfortable he* is in dealing with sex, how knowledgeable he is, and how much time he has available. All sex counseling, whether very brief or intensive, requires the practitioner to be reasonably well informed about sexuality and comfortable in dealing with sexual concerns. The popular image of sex counseling is of intensive or long term couple therapy, but more commonly it involves a procedure as simple as answering questions raised during annual or prenatal exams. It may entail having recent reading material on sexuality available for patients, including references regarding sexual dysfunctions, or being aware of suitable referral sources in the community.

The process of sex counseling can be divided into four levels: (1) validation, (2) education, (3) suggestion, and (4) therapy. If the first is not sufficient to alleviate the problem, the second is invoked, then the third, and finally the fourth.

The first level, validation, is one of the major elements of counseling. Validation refers to the process whereby the interest or discussion you provide about a sexual area reassures the patient that sex is a natural function and thus allows her to be comfortable in dealing with that area. For example, discussing oral sex with a patient implies that engaging in oral sex is normal or expected. It is also important to validate the patient's individual practices, attitudes, and feelings, including her concern or dysfunction. It is reassuring to a patient to learn that sexual

---

* Our use of the word "he" to describe physicians of both sexes reflects the unavailability of a term in our language that recognizes that physicians can be "he or she."

dysfunctions are natural outgrowths of common life situations and backgrounds.

Why should physicians do sex counseling?

The most striking reason is that sexual dysfunction, because of its high incidence in the general population, may be the most common problem encountered in general office practice. According to Masters and Johnson, over 50% of married couples have some form of sexual dysfunction. Because patients are often reluctant to broach sexual problems, many physicians may underestimate their incidence. Because sex therapy is brief therapy and because most patients with problems respond well to the validation and education provided in office counseling, the average physician can be a highly appropriate counselor.

The physician is in a favored position to provide counseling because he has a unique relationship with his patients. Many women will reveal problems to their doctor because of this unique, intimate relationship. For many a woman, the visit to her doctor is the one time she can reveal or discuss problems she feels uncomfortable sharing with even her husband or friends. Too many physicians fail to facilitate this process.

It is particularly important that the patient receive accurate and understandable information since many women know very little about how their bodies look and how they function. When discussing sexuality with a woman, it is necessary to provide information and suggestions that will be useful to her and appropriate to her sexual lifestyle. Although many physicians have acquired sophisticated information about contraception, infertility and pregnancy, many have not attained the same level of knowledge about sexuality.

The following sections include a review of human sexuality, the identification of sexual problems (office management), and a brief discussion of sexual aids.

SEXUALITY

Much of our knowledge about human sexuality has been provided by the research of Masters and Johnson. Their work included clinical observation and examination, as well as individual and couple interviews. Masters and Johnson emphasize that although there are general patterns of sexual response a wide range of normal variations exists. Therefore, every healthy individual's response is unique and valid.

Female Sexual Response

The major physiologic changes that occur during the four stages of the sexual response cycle are vasocongestion and muscle tension. Specific changes can be viewed as effects of these two major processes. For descriptive purposes, Masters and Johnson distinguish four phases of sexual response, which are not sharply differentiated.

Excitement Phase. During excitement phase the vagina becomes lubricated by a transudate and begins to lengthen and widen. The unstimulated vaginal barrel measures 2 cm, while with excitement, vaginal wall expansion averages 6 cm. The length increases from 7 or 8 cm to 10 cm. The expansion occurs mainly in the inner two-thirds. Toward the end of excitement stage, the vaginal mucosa flattens.

With stimulation, the uterus elevates from the true pelvis into the false pelvis. The cervix, as a result, retracts out of the vaginal barrel.

The labia majora become distended with blood, and the labia minora expand in diameter. The clitoris usually increases in size in a time sequence similar to the labia minora.

Plateau Phase. During plateau phase, the vaginal wall distends in the outer third owing to vasocongestion. This distention produces a reduction by a third in the diameter of the vagina, an effect which forms the basis for what is called the *orgasmic platform*. The vagina increases minimally in width and depth. Interestingly, lubrication reaches its peak and subsides during plateau. As lubrication diminishes, it may become necessary to use a hypoallergenic massage or body oil during intercourse.

The uterus completes elevation and lifts the cervix farther out of the vaginal barrel. With stimulation, the clitoris withdraws and retracts against the pubis. The clitoral shaft retracts by 50% in overall length, withdrawing the clitoris under the protective clitoral hood.

Labial engorgement continues during plateau phase. The labia minora during plateau undergo a remarkable color change, from pink to a deep red. The more effective the stimulation, the deeper and more brilliant is the color change. According to Masters and Johnson, orgasm never occurs without these color changes.

Orgasmic Phase. The vaginal expansion remains the same as during plateau. The vagina responds to orgasm in the outer third, in the orgasmic platform. The platform contracts rhythmically at 0.8-second intervals, with the contractions recurring within a range of 3–5 times to a maximum of 10–15 times.

During orgasm, the uterus undergoes no further change. The labia majora and minora remain as in plateau stage.

The clitoris remains retracted under the clitoral hood during orgasm.

Resolution Phase. In general, resolution results in the returning of the pelvic organs to a resting state.

The vagina increases in diameter as the vasocongestive reaction disperses. The deep purple color of the vagina returns to normal level and the normal pattern returns. The uterus begins to return to its resting position, and the cervix drops into the vaginal barrel and into the seminal pool if the partner has ejaculated.

After orgasm, the clitoris returns to its unstimulated state within 5 to 10 seconds, and the labia majora return to their previous thickness. After orgasm, the color in the labia minora lightens.

It is important in discussing sexuality with a patient always to emphasize the individuality of her sexuality. Every woman responds to sexual stimulation in her own way. Each response is valid; there is no correct or normal way. Many women, especially those who are nonorgasmic, have fixed and unrealistic expectations of how they should respond sexually.

Orgasm. Orgasm is a unique experience for every woman. For women who have never experienced it, orgasm remains a mysterious happening. Many of these women fake orgasm, having never experienced one. These women will read books describing orgasm and then attempt to mimic one in an effort to convince their partners they are sexually responsive. Subjective descriptions of orgasm are varied. Not only do subjective sensations vary from woman to woman, but in each individual from one episode to another. The most consistent features are initial sensual feelings in the clitoris that radiate into the pelvis. Accompanying this sensation is a focusing of sensory awareness on the pelvis and a decreasing awareness of external sensations. Some women experience a sensation of bearing down as they reach orgasm. Later many women report a feeling of spreading warmth that originates in the pelvis and radiates throughout the body. The final stage is that of involuntary contractions in the vagina. This is often accompanied by general body tremors. Most women report resolution phase as the feeling of being finished, of release and of complete relaxation.

Various amounts of stimulation are required to initiate the sexual response that results in orgasm. Many women can attain orgasm with brief stimulation lasting 1 to 3 minutes, or occasionally through fantasy alone; others may require an hour or more. Some require stimulation directly on or near the clitoris; others can respond to more diffuse stimulation of the genital or other body areas. Many nonorgasmic women have expectations that self-manipulation should create pleasurable experiences within a few minutes. The reassurance that stimulation for much longer periods is normal is all the information many women need to achieve orgasm. Encouraging women to experiment with various forms of stimulation gives them permission to expand their sexual experiences.

Clinical Suggestions. 1. Pain may occur during intercourse if the woman is still in early excitement phase and the cervix has not been elevated. Deep penetration may result in pressure on the cervix with resulting discomfort. To avoid this discomfort, suggest that the woman and her partner prolong *pleasuring*† prior to entry. Many men believe that once their partners begin to produce lubrication they are strongly aroused. In fact, vaginal lubrication is a very early sign of arousal, generally preceding a woman's subjective readiness for intromission.

2. Since lubricant production peaks and then is reduced during plateau phase, many couples require additional lubrication at this time. Unfortunately, many women interpret diminished lubrication as a sign that they are not receiving adequate pleasuring. They may try altering stimulation to increase their arousal. Suggesting the use of hypoallergenic massage oil may increase the woman's pleasure and reduce her concerns about how responsive she is.

3. In late excitement phase or early plateau, the clitoris shortens and retracts under the clitoral hood. This "disappearance" can be a frustrating experience for a sexual partner. The clitoris, which originally was firm and easily manipulated, has now become hidden and inaccessible. This may require more direct stimulation on the clitoris, rather than the indirect stimulation that previously was effective. Because of individual differences, it is important that each woman become aware of her own response pattern and keep her partner informed of the kind of stimulation she prefers at the moment.

Male Sexual Response

Excitement Phase. The physiologic changes during the male response, as in the female response, result from vasocongestion and muscular tension. The male's first

---

† This term is used by Masters and Johnson to denote noncoital sexual or sensual stimulation, e.g. through oral or manual contact.

response to effective stimulation is usually erection of the penis. However, secretion of pre-ejaculatory fluid from Cowper's gland can precede or occur simultaneously with erection. This response may occur with very minimal stimulation or may occur only after prolonged stimulation. With stimulation, the scrotum tenses and thickens as the dartos muscle contracts, and the testes elevate because of shortening of the spermatic cord.

Plateau Phase. The penis increases in diameter with increasing vasocongestion. Accompanying these changes is a deepening in color of the penis, especially around the coronal ridge, an analogue to the color change in the labia minora. The scrotum and testes remain elevated, as in the excitement stage. Full testicular elevation and further deepening in color herald orgasm.

Orgasm Phase. During orgasm, rhythmic contractions of the penile urethra and seminal vesicles create pressure which releases seminal fluid. The contractions occur at intervals of 0.8 seconds, as is true of the orgasmic platform in the female. The scrotum and testes remain as in plateau stage.

Resolution Phase. Resolution occurs in two stages. Within a few moments after ejaculation, 50% of the engorgement disappears. The remaining involution may take an extended period of time. The scrotum returns to its pre-excitement stage, with the scrotal folds returning to their previous pattern. For some men this is a rapid return, for others more prolonged.

The testes also have an individualized response. The testes may rapidly or more slowly return to their position in the scrotum.

Sexuality and Aging

The effect of aging on sexuality is becoming an increasingly important area of study. More and more women are expressing concerns about how they will function sexually after the menopause. Of course, each woman is unique and each will respond differently to the changes that occur with the aging process. In general, however, Masters and Johnson observed certain physiologic and behavioral changes that frequently occur for both men and women following the male climacteric and the female menopause.

The following commonly occur in women after menopause.

Excitement Phase. The vaginal response to sexual stimulation is similar in postmenopausal women and younger women. The major difference is the degree of vasocogestion. After menopause, vaginal lubrication is reduced in amount and more time is required for its production. The vaginal barrel lengthens and broadens, but to a much lesser degree.

Uterine elevation occurs but is not so marked. There is no vasocongestive uterine enlargement.

The labia majora in older women do not elevate and separate. The labia minora similarly do not engorge as much as in younger women; color changes are also less marked.

Plateau Phase. With age the vaginal barrel is slower to expand. Expansion may occur during the plateau, rather than excitement phases. The orgasmic platform forms, but to a lesser degree.

The uterus, cervix, labia majora, and labia minora remain the same as in the excitement phase.

Orgasm Phase. All the physiologic changes that occur in younger women occur in postmenopausal women. However, there are fewer orgasmic contractions and, hence, the duration of orgasm is less. The uterus maintains its contractions during orgasm.

Resolution Phase. The vaginal barrel returns more rapidly to pre-excitement levels, probably because of decreased elasticity of the vaginal tissues. Similarly, the rest of the pelvic organs return to the preorgasmic state.

The Aging Male. As part of counseling a woman or a couple, it is useful to have an understanding of the changes that commonly occur in men as they age. Many women are concerned about the sexual changes in their partners. In counseling middle-aged couples about their sexuality, it is important to acquaint them with the changes that commonly occur with aging.

The major difference in physiologic response for the older man is the duration of the four phases of the sexual response cycle. Erections which previously occurred in as little as 3 to 5 seconds now may take two to three times as long to achieve. It is not until just prior to ejaculation that the penis is fully erect. Erections can be maintained for prolonged periods without ejaculation. After an ejaculation, the refractory period for erection may be 24 hours or more. A major change in ejaculation is a reduction in the distance the ejaculate can be expelled. For many men, the ejaculate dribbles from the urethra.

In older men, as in older women, the resolution phase becomes more rapid.

As men become older, their sex drive and their interest in frequent sexual contact may decrease. However, Masters and Johnson emphasize that men (and women) who enjoy frequent sexual activity and have a compatible partner may maintain sexual activity into advanced age.

Clinical Suggestions. *Dyspareunia.* Dyspareunia frequently occurs with intercourse and can last for several hours. It is often accompanied by dysuria and urethral irritation. Postmenopausal hormone replacement and local application of estrogen creams in the vagina decrease discomfort. Unfortunately, for many aging women, orgasm can produce painful contractions of the uterus. Usually, this pain also responds to hormone replacement.

Insufficient lubrication can cause dyspareunia. More prolonged stimulation prior to coitus may increase the amount of lubrication and reduce the discomfort of early penile insertion.

Sexual Frequency. After menopause a woman may decrease her sexual contact; as a result, when she does have intercourse, her tissues are less responsive and coitus may produce discomfort rather than pleasure. The more frequent the sexual contact, the more completely and easily can the tissues respond. For women who enjoy masturbation, continuing regular masturbation may help preserve their sexual pleasure with intercourse.

Change in Sexual Pattern. Many postmenopausal women undergo changes in their sexual drive. With fear of pregnancy removed and reduced demands from family etc., many women find that their sexual drive increases. Kinsey reported that women who have active sexual lives prior to menopause continue to do so after menopause. As many women's sexual drive increases, their partners may be experiencing declining drive. In such cases the woman would enjoy having more frequent sexual contact while her partner is experiencing the opposite. Furthermore, many older women do not have regular partners and they may choose not to have any further sexual contact. At this time, some women may resume masturbating, something they have not done since childhood. Others may find the idea of masturbation disgusting or unnatural. Discussing masturbation with older single women may give some permission to experiment with self pleasuring.

IDENTIFICATION OF SEXUAL PROBLEMS AND DYSFUNCTIONS

By way of definition, a sexual problem exists when a patient complains about her sexual functioning or relationship. The problem can be labeled a dysfunction when there are disruptions of the response cycle. Before deciding whether or not to counsel the patient, the physician will need to make some determination of the nature and complexity of the complaint.

Sex History

As with all other problems, the identification of a sexual problem requires adequate history taking. The sex history can be taken as part of a general medical history. It can be done verbally or in written form. Any sex history should be thorough and aimed at identifying sexual dysfunctions or sexual misinformation. The history should include specific questions and should provide an opportunity for comments and questions from the patient.

Figure 9.1 is a sample sex history form.

For some physicians a written history filled out by the patient privately can be useful and time saving. However, it is essential that the doctor review the history and discuss with the patient any questions she may have, allowing her time for questions of her own. For many women, giving a sex history is a new experience; for some, it is uncomfortable and embarrassing. At this point, it is very important for the physician to acknowledge these feelings and provide reassurance. It is also important for the physician to listen objectively and to avoid responding subjectively or imposing his personal values upon the patient.

The sex history can be used as a point of departure for discussion between patient and physician. It can also provide a basis for the identification of a sexual dysfunction. Whether the information is obtained with a formal sex history or a more informal question and answer session, the material obtained can be useful in learning more about the particular patient and her problems. Problem identification in itself can be of value, even though many women or couples will choose not to have counseling. For many women the changes necessary as part of sex therapy seem too disturbing or difficult to undergo; therefore, they choose not to follow through with counseling. As long as the patient is aware of the options in terms of counseling, then the problem identification has been of value.

Sex History

Early Sex Information
  Sources:
      Family_____
      Friends_____
      School_____
      Books_____
      Other_____
  When did you first have an understanding of what
      Menstruation is_____
      Sexual intercourse is_____
      Orgasm is_____
      Homosexuality is_____
      Masturbation is_____
Orgasm Pattern
  Do you have orgasms?
      _____No
      _____Yes, regularly (more than 50% of time)
      _____Yes, rarely (less than 50% of time)
  If yes, method:
      _____With manual stimulation
      _____With vibrator
      _____With partner stimulation
      _____With intercourse only
Masturbation Pattern
  Do you masturbate?
      _____No _____Rarely _____With some regularity
  Method of stimulation
      _____With hand/hands Yes_____ No_____
      _____With vibrator   Yes_____ No_____
      _____With water   Yes_____ No_____
      _____With towel/sheet Yes_____ No_____
      _____Other_____   Yes_____ No_____
Intercourse Pattern
  Frequency:
      _____Three times a week or more
      _____Twice a week
      _____About once a week
      _____About once in two weeks
      _____About once a month
      _____Less than once a month
  Orgasm with intercourse:
      _____Never
      _____10–25%
      _____25–50%
      _____50–75%
      _____75–100%
Partner
      _____Functions satisfactorily
      _____Functions unsatisfactorily
  If unsatisfactory, nature of problem:
      _____Problems with erections
      _____Problems with ejaculations (coming) early
      _____Lack of interest in sex

Fig. 9.1. Sex history

Other _____ _____

Comments, Questions
_____
_____
_____
_____
_____

Fig. 9.1 (*cont.*)

Patient Suitability for Counseling

Identified Sexual Problem. In order for sexual counseling to be a worthwhile venture for both the patient and the counselor, it is important to establish that counseling is likely to meet the needs of the patient or couple.

To be considered suitable for sex counseling, the patient should have an identified sexual problem, e.g. anorgasmia. It is very difficult to provide suitable counseling if the problem is not clearly defined, e.g. "I'm not turned on any more." Before treating such a complaint, the physician would need more details. When a patient can be clear about how she sees her problem and how she wants to change, then counseling can proceed suitably. However, if the problem is ill defined initially, a more detailed assessment may clarify it.

Problem Suitable for Short Term Therapy. In selecting patients for counseling, choose those who you feel could be helped through short term therapy, which usually consists of 5 to 8 sessions. Patients with more involved sexual dysfunction should be referred to outside resources who are set up for long term therapy.

Select patients or couples whose problem seems mainly confined to their sexual functioning. Patients or couples with long term emotional or communication problems are best referred to psychiatrists, psychologists, or family therapists.

Commitment to a Contract with a Counselor. Finally, it is important for the patient or couple to commit themselves to a contract. This contract allows you to set up appointments for a given number of weeks on a designated day. The couple's willingness to set up a contract in advance provides an indication of their level of motivation.

Mechanics of Setting up Counseling

Where to Do Counseling? The counselor should select an area that is quiet and relatively free of interruption. A deliberate attempt should be made to create an atmosphere conducive to patient comfort and relaxation. Being able to face a patient or couple directly without a large desk as a barrier can aid in establishing a relationship more rapidly. The physician may prefer to be dressed in street clothes rather than operating room greens or whites, if that is practical.

When to Do Counseling? When is the most suitable time for doing counseling? The giving of information and reassurance, which is the essence of most counseling, is usually most appropriate at the time the question is raised rather than at a later time. However, if the problem seems sufficiently complex to require a longer session, then a specific time should be set aside. Many physicians are now scheduling half-days in which to do counseling. It is best to set a specific time allotment, such as 15 to 30 minutes, in order that both you and the patient can deal with the problem in a limited period. When the patient knows that her time with you is limited, she is more likely to organize her ideas and priorities and move directly to her concerns.

Who Does Counseling? There are several possible options in terms of who does the actual counseling. Once a suitable patient or couple indicates an interest in counseling, the appropriate counselor should be selected. The counselor can be the physician or one of the paramedical persons in his office, such as a nurse or a nurse practitioner. Many nursing education programs are beginning to provide formal instruction in sexual health. If she is not already trained, your nurse can receive basic training that will enable her to do certain limited areas of counseling. She can be trained by you or can take continuing education courses. For example, the nurse or nurse practitioner may be able to provide excellent guidance for the adolescents in your practice. She may also be available to discuss sexuality during specific prenatal visits. Many nurses are already doing routine prenatal visits in many practices. It would be entirely appropriate for the nurse to discuss changes in sexual patterns during pregnancy as part of a routine visit. However, it is important that the nurse be comfortable with the subject and able to avoid projecting her biases upon the patient if she is to be an effective counselor.

In many cases, if a problem is complex or would involve long term therapy, referral to a sex-counseling unit or private sex therapist would be preferable. The number of clinics, private psychologists, or psychiatrists who do sex counseling is increasing; therefore, it pays to check out local resources.

In some places physicians, especially in group settings, have a psychologist associated with their practice, on a full time or part time basis, depending on the volume of referrals.

All these options are readily workable. Again, the most important consideration is that the patients be comfortable with their counselor and, conversely, that the counselor be comfortable dealing with the patients.

What Are the Qualities of a Good Counselor?

Any person doing counseling must be informative, factual, and familiar with recent work on sexuality. The counselor should have access to clear, descriptive references and reading materials. It is equally important for the counselor to be nonjudgmental. A counselor must be able to deal calmly with various sexual lifestyles. To do this, he should be comfortable with his own sexuality and should be able to understand other lifestyles and accept them for what they are. A good counselor must be flexible in his approach to patients and their problems.

Despite the fact that 50% of married women have sexual problems, many physicians indicate that their patients do not report any sexual problems. This apparent reticence on the part of the patient is probably due to a traditional reluctance to discuss intimate sexual details as well as to the former unavailability of professional help for sexual problems. Of course, it is difficult for a woman to initiate any discussion about sex unless she can trust her physician to be accepting and receptive to discussing sexuality.

Are You Receptive? In order to assess your level of receptiveness to discussing sex with patients, you might ask yourself the following questions:

1. Do you have reading or educational material on sexuality in your waiting room, along with other health care materials?

2. Is a sex history or sex questionnaire a part of your general history taking?

3. If you do have a sex history taken, is it done by a nurse or secretary in the center of a busy office?

4. When sex is being discussed, what form of language is used? Do you use terms used by the patient, or do you hide behind technical or anatomical names?

5. When discussing sexuality or a sexual problem, what is your manner? Are you relaxed, attentive? Do you overreact? Are you in a hurry? Do you acknowledge that you have heard and understood? Do you remember you have to make a phone call? Are you too quick to reassure? Are you hanging on the doorknob trying to leave?

6. During counseling, is the patient comfortable? Is she dressed, or clinging to a gown? Are you on the same eye level? Are you hiding behind a desk piled with dictation, journals, and a statue inscribed "Best Lover, from the nurses of 4th floor Gyn"?

7. How correct is your information? When did you last read Kinsey, or Masters and Johnson? Or is your sexual information from *Playboy* and *Penthouse?*

8. Is your concept of women's sexuality relevant to the times? Is it relevant to the various lifestyles and attitudes of the women who seek counseling or information? Does it acknowledge the wide range of variations that occur among women? Do you recognize that sexual functioning is related to other aspects of a woman's life?

9. What is your usual response to "I'm no longer interested in sex, doctor"? Do you reassure the patient? Relate it to a previous problem, e.g. surgery, problems with birth control pills, infection, etc? Suggest that she grin and bear it? Prescribe a romantic weekend in the mountains with her partner? Take a sex history?

10. Do you discuss changes in sexuality during pregnancy—changes in sex drive, alternate positions for intercourse, and alternates to intercourse?

11. Do you discuss changes in sexuality with aging? Do you give practical suggestions to enhance sexual pleasure in older women?

12. Do you routinely discuss sexuality with adolescents? Do they know that they can discuss sexuality with you, now or later, if they have questions? Do you provide information about birth control without discussing how the adolescent feels about being sexual? Do you avoid imposing your values?

NATURE AND MANAGEMENT OF COMMON PROBLEMS

In general, the common sexual problems seen in office practice can be organized in four areas: problems requiring validation, education, and reassurance, problems involving sexual dysfunction in the female partner, problems involving sexual dysfunction in the male partner, and problems involving sexual dysfunction in both partners.

Problems Requiring Validation, Education, and Reassurance

General Information. Many women have unrealistic expectations of how they should perform sexually. Often their partners suggest they are abnormal. One of the most common areas of misinformation is that of orgasm with intercourse. Most women and their partners are not aware that only 35 to 40% of women regularly reach orgasm with intercourse alone. This leads to the complaint that the male does not last long enough for her to have an orgasm. Some women may have exceptionally high thresholds for orgasm during intercourse, although no definitive research has been done on this question. Others simply do not receive much effective stimulation during intercourse.

Another common myth is that women are not sexual. This stereotype implies that they do not masturbate, they do not initiate sex, and they do not have sexual fantasies. Many women with strong sexual urges will seek medical advice, feeling that their sex drive is abnormal.

Women can approach sex with very limited information. Often a woman has been guided by a partner whose own fund of information is scanty or distorted. She may be very concerned about the normality of what she is doing and how she is doing it. This concern gives rise to such questions as, How often is it normal to have intercourse? How quickly should I be aroused? What are the normal positions for intercourse? Is it okay not to want to have sex every time my partner asks?

This type of question can usually be answered by emphasizing the individuality of sexual response. Since many women do not discuss sexuality with family or friends, they have no concept of the wide range of sexual behavior. It is important to point out that the oft-quoted averages are statistical concepts composed of a range of people differing widely in behavior.

Postpartum or Postoperative Information. After surgery or during pregnancy, many new questions are raised. In general, women who have had surgery are concerned about when they can safely resume intercourse. This is also true of most postpartum women. In general, it is best to individualize for each woman that which suits her best. This provides an excellent opportunity to discuss alternates to intercourse, such as oral sex and mutual sex play. The physician may sometimes encounter women who would like to use an illness or operation as an excuse for discontinuing an unsatisfying sexual relationship. Such women may be willing to consider counseling as an option, once they learn that it is available.

Some women are concerned that after hysterectomy they will no longer have orgasms, they will no longer be able to lubricate, or they will lose sexual desire. Providing these women with an accurate explanation of the typical sexual response cycle will demonstrate their continued ability to respond as before, including having orgasms.

Adolescent Information. A special effort should be made to provide education and information to adolescents and young women. Many young women in their early teens regard sex and sexuality as mysterious areas. Their information is often inaccurate and unreliable. Their fund of information garnered from friends or from popular magazines for men and women is often incomplete or erroneous. Teenagers should be permitted to enjoy and express their sexuality, in the sense that sexuality means taking pride in their bodies, in the way they look and feel. For many young women, this means becoming familiar with their bodies and starting to enjoy them. Teenagers receive strong messages about sex, mostly from parents who have some discomfort in discussing sex with their daughters. What information they provide is often negative or repressive, giving little support for young women to feel accepting of their bodies and their sexuality. For many girls, sex is equated with pregnancy, birth control, and V.D. That sex can produce pleasure is rarely a part of the information they receive.

Two of the most common messages given to young women are, "Sex is dirty" and "Save it for someone you love." Putting these two phrases together yields a very confusing message.

Fed on misinformation, young women do not have accurate knowledge of their sexuality. They require specific detailed information about anatomy and physiology, about sexual practices, and about the individuality of sexual responses. It is important for the young woman to know that she has the option not to be sexual, if that is her preference. An important area to discuss is the woman's expectations, her ideas of what being sexual means. Many young women have stereotyped ideas of what being sexual involves. They expect to be sexual in the same way as the women they read about in *Playboy* or *The Happy Hooker*. Others are convinced that there is a correct or proper way for them to behave sexually. They should be seductive but not easy, or they should be flirtatious but not aggressive.

Young women need to be told that their sexuality is unique. They do not have to fit into specific sexual roles. Instead they can allow their personal feelings, values, and honest good sense to guide them.

Incredibly, many young women have never looked at their genital area. In such cases, validation and education can be supplemented by a third level of counseling: suggestion. The physician can suggest a specific procedure. He can encourage a woman to touch and look at all parts of her body. During the physical examination he can hand her a mirror so that she can become familiar with the different parts of her genitals: the external genitalia, the vagina, and the cervix. He might suggest self-examination of the vulva at home using a mirror. Giving permission to look at and touch the genitals by suggesting a self-examination may be very helpful to a young woman in terms of her self-awareness and self-acceptance. This may help to balance the many negative messages transmitted to young women about their bodies, as typified by commercials for feminine hygiene sprays, douches, or padded bras.

Among the good reading material available for young women who are interested in learning more about themselves are such books as *Our Bodies Ourselves* and *The Sex Handbook*.

Throughout this chapter, it is emphasized that the first three levels of counseling, validation, education, and suggestion, may often suffice for problems encountered in office practice. However, therapy requiring more complex and more sustained intervention should be undertaken when the other approaches do not produce the desired change.

Problems Involving Sexual Dysfunction in the Female

Primary Anorgasmia. According to Kinsey, 23% of all women age 25 have *rarely or never* experienced an orgasm. These women are categorized as presenting primary anorgasmia. For the purposes of counseling, women who cannot masturbate to orgasm with their hands but can *only* reach orgasm through streams of water, rubbing against objects, or using a vibrator are included in the primary group. Many women expect orgasm to occur "naturally," that is, without clitoral stimulation. They expect the stimulation of intercourse to produce orgasms. A woman may be convinced she is anorgasmic because her clitoris is in the wrong place or because it is too small. Or she may blame her partner: his penis is not large enough or it is too large.

Unless there are strong emotional blocks preventing change, the majority of these women will learn to have orgasms when they have been given permission to explore and touch their bodies. For women who have never masturbated or for women who are uncomfortable looking at or touching their bodies, suggest a homework assignment called the Bath/Mirror.

Bath/Mirror. Ask the woman to take a bath. The purpose of the bath is not to get clean, but rather an opportunity to get to know more of her body. Suggest using oils, scents, or bubble bath to make the bath more pleasant. Ask her to bathe without a washcloth so that she is touching her body at all times with her hands. As she explores her body with her hands she is to find out what parts of her body she likes and what parts she dislikes. Emphasize the importance of touching all parts of her body and the use of different types of touch such as soft strokes, hard strokes, long and circular strokes.

Following the bath she is to towel herself dry, again experimenting with different touches. In front of a full length mirror, the woman is to examine her body. After looking, she is then to touch all parts and different areas to find out what kinds of touches she likes and dislikes. The whole bath/mirror exercise should take 1 hour, with the majority of the time in front of the mirror.

Some women may need or want to repeat this exercise several times, learning more each time.

When the woman has done the bath/mirror assignment, she can then do a genital examination on a separate occasion.

Genital Self-examination. This should be done with a hand mirror and a picture of the external genitals, such as the one provided in the *Yes Book: Female Masturbation* of the National Sex Forum. The purpose of the exam is for a woman to begin to explore her genitals. This may be the first time she has been told that it is okay to touch and look at her genitals. Despite having delivered children and inserted tampons, etc., many women have never looked at themselves; they may feel that their genitals are dirty and untouchable. As part of the assignment, ask the woman to find out what she likes or dislikes in terms of looks and touch.

While the woman is doing the genital exam, she can practice her Kegel exercises.

Kegel Exercises. (As adapted from the Sex Advisory Counseling Unit.) The original purpose for which the late Dr. Arnold Kegel prescribed these exercises was to improve control of urination. The exercises are designed to identify and strengthen the pubococcygeus (PC) muscle, which runs from the pubic bone in the front to the coccyx in the back and surrounds the urinary, vaginal, and rectal openings. Kegel found that many women who practiced the exercises reported increased sexual awareness in the genital area and increased sexual responsiveness.

Identifying the PC muscle: Ask the woman to sit on the toilet with legs spread apart and start the urinary stream. She should then attempt to stop and start the stream. The muscle that does this is the PC.

Exercises: Slow—tighten the PC muscle and hold it for a slow count of three, then relax. Quick—tighten and relax the PC as rapidly as possible in bursts of ten contractions. Pull-in/Push-out—Pull in the entire pelvic floor as though trying to suck water into the vagina, then push out the water. (This will require use of the abdominal muscles.) The woman should practice these exercises at intervals throughout the day with whatever frequency is comfortable and practical. They can be done while driving, sitting in a chair, or standing.

Masturbation Homework. The masturbation or self-pleasuring should take 1 hour. Many women like to do the bath and mirror exercise prior to doing this homework. Suggest using a mild massage oil to reduce friction and increase sensation. Once the woman has found a comfortable relaxed place to masturbate, then, using the oil, she should slowly start touching various areas of her entire body and of her genitals. Often using the hand mirror during genital stimulation provides reassurance about where she is touching. The exercise is designed to allow women to start masturbating; many women who would never consider masturbation will start pleasuring themselves because of the permission inherent in having the exercise assigned by a doctor.

During the first few masturbation sessions, many women experience very little pleasure. It is important to reassure these women that, like many other exercises, masturbation takes practice. If they do experience some pleasurable feelings, then instruct them to focus on these feelings, no matter how small the feelings may be.

Once a woman is masturbating regularly and experiencing pleasure, suggest that she masturbate to a peak of pleasure and then interrupt stimulation. In a few seconds, she is to resume stimulation and build to a second and then a third peak of pleasurable sensation, stopping short of orgasm. It is reassuring to many women that they can stop stimulating themselves and then resume without losing all pleasurable feelings. Many women are convinced that any interruption of stimulation during masturbation or intercourse will destroy any chance they have for achieving orgasm.

This technique of teasing is valuable for women who feel their orgasms are too weak. Prolonging stimulation often results in a more intense orgasm.

Many women report that fantasizing during masturbation enables them to reach orgasm. Any fantasy that a woman finds stimulating is acceptable. Many women feel guilty about their fantasies because they involve other women, animals, rape, etc. It is important to reassure women that fantasy is a separate and legitimate element of experience. They should be told that fantasies are syntheses of things they have read, heard, or imagined. They are not signs of emotional disturbance, symbolic infidelity, or precursors of deviant behavior. *My Secret Garden* by Nancy Friday is a collection of fantasies that includes many different types of fantasies and shows the broad range that women experience.

Many women enjoy reading pornographic books as they masturbate. There are many erotic books available, such as *The Pearl* and *The Story of O*. It is helpful for each woman to find a book or part of a book that she enjoys for herself.

Table 9.1 is a schematic representation of the program followed at the Sex Advisory and Counseling Unit for the treatment of primary anorgasmia in women. This approach is based on the work of Lonnie Barbach, and is described in detail in her book *For Yourself*.

TABLE 9.1
Program for Treatment of Primary Anorgasmia

Session	Content	Homework
Session I		
What are her goals?	What is it like not to have an	Bath/Mirror
What are her chances of	orgasm?	Buy body oil
success?	How does she handle not having	Kegel exercises
What is the worst thing that	an orgasm?	*Our Bodies Ourselves*
could happen if she does		Orgams with intercourse
not have an orgasm?		temporarily prohibited
Session II		
Specific report on homework	Anatomy and physiology	Genital self-examination
(deal with reaction from	Sexual response cycle	*Yes Book: Masturbation*
women, e.g. anger)		Communication exercise
Session III		
Specific report on homework	Masturbation myths, e.g. causes	Masturbation with no orgasm
	insanity, is for lesbians or	Focus on feelings
	nymphomaniacs	
	Fear of orgasm, e.g. too	
	intense, painful, loss of	
	bowel, bladder, or emotional	
	control.	
	Reaching Orgasm	
	(masturbation film)	
Session IV		
Specific report on homework—	First orgasm—celebrate, confirm	Masturbation for one hour
feelings, sensations,	How she got orgasm	Erotic literature
Where, when, how		Teasing to 3 peaks
Why did you stop?		Yes/No
Emphasis on small feelings		
Session VI		
Specific report on homework—	Fantasy discussions	Masturbate in position of
find out expectations of	Exaggeration of responses	intercourse
orgasm	during masturbation	Repeat earlier homework
		Individual homework, e.g. shorter
		times for women who are
		frightened
Sessions VI to X		
Specific report on homework	Discussion of resistances, e.g.	Partner homework
	"I'll never have an orgasm"	Masturbation with partner
		present
		Pleasuring for one hour with
		no intercourse
		Man pleasuring woman during
		intercourse

The schematic account of the program is useful as an outline of the areas that often must be dealt with. This approach may not be consistently successful in a one-to-one counseling situation. When it is used with groups of women led by women counselors, the support generated by the group helps produce a high rate of success. In busy practices, it might be feasible for female counselors in the office to receive training to equip them to run periodic groups.

The experience of groups has provided a great deal of information about women's sexuality. It is common for a woman to enter sex counseling because her partner is pressuring her to get her sexual problem cured. Many fear they will lose their partners if they do not prove their sexual responsiveness by having orgasms. Many feel they are physically or emotionally abnormal. There is usually no need to explain to a woman why she is not having orgasms. The reassurance that she is like many other women and that, like the majority of women, she can have orgasms is usually explanation enough.

When assigning sexual homework, emphasize the importance of doing the homework regularly. Homework is usually the major portion of counseling nonorgasmic women. The basic concept of all the homework assigned is that the woman find 1 hour a day for herself. This hour must be private, uninterrupted, and quiet.

In reviewing homework, the report must be specific. It is important for the woman to find out specifically what she liked and what she did not like. For some women, doing homework such as bath and mirror work is the first time they really look at their bodies. Many have taken quick, critical glances in the past, comparing themselves to fashion models. It is a surprise to many that their bodies have many textures and contours. For some women, the exercises merely reinforce the negative image they have of themselves. Whatever experience they have is valid. No attempt should be made to alter a woman's interpretation of what she experienced. But she may be asked to look again and be aware of any change in response.

For some women, the idea of looking or touching their bodies has many negative aspects. They may question your reasons for suggesting such homework. The best response is not to dispute their feelings but to accept them. You can agree that the homework may be distasteful or boring but emphasize that it is nonetheless necessary, if they want to have orgasms. When women start with low expectations about the assignments, it is easier to avoid disappointments. Telling them that they will enjoy the exercises may have the opposite effect.

Many women in the women's groups initially were unable to set aside time and space for themselves. This inability appeared to be a common problem among the women who were unable to assert themselves with their partners. Two specific nonsexual exercises were helpful. The first is called Yes/No exercises. A Yes is doing or saying Yes to something one would normally say no to, for example, buying an extravagent item. A No is saying No to something one would normally say yes to, for example, intercourse.

The second exercise is a communication exercise to be done with a partner. One person in the couple is the speaker and the other the listener. Both must agree to the length of speech, e.g. 2 or 5 minutes, and the time to do the speech. The speaker discusses his/her feelings. The listener is not permitted to discuss or interrupt the speaker. Following this exercise, the speaker and listener reverse roles.

As part of a woman's counseling, it is important to help her deal with her partner's reaction. Many a man is curious or distrustful about what may be happening to his partner. It may be helpful to find out how much information the woman intends to share with her partner. She may want to share all or none of her homework with him. Any combination is all right. If she chooses to share, you may suggest using a positive approach such as, "I'm learning more about myself, to share with you."

Secondary Anorgasmia. The term secondary anorgasmia describes women who have orgasms by some means and who would like to increase their range of orgasm potential. For most women, the term denotes that they are orgasmic through masturbation and are hoping to start having orgasms with intercourse. However, a woman may be orgasmic through intercourse and want to learn to reach orgasm through masturbation or oral stimulation. What is important is that she is seeking alternate means of reaching orgasm. Before any woman starts a program for secondary anorgasmia, she should be aware that a large proportion of women do not regularly have orgasms during intercourse, especially if penile thrusting is the only mode of stimulation. The program will probably enable them to have orgasms during intercourse, but this may include clitoral manipulation simultaneous with penile thrusting. Again, applying this approach in the context of women's groups is likely to improve chances for success.

Session I. This session allows you to get to know the woman and to discover her expectations. It is important to restate to her that there is no way to determine at this time whether she will ever have orgasm during intercourse with penile thrusting alone or ever experience orgasm during intercourse. Nonetheless, many women can widen their abilities to have orgasm and find pleasure in other forms of sexual play.

Homework Assignment: Bath/Mirror. This is the same exercise that is assigned for primary anorgasmia. It is designed to provide the woman with a positive body experience. Many perfectly normal women see themselves as deficient or abnormal. When woman examine their bodies and reassure themselves that they are in fact normal, they often become more comfortable in sharing their body with a sexual partner. In addition to doing the general body examination, the woman should also include a genital examination, using the diagram in the *Yes Book of Female Masturbation* as an aid in identifying the different parts of the genitals.

Masturbation. At first, the woman should masturbate in her usual manner for a full hour with her hands. During the hour, the woman can stimulate herself to a high level, then decrease stimulation. She should repeat this exercise of building and then reducing stimulation two or three more times each hour. This procedure will require longer than usual masturbation time and may also increase the intensity of the orgasm. If the woman has a sexual partner, she might want to consider telling him that she is masturbating. Often a woman may be apprehensive about letting her partner know that she masturbates. However, many partners respond positively to the information. Some men may initially respond negatively but may become more accepting of the idea later. Many men find the information arousing. It rests with each individual woman to decide whether to inform her partner and to select the most appropriate way of doing so.

Communication Exercise. This exercise is designed to help improve the communication pattern between partners. This first step is to establish a time for the exercise and how long it will last. The speaker and listener must negotiate a time and duration that suits them both. The speaker should select a short duration, usually 2 or 5 minutes is ample. The listener is in charge of making sure the speaker stops at the correct time. The speaker should talk about a topic that is important to her or him. The topic should deal with how the speaker feels; the exercise should not be used to debate the merits of a political candidate. One further idea is that the speaker should keep to one topic.

During the talk, the listener listens. He has no right to argue or rebut.

Following the talk, the speaker thanks the listener for listening, and the listener thanks the speaker for sharing his or her feelings. This small formality helps to end the exercise on a friendly basis.

The entire purpose of this type of formalized ritual is to help improve the listening abilities of both partners. The speaker has to learn to be specific and keep to one topic. The listener has to learn to listen and not interrupt.

After the speaker has finished, the listener should be given an opportunity to speak at a later date. It is important to separate the speeches by at least 30 minutes to an hour. This separation helps prevent the beginning of an ongoing argument.

Suggestions for topics are numerous but might include how the woman feels about having counseling. The husband in turn may want to share some of his feelings about his wife masturbating. For many men, sharing feeling is difficult but with the aid of a formalized ritual, many men do become more comfortable.

Session II: Homework Report. Request a specific report on the bath and mirror exercise. Find out what areas of her body she likes and what areas she dislikes. What is her general impression of her body: What does she think her partner thinks about her body?

In a similar manner, have her describe her reaction to looking at her genitals. Although many of these women have masturbated for years, they have done so quickly, without ever looking. It is as important to them to have complete knowledge and self-awareness as it is to the primary women. Many women consider the genitals disgusting or unpleasant. Because of their disappointment in not having orgasms, these women may have come to feel that their bodies are defective. The woman may feel that her clitoris is too small or too far away from her vagina.

Get information about her typical masturbation. Does she masturbate on her back or on her stomach? Does she use one or two hands? How long does it take her to reach an orgasm? Many women have very rigid, almost ritualistic patterns for masturbating. In general, the aim of homework is to broaden her ability to masturbate in different positions so that she can incorporate her masturbation into sexual play with a partner, if her goal is to become more responsive during sex with him.

Was she able to do the communication exercises? Did she feel that her partner heard her? Were they both able to be quiet listeners? The information obtained from this exercise is often very revealing. Couples discover during the exercise how poorly or ineffectively they communicate and learn ways of dissolving resentments and misunderstandings that prevent intimacy and trust.

Homework Assignment: Sexologic. With her partner present, the women identifies the various parts of her genital area. The purpose of the sexological examination is to make both partners comfortable with looking at, touching, and talking about one another's genitals. After both partners are familiar with the different parts of the woman's genitals, they can then begin to experiment with different types of touching. The woman can begin to tell her partner the different types of touching she enjoys. After the couple has practiced examining and touching the woman partner, they can then trade places so that the man can receive the examination.

Masturbation. In this session, the woman begins to learn new positions for masturbating. Many women have rigid patterns for self-stimulation; they may feel that they cannot have orgasms unless they do exactly the same things each time.

Attachment to a sequence of conditioned responses inhibits orgasm during coitus, because the coital position often differs from the preferred positions used in masturbation. To break away from these patterns, they should practice masturbating in positions that are similar to their positions for intercourse. The masturbation should be practiced daily for at least an hour. If the woman becomes fatigued, she can pause and resume. Again, a lubricant is advisable to prevent irritation.

Session III: Homework Report. The woman should briefly discuss her reaction to doing the sexologic assignment. What feelings did she experience while showing her genitals to her partner? How did he feel about looking at and touching her? Did they become more comfortable after repeating the sexologic assignment?

Find out whether she has learned to reach orgasm in some new positions.

Homework: Masturbation. This exercise requires the woman to stimulate her genitals with her hands while having intercourse. The woman may feel very uneasy about masturbating with her partner aware of what she is doing. If so, she may want to start by just touching her genital area during intercourse. With more practice and confidence, the woman can then add more sustained and intense stroking.

The primary purpose of this masturbation exercise is not to have an orgasm but to develop comfort with masturbation. The woman should be told not to strive for orgasm but rather to find ways of intensifying her enjoyment.

Communication Exercise. Following the model of the communication exercise in Session I, one member of the couple should become the speaker, and the couple should agree on a time and a length for the talk. The speaker should then talk about what he/she likes and dislikes about the partner. In doing the exercise for the first time, the speaker should state only one like and one dislike. A like is an appreciation of something the partner does that pleases the speaker. A dislike is something that displeases or hurts the speaker.

Sharing likes and dislikes gives a couple the opportunity to talk about areas of their lives that they usually avoid. Sharing a dislike during a communication exercise is a safe way of telling a partner about a problem. Similarly, sharing an appreciation with a partner can help reinforce the positive changes that are occurring. These basic communication exercises teach skills that can help to resolve or prevent pent-up feelings and misunderstandings. Positive feelings and trust between the partners are often prerequisites to the intimacy that enables partners to relax and respond to one another sexually.

Session IV: Homework Report. Review how the woman is masturbating, in which positions, and how comfortable she is in sharing her masturbation with her partner. Find out how the communication exercises are progressing.

Homework: Masturbation. At first, ask the woman to arrange with her sexual partner to masturbate in his presence. For many women, this is a new experience. Many are very uncomfortable with the knowledge that they can have orgasms by themselves but not with their partners. Many women have never told their partners that they masturbate. They are concerned that their husbands will feel that they are poor sexual partners. Sharing the information that they masturbate, that they are sexual without a partner is a very large step for many to take.

Once women are comfortable with having told their partner, they are then to start doing a 1-hour masturbation exercise with the partner as near to them physically as possible. In some instances, the partner may have to start quite far away, perhaps out of the house. However, he will probably be able to move fairly quickly to a closer position in the bedroom. Having the partner in the room, even well across the room, is a very important step for a woman to take and a sign of increasing comfort.

New Positions. When the woman can masturbate with her partner present, she can try different positions for intercourse. These new positions should be ones in which she or her partner can stimulate the clitoris.

Session V. During this session, find out how all the homework has been going. If a woman is having problems with earlier homework, have her repeat these exercises. Many of the exercises require repeated practice and experimentation.

After the woman has been seen for five sessions, it may be useful to space out any further visits so that she can have additional time to practice the various exercises.

By this time, most women are having orgasms with stimulation of the clitoral region during intercourse. Many women find this new ability exciting, and their determination to have an orgasm without stimulating their clitoral area diminishes. At this point, many women report that their approach to intercourse has become more positive. They enjoy sex more and feel more confident in their ability to experience pleasure.

Vaginismus. Vaginismus is not one of the more common sexual dysfunctions, although one does encounter it in practice. A woman with vaginismus may experience sexual interest and arousal but will find intercourse painful and impossible, even with a gentle, patient partner, because involuntary contractions of the PC muscle prevent penile penetration. The partner of a woman with vaginismus should always be included in counseling. For many couples, simply to reassure them that their problem is not unique and can be reversed goes a long way toward solving the problem itself.

Session I. After the problem has been assessed in an office visit, arrange to see the couple together. During this session, a brief pelvic examination should be done with the husband present. The purpose of the physical examination is to demonstrate to both partners how the contractions of the PC muscle obstruct entry. For the husband, this will provide physical proof that his partner has not imagined the problem. In the examination, emphasize the involuntary nature of the contractions and the overall normalcy of the woman's other responses.

Following the examination, with both partners present, explain that the problem can be corrected in a brief time with relative ease. It is usually better to avoid an analytic discussion of the cause of the vaginismus. Although many women have, in fact, had traumatic experiences that have created anxiety about sexual contact, many women have no apparent cause for their problem.

Homework Assignment: Mirror/Bath. Assigning body exploration and examination allows the patient to learn more about her body. For many women, this is an opportunity to become more aware of how they feel about touching and examining their bodies. A woman who has been unable to experience pleasure with her body may have regarded her body as useless. After all, she may have told herself, who has ever heard of a normal woman who could not have sex?

Following the general body and mirror exercises, instruct the woman to do a genital examination, using a hand mirror. After the woman has done her examination privately and has become comfortable with the procedure, she should do the examination with her husband present.

Kegel Exercises. As part of learning more about her body, assigning Kegel exercises allows the woman to become more aware of her vaginal area and of her voluntary control of vaginal muscles. Encourage her to do all types of Kegels, but especially emphasize the pull-in and push-out exercise.

For many women, doing the Kegels can be part of the bath exercise. With practice, women can learn to displace water in and out of the vagina. During the bath, have the woman insert her little finger in the vagina as part of the Kegels. She may be amazed at the strength of muscles in the vagina, muscles she may not have known she possessed.

The Kegels can also be done as part of the genital mirror examination. Seeing the muscles tense and relax helps demonstrate to the patient and her partner the possibility of voluntary control of these muscles.

Dilators. Following the bath and Kegel exercises, the woman can begin inserting vaginal dilators into her vagina. Practicing with dilators of increasing diameter gives the woman an idea of how her partner's penis will feel.

Session II. The homework report should be brief and should emphasize experiences that were new for the couple. The couple may express fairly mixed reactions to their homework, ranging from excitement to disgust. Check to see that the woman is doing her Kegel exercises correctly.

Homework Assignment. Genital pleasuring without intercourse, allows the partners to receive pleasure, one at a time, and allows the partner receiving pleasure to direct the other partner. With the man sitting with his back against the headboard of the bed, his partner sits with her back to him and leans against him. This position allows the male to place his hands on different areas of his partner's body. The female, using both her hands, touches and pleasures her breasts and genitals. When she feels comfortable, she can then place her partner's hands on top of hers. The male simply rests his hands on hers without exerting pressure. In this position, the woman can maintain control of pleasuring while demonstrating to her partner what she enjoys.

Session III. Briefly determine that the homework is being done properly. With no pressure for intercourse, the woman may be able to relax sufficiently to enjoy the pleasuring. A couple may need repeated practice of these kinds of exercises before the man and woman feel competent in touching and pleasuring each other.

Homework Assignment. Pleasuring with Dilators: If the couple are doing well with the previous homework and the woman is learning to use the dilators, then include the dilators as part of the pleasuring. The woman may initially want to insert the dilators with her own hands or have her husband's hands near her genitals but not on the dilators.

Pleasuring variations: in addition, suggest the couple try other positions for pleasuring which are more similar to positions for intercourse.

Session IV. By this session, pleasuring is becoming more natural and more pleasing. The dilator exercises are part of pleasuring, and the couple is pleasuring in positions of intercourse.

Homework Assignment. Assign pleasuring with the dilators. When the woman is tolerating the large dilators, she is ready to insert her partner's penis. For some women, this can be facilitated by using a lubricant. Many women find that if they push their PC muscle out as the penis is being inserted, they are able to allow entry. Once the penis is slowly inserted, there should be a minimum of movement until the woman feels comfortable. If she indicates that she would like more movement, then her partner can slowly initiate shallow thrusting or a gentle rotary motion.

With initial success it is still important that the couple follow the same procedures on successive occasions. Once the woman can enjoy intercourse this way, suggest that she allow her partner to insert his penis. With patience and practice, gradually intercourse can become more spontaneous and varied.

Problems Involving Sexual Dysfunction in the Male

If a woman feels that her partner has a sexual dysfunction and that he alone requires counseling, you may choose to refer the couple to the man's physician. Many women prefer not to beome involved in counseling if their partner is dysfunctional. It may be appropriate to provide the woman with the name of a sex counseling unit or a psychologist who deals with sexual problems.

It is always difficult to form an understanding of a couple's problem if only half the couple is present. If you feel that it would be of value to the couple, you might suggest a short assessment visit to help sort out the problems. It is important to emphasize that sex problems, no matter how defined by one or both marital partners, generally affect both partners. Although she may say, "It's his problem," the problem has consequences for her. Besides, the other partner may be quite unaware of how his or her role in the relationship influenced the onset of the problem or is helping to maintain it. Therefore, it usually makes sense to involve the partner of the identified patient in all or part of the counseling.

Problems Involving Sexual Dysfunction in Both Partners

Masters and Johnson have provided a model for short term couple counseling. The couple meet daily with a male and female cotherapy team for an intensive 2-week program. Although this has provided an excellent model, there are other models more suitable for office practice. Other counseling units see couples on a once-a-week basis, rather than daily. A very practical model for private practice is a single counselor seeing couples on a weekly basis.

When both members of a couple have a sexual dysfunction or when both seem involved in a problem presented by one of them, they should be considered for couple counseling. In order to have a framework for counseling, it is essential to form a contract or an understanding with the couple. The contract should specify the number of sessions you feel will be necessary to deal with the couple's problem. For example, three or four sessions may be appropriate for couples who require mainly education and reassurance, while couples with more involved dysfunctions may require nine or ten sessions or more. The contract should include the length of each session and the fee. In addition to the time the couple sets aside for the actual counseling, they must also be prepared to set aside time for homework assignments—usually 4 hours spread out over each week.

The first session should be used as a time for the counselor to make an assessment of the couple and their problem. During this session, there are several areas that should be explored. The first is identification of the problem. The couple should state how they individually see their problem, when they first believed that a problem existed, and what their specific goals are. In helping make an assessment, it may be of value to have the couple discuss a typical sexual experience in precise detail. This account might include who initiates sex, the kinds and length of precoital stimulation,§ and what happens after intercourse. Does this couple have a fairly rigid pattern of sexual contact, or do they have a more varied sexual lifestyle?

The second area to be explored is the way in which the couple has dealt with their problem. Learning how they have dealt with their problems in the past can provide you with information about the systems that exist in their relationship. Every couple develops their own method or system for dealing with problems. For example, the systems may involve the woman covering up for the husband's dysfunction, or the woman may exaggerate her husband's dysfunction in an effort to camouflage her own.

The third area to explore is whether the problem the couple presents can be helped by sex therapy or whether the problems are better handled by family or marital therapy.

The final area is whether you, as the therapist, can be an effective therapist with this particular couple. A therapist is not equally effective with all couples. Respecting your limitations as a therapist allows you to deal appropriately with all your patients. If, after the assessment visit, you feel that you personally are not the proper therapist for this couple, you can then refer them to other counseling services.

During the first visit, it is important to find out the expectations held by the couple concerning what will happen during therapy. Are their goals unrealistic? Are they prepared for the possibility that their overall relationship may change as their sexual relationship changes? Is one partner anticipating that you, as the therapist, will side with him/her and "fix" his/her partner?

When you have completed your assessment you may want to discuss with the couple two basic relationship concepts defined by Masters and Johnson.

The first, the principle of *vulnerability*, states that intimate relationships are built through sharing weaknesses rather than strengths. In other words, couples can form a firm foundation for trust not merely by showing their strengths but also by disclosing to one another the areas of their personalities about which they have misgivings, and informing one another of their sensitivities. Such disclosure allows them to relax more with one another, rather than living in fear that the other will discover their presumed weaknesses and reject them or inadvertently "step on their sore toe." When partners seek therapy, it is assumed that they are sincere in trying to improve their relationship and will avoid continually trying to undermine one

---

§ The commonly used word "foreplay" connotes that coitus is the "main event" and that noncoital types of sex play are only the means to an end. Many couples do enjoy manual and oral stimulation for its own sake. By not referring to such stimulation as foreplay, but instead by encouraging couples to enjoy all forms of stimulation for what they are, the practitioner may help them to appreciate more aspects of their sexual activity.

another. Therefore, if one person uses a disclosure of vulnerability as a weapon against the other, that person's intent to hurt the other is clear. He/she can no longer say, "I didn't think you were sensitive about that." Instead he/she must acknowledge that the intent was to wound. Typically, when an individual has disclosed some vulnerable area to the other, there is a sense of relief on both parts. More often than not, the disclosure does not come as a surprise to the other partner, and both are relieved to have it out in the open. Partners often learn that it is much less stressful to expose a vulnerable area than to put constant vigilance into guarding it.

The second principle, that of *neutrality*, states that the future need not be an inevitable repetition of the past. For example, just because the male partner has complained when his partner tried to initiate sex in the past, she need not predict that he will not react differently in the future. Failure to believe that change is possible is a self-fulfilling prophecy that negates the effectiveness of therapy. The principle of neutrality allows a couple to wipe the sexual slate clean. The significance of vulnerability and neutrality is that they allow changes to occur in the relationship. Freed of old constraints, couples can begin to experiment and to make changes in old patterns that have not worked for them.

In assigning homework exercises, the physician should anticipate problems, avoid areas of anxiety, and give permission or reassurances. In order to anticipate sexual difficulties that might occur, one needs an understanding of what the couple's basic problems are. For example, if one partner experiences displeasure touching the other's genitals, then assign homework that involves nongenital touching. This approach will allow the partner first to gain confidence in touching nonsexual areas so that he or she will eventually have more confidence in touching genitals.

Assigning homework in a progression from less- to more-anxiety-laden tasks will help couples deal with specific areas of anxiety. By gradually desensitizing the anxiety in each area, the couple can move through the hierarchy of situations that comprise the problem. Finally, assigning sexual homework gives couples permission or reassurance to be sexual. Many couples are fixed in rigid sex roles and patterns. For example, many men are convinced that they must always initiate sex and be aggressive. This emphasis on performance may detract from their sensual experience. Assigning an exercise in which the man is totally passive, the receiver of pleasure, allows the couple to experiment with other sexual styles.

The aim of most homework is to learn to receive pleasure. Many couples are expert at giving pleasure but must learn to receive pleasure. When assigning homework, the instructions should be specific and detailed. Giving the couple specific instructions facilitates the process of learning how to receive pleasure.

The physician can help an inveterate giver (as are many men) to become a good receiver by redefining the concept of giving. For example, if it is the man who is focused only on giving, he can be instructed to stroke and caress his partner and to focus only on what it is like for him to touch her body. He does not attempt to program or evaluate her responses. Instead, if he can allow himself to enjoy the touching of her for its own sake, he can realize that her receptive body is a source of pleasure to him. Her willingness to receive is necessary for his pleasure in touching.

The physician can then ask him whether he would be willing to *receive* touch from his partner in order to give her pleasure. Masters and Johnson call the concept that giving and receiving occur simultaneously *give to get*. Additional exercises to teach this concept are described below.

Although homework is highly individualized and flexible, there is a rationale for assigning it in a general order. The initial homework should be aimed at having each partner become more at ease at looking and touching his or her own body. Such exercises as bathing and mirror work provide opportunity for the couple to look at and feel their own bodies. This may allow the couple to re-examine their ideas about themselves. Once the partners have developed comfort with their own bodies, they can then begin exercises involving touching each other. One good type of touching homework is sensual massage.

The massage homework is assigned so that each partner gives two massages and each receives two massages. The first time the partner gives a massage, he or she gives it with the goal of giving his/her partner a sensual relaxing massage. The second time the massager gives the massage with the goal of receiving pleasure from doing it. Then on a different occasion, the partners switch roles.

In assigning this four step massage for the first time, suggest that each partner select one part of his/her body that he/she would enjoy having massaged. Good areas are the foot, hand, or head. It is often useful to suggest that they alternate giving and receiving massage.

For example, on the first night the woman may choose to give the massage and do it for her partner's benefit. (The word "benefit" is used rather than "pleasure" in order to keep expectations low. If an individual anticipates high pleasure at first, he/she runs the risk of being disappointed.) With her partner giving specific directions, she massages for a limited time period, usually one-half hour. During the massage, the man must direct the caressing so that he receives the preferred kinds of strokes and the right pressure, etc. It is important to tell the couple that the aim of the exercise is sensual pleasure, *not* sexual arousal. If arousal occurs, that is fine; however, it is not the goal. After the massage, the couple should discuss how they each experienced the exercise. On that same occasion or, better, at a later day, the couple should reverse roles so that the man massages the woman for her benefit.

On a separate occasion, the woman massages her partner for her own benefit. This means she uses the kinds of strokes she enjoys. During this exercise, the one being massaged may inform his partner if he is experiencing pain or displeasure; otherwise there is no communication while massaging. After the massage, each partner discusses the massage from his/her point of view. Again, on the same day or a later day, the partners reverse.

When the couple is able to massage one area of the body, using the four steps, they can then include the whole body, briefly touching the genitals in passing but not focusing on them. Using massage oil greatly enhances the pleasuring. If the couple are interested in learning more about massage, *The Massage Book* by George Downing provides an excellent guide.

The massage instructions are very specific and structured in such a way that each partner has to take responsibility for guaranteeing his or her own pleasure. Once each partner develops the ability to be selfish, to look after himself or herself, one of the basics for better sexual functioning has been learned. Being selfish means doing what is needed to get one's own needs met; it does not mean ignoring the expressed wishes or feelings of the other. When communication has been established with massage, then focused genital touching is added to the homework.

Massage oil can be used on the genitals, but it should be unscented and nonirritating. Following this total body massage, if the couple wants to have intercourse, they should refrain from consummating it for a specified time period, usually 1 or 2 hours. Postponing intercourse after body massages encourages the couple to enjoy sensual and sexual pleasuring without pressure for intercourse. Many couples rarely touch or pleasure one another unless they are anticipating intercourse. Often the pleasuring becomes overlooked in an attempt to get to the "real thing." Overlooking noncoital pleasuring, especially for women, decreases their overall enjoyment. Many women are reluctant to ask their partners to pleasure them for fear they will appear too aggressive or they will tire their partners.

There are several positions that can be suggested for genital or full body pleasuring.

Often the woman will enjoy being pleasured with her partner sitting on the bed behind her, with his legs outside hers. In this position, her partner can stimulate her genitals as well as the rest of her upper body, both back and front. If the woman is uneasy about having her partner touch her directly, she can have him place his hands over hers while she pleasures herself.

The man can be pleasured while he lies on his back with his partner seated between his legs and facing toward his upper body. The woman can slide her legs under his, if this is more comfortable. In this position, the women can stimulate her partner's genitals and, if he wishes, his abdomen and chest. When the couple has learned to stimulate genitals effectively, homework designed to deal with specific dysfunction can then be added. Individual homework can be continued in addition to this mutual homework.

Prior to assigning genital touching, it is often of value to spend a session doing a sexological examination. This procedure is an educational examination of one another's genitals by both partners under the guidance of the physician. The purpose of the examination is to teach the partners about their bodies, to increase comfort in viewing the genitals, and to improve feedback between partners about touching. This exercise is always optional. Many couples report that the sexological examination was one of the most significant aspects of therapy.

The sexological examination is not a medical examination intended to discover pathology. Because of the physician's familiarity with the medical model, which requires a methodical, efficient, and definitely nonsexual examination, this procedure usually requires practice on his/her part. The equipment required is an examining table, a pillow, a full length mirror, a hand mirror, and a plastic (see-through) speculum.

During the examination the partners can identify the different parts of the body by name. It is not necessary that they learn the correct anatomic names. Once the identification is done, then one partner should systematically explore the external genitals of the other partner. The exploration should include communicating how to touch with different pressures, in different directions and strokes. Suggest that the partner try touching with one or two fingers on small areas, experimenting with different touches. Often comparing one side to the other demonstrates differences in sensation. Many couples report that using oil increases the sensations. During the exploration, determine which areas are pleasurable and which experience discomfort.

Each time the couple repeats the sexological, they will discover new areas of pleasure, different techniques and improved methods of communicating likes or dislikes.

Method. Ask the partners to decide which one will volunteer to go first. For example, if the woman goes first, she should be asked whether she wants her partner and you present while she undresses. Position the woman comfortably on the examining table so she is sitting up and able to see her pelvic area in the full length mirror. Her partner should be positioned either sitting or standing at the foot of the examining table. The physician should be at the side to provide directions.

Allow the male to do the anatomical identifications with help as needed from you or his partner. The partner should then start carefully exploring the genitals. The physician can provide suggestions on different touches and techniques. Pay attention to how well the woman is able to direct her partner to touch her in ways that she likes. It is best to encourage direct verbal communications, so that misunderstanding is kept to a minimum.

Following the external examination, the physician should insert the speculum, allowing both partners a clear view of the vaginal mucosa and cervix. A gooseneck lamp or flashlight may be helpful. Demonstrating the lack of sensation in the inner vaginal wall and comparing it to the sensitive outer third is often dramatic. It is reassuring to men who remain concerned about penis size that only the outer third of the vagina responds to pleasurable touch. The entire vagina may respond to the pleasurable experience of distention, however.

When both partners feel satisfied that the exam has been helpful, then the second partner can get ready for his examination.

Premature Ejaculation. Before starting a specific therapy program, it is important to agree upon a definition of premature ejaculation. The definition varies according to the source; however, the most useful one defines premature ejaculation as ejaculation that occurs before either partner wishes. According to Kinsey, the average male lasts 2 minutes before ejaculation after insertion of the penis in the vagina. Many couples feel this is not long enough, particularly if the woman needs more time to achieve orgasm.

At present, the specific cause for premature ejaculation is not known. Two common factors seem to be associated with men who ejaculate early. The first is a history of hurried masturbation or hurried coitus during the adolescent years. Many men's first coitus typically occurred under time pressure in the back seat of a car or in the partner's living room. This pattern of ejaculating rapidly apparently transfers to their later sexual life. Also, rapid progress to ejaculation might well be the natural pattern of the body. Inhibiting ejaculation may be a learned behavior—a product of social conditioning.

The second factor related to ejaculation that occurs sooner than desired is anxiety. Anxiety, mediated via the sympathetic nervous system, facilitates ejaculation. Most men experience fears or concerns about how they will perform, how long they will last, or how they will satisfy their partners. Because of their anxieties, many men experience little sexual pleasure during intercourse. These concerns also impair thorough vasocongestion and muscular tension, the hallmarks of the plateau stage. Men in this stage of arousal appear better able to control ejaculation than those in earlier stages of arousal.

The basic aim in counseling men with premature ejaculation is to increase their ability to focus on the pleasure they are experiencing in their genitals. Thus they can increase arousal and counter anxiety. Focusing involves concentrating on the sensations in the genitals.

At the Sex Advisory and Counseling Unit, an eight-step program has been adapted from the method originally described by Semans. The eight-step method is based on the man's ability to focus on his genital sensations. With practice, most men can learn to identify their location on the sexual response curve at a given moment. They can identify various points on the curve as they approach the point of inevitability and ejaculation.

Step One. The man masturbates with a dry hand until he can comfortably forestall ejaculation for 15 minutes. During his masturbation, he is instructed to focus on the feelings he is experiencing in his penis. As he becomes more aroused and senses he is approaching the point of inevitability, he alters his masturbation until he feels that he has regained control. Most men find that stopping or slowing down the rate of stimulation, lightening the touch, or cutting out a fantasy enables them to regain control within a time period of a few seconds to 1 or 2 minutes.

Step Two. Using massage oil or lotion, the man masturbates for 15 minutes. For many men, adding oil is much more stimulating, which may result in more frequently stopping and resuming stimulation in order to forestall ejaculation for 15 minutes.

Step Three. When the man is able to masturbate reliably without ejaculation, he goes to a third step, in which his partner stimulates his penis and other responsive areas for 15 minutes. The man continues focusing and when he feels that he might lose his control he instructs his partner to change her stimulation until he feels he has regained control.

Step Four. When the man feels he has sufficient practice with Step Three, he then has his partner stimulate him after putting lotion on her hand. He may require more stops and starts to achieve the full 15 minutes than were necessary when his partner used a dry hand.

Step Five. When the partners have learned to perform the masturbation and partner stimulation homework reliably, the couple is ready for homework involving intercourse. With the male on his back and the female kneeling astride and facing, the male slowly inserts his penis in the vagina. The woman is to remain quiet without pelvic movement. For many men, the female astride position makes focusing easier since it enables them to keep muscles relaxed. Simple vaginal containment for many men is very stimulating. When they feel that they are approaching the point of inevitability, they instruct their partner to remove the penis until control can be maintained. For others, containment is not sufficiently stimulating to enable them to maintain full erection. If an erection partially subsides, a small amount of movement usually brings it back.

Step Six. When the man is able to tolerate vaginal containment for 15 minutes without ejaculation, he instructs his partner to start thrusting gently. This usually requires many practice sessions, because many men will have increased difficulty focusing on their genital sensations.

Step Seven. After practicing with the female partner thrusting, the male gently begins thrusting while his partner remains still. When he is able to last 15 minutes without ejaculating, he can proceed to the last step.

Step Eight. In the last step, both partners thrust for 15 minutes. With practice, most men become able to last 15 minutes with a decreasing number of stops and starts.

For most couples, the entire eight steps may take several weeks or several months to complete. In general, there will be times when the problem recurs, usually when the man is under additional stress. If the couple is prepared for this possibility, they are able to adjust themselves when it does occur. It is useful to suggest to them that when problems occur, they can return to earlier steps in the program and work their way through the remaining steps.

Another method recommended by Masters and Johnson for forestalling ejaculation is called the squeeze technique. This procedure requires the woman to use her thumb and opposing finger to exert pressure on the coronal ridge before the male approaches ejaculatory inevitability. It is believed that the distraction of the squeeze reduces excitement and enables the man to regain control. Squeezing serves the same purpose as the stop-and-start tactics of the original Semans technique. Both methods rely on the man's ability to focus on his sensations and reduce his arousal to regain ejaculatory control.

Impotence (Erectile Difficulties). Impotence is the second most common male sexual dysfunction. The word itself, with its connotation of powerlessness, evokes a negative response. A more precise and less loaded term is *erectile difficulties*. This term describes the following categories: men who never have erections, men who have erections only with masturbation, men who lose erections during insertion, and men who lose erections during intercourse. Situational erectile difficulty refers to men who lose their erections only in certain situations, for example, only with their wives or only with their lovers. *Primary erectile difficulty* refers to the man who has never experienced erection; *secondary erectile difficulty* refers to the man who has lost his erectile capability to some extent. Before a couple enters sexual counseling for erectile difficulties, the man should have a complete physical, including neurologic examination. Finding a possible medical cause for impotence, such as diabetes, should not necessarily preclude sexual counseling. Often organic and psychological factors interact to produce the difficulty. The man's awareness that his disease might affect sexual response or his experiencing some alteration in his capacity to react to sexual stimulation are among the disease-related factors that can produce psychological blocks to erection.

The basic principle in counseling a couple when the man is having erectile difficulties is to remove pressure for intercourse. To most couples, sex and intercourse are synonymous. They do not include self pleasuring or mutual pleasuring as part of "real sex." The man relies on his penis as the sole means of experiencing and giving pleasure. He excludes his mouth and hands as part of his sexual equipment. The woman often supports this view that intercourse is the only way for her to enjoy sex with her partner. Although they enjoy being pleasured by their partner's hands or tongue, many women feel discomfort in asking their partners for this form of stimulation. The aim of homework is to dispel the myth that intercourse is the only valid mode of sexual expression and to allow couples to widen their range of sexual activities.

The progression of homework is similar to that used with premature ejaculation. The initial homework involves individual exercises for each partner. For the man, homework involves masturbation for 15 minutes, focusing on sensations in the penis. Most men with erectile difficulties can achieve erections spontaneously or with masturbation. However, even for men who do not achieve erections, the masturbation homework can be done with a flaccid penis.

When the man begins to attain erections with masturbation and is able to master the focusing technique, he should then deliberately stop stimulation two or three times during the 15-minute session. With the cessation of stimulation, most men will partially or totally lose their erections. After 30 seconds to 1 minute, stimulation can be resumed; with refocusing, the erection will usually return. For a man who has had protracted problems with erections, the ability to produce erections two or three times in a short period of time can be very reassuring.

When the man is able to focus and have erections by himself reliably, he can then have his partner stimulate him for a 15-minute period. It is important to encourage the couple to do this pleasuring exercise even when an erection is absent. With practice focusing, it is likely that the man will begin to have erections. Even if pleasuring regularly produces erections, the couple should refrain from intercourse until the man feels comfortable with the idea.

Many couples enjoy doing the genital pleasuring as part of a massage or separately. A good position for the woman to take to stimulate her partner's genitals is to have him lie on his back with her sitting between his legs and facing him. With the man providing the directions, the woman stimulates her partner. During the period when intercourse is prohibited, the man may experience sexual tension. He can relish this for its own sake and allow it to subside gradually. Alternatively, if the couple wishes, the partner can continue stimulation until the man ejaculates or until he feels satisfied.

When genital pleasuring reliably results in erections and when the male feels confident, intercourse can then be added to the homework.

Almost all men experience erectile difficulties in certain situations or at certain times in their lives. For a man who has a history of erectile difficulties, the occasional lack of an erection can be devastating if he is not forewarned. Men can learn to recognize circumstances that create erectile difficulties and enjoy sex play without intercourse under these circumstances. Alcohol, fatigue, and work stress are common examples of influences that can impair sexual functioning.

Homework designed to reduce erectile difficulties can be readily combined with homework for women with sexual dysfunctions. For example, the couple can take turns pleasuring. The woman can pleasure her partner for 15 to 30 minutes to help him learn how to focus. When he is satisfied or has ejaculated, he can then pleasure her as part of her homework. The partners may want to alternate in doing individual homework. For example, the female partner can practice masturbating with the male present and then the male partner can do his 15 minute self pleasuring.

Any combination of homework is acceptable as long as the partners negotiate ahead of time the nature of the homework and what they expect from one another. Because one partner decides to do his/her homework with the other partner present, it cannot be assumed that he or she intends to progress to mutual sexual play. By making the intent of the homework clear, the couple can avoid disagreements over what could have happened or was expected to happen.

SEXUAL AND EDUCATIONAL AIDS

Lubricants

Many couples use lubricants to enhance sexual enjoyment. There are many types of lubricants available. In general, when recommending a lubricant, suggest one that is water soluble, hypoallergenic, and mildly scented or unscented. The purpose of a lubricant is to decrease friction and improve pleasurable sensations. Moist tissues appear to experience more sensation than do dry. Unscented massage oil is a good choice, because it can be used for total body pleasuring, including the genitals. Unscented Albolene, a cosmetic cream, is also good. It is best not to suggest heavy gels such as Vaseline, as they tend to cling to tissues and are difficult to remove.

Vibrators

The vibrator is an increasingly popular form of sexual aid. They are more commonly used by women; however, some types are used by men. The vibrator provides localized, intense stimulation to the clitoris or glans penis and enables many women to experience orgasm for the first time. At present there are many models of vibrators. Many models have several detachable heads that can be used on different areas of the body. In general there are three classes of vibrators: an over-the-hand model, a phallus-shaped model, and a hand-held model. The over-the-hand model slides onto the hand and vibrates the hand, which in turn stimulates the genital area. The major inconvenience with this model is its awkwardness and appearance. The phallus shaped model can be inserted in the vagina or used directly on the clitoral area. Some women do not find stimulation of the vagina in this way particularly pleasurable; others enjoy intravaginal pressure or stimulation, usually close to the introitus. The third model, the hand-held type, can be used for body massage. Vibrators are generally available in the larger cities in book stores selling erotic literature. The types used as massagers can be bought in small appliance departments. Various types are also available via mail order from the Sears catalog.

Literature

Patient Reading Literature. For many women and couples, counseling may involve the providing of information and education. This can be done during office visits as part of the examination. Information can also be provided through up-to-date reading material that patients can buy or borrow. The following is a short list of books many women have read and enjoyed.

Our Bodies, Ourselves. This book—written by the Boston Women's Health Collective—provides basic information about female sexuality. It is an excellent, inexpensive book for both men and women to learn more about sexuality.

The Joy of Sex, by Alex Comfort. This book provides detailed information about many aspects of sexuality. It discusses many different sexual techniques and styles.

Intimate Enemy, by George Bach and Peter Wyden. This book provides suggestions for improving communication between partners. Bach describes how couples can learn to handle anger and develop improved techniques for fighting—a technique he calls Fair Fighting.

The Massage Book, by George Downing. This book is a manual for learning how to do massage. The diagrams illustrate different types of massage strokes that can be used.

Getting Clear, by Anne Kent Rush. This is a book on women's body work. It is designed to improve a woman's ability to be more in touch with her body.

Boys and Sex and *Girls and Sex*, by Wardell Pomeroy. These books are designed to provide sexual information to teenagers. Adults also will be able to benefit from reading both of these books.

The Sex Handbook, by Handman and Brennan. This book is for teenagers and provides detailed information about sexuality, with an emphasis on birth control and venereal disease.

Liberating Masturbation, by Betty Dodson. This book discusses self pleasuring and self sexuality for women. It also contains sketches of different women's genitals, demonstrating their beauty and uniqueness.

For Yourself, by Lonnie Barbach. This book is designed to teach women methods for reaching orgasm.

My Secret Garden, by Nancy Friday. This book is a description of sexual fantasies reported by women.

The Yes Book: Female Masturbation, by the National Sex Forum. This book discusses masturbation and self sexuality for women.

Physician's Reading List. *Human Sexual Response*, by Masters and Johnson. This is the only book that contains clinical research on sexual behavior and sexual response. This book provides a background of information necessary for counseling.

Human Sexual Inadequacy, by Masters and Johnson. This book deals with various sexual dysfunctions. Many patients will also benefit from reading this book.

The New Sex Therapy, by Helen Singer Kaplan. This book discusses sexuality and sexual counseling. It is based on the counseling program at Cornell University.

Creative Aggression, by George Bach. This book deals with the techniques of fair fighting. It explains the various rituals used by Bach to help couples deal with anger and improve their communications.

Films. *Reaching Orgasm.* This 20-minute film, produced by and available from the Human Sexuality Program at the University of California School of Medicine in San Francisco, presents the home assignments used in their program to help women reach orgasm.

Multi-Media Corporation provides a catalog of sexual films that depict various aspects of sexuality and sexual life styles. The films may be purchased or rented.

SUMMARY

The preceding chapter is a review of techniques for office sex counseling. Included in this review are a summary of human sexual response, male and female sexual dysfunctions, and couple sexual dysfunctions.

The chapter discusses the four levels of intervention: validation, education, suggestion, and therapy. Selection of the appropriate level of intervention is discussed, as well as selection of suitable patients or couples.

Providing a setting which will encourage women to discuss their sexual problems is important. Some suggestions are made of ways the physician can be more receptive to discussing sexuality.

Often, because of limited time or opportunity or because the physician is not comfortable dealing wih sexual problems, it is more appropriate to refer the patient to other counseling services in the community.

Specific counseling methods are applied to the common sexual dysfunctions of both men and women. The final section describes a variety of educational and sexual aids.

This chapter is presented to help physicians deal with patients who have sexual problems. Sexual problems are common in office practice, and physicians need to develop their abilities to deal with patients who have these problems. The most important aspects of counseling are validation and information giving. With practice, the techniques discussed in this chapter will become more familiar and can be utilized more comfortably and more effectively.

It is hoped that this approach will be helpful both to physicians and to their patients.

10

WOMEN'S VIEW OF THE GYNECOLOGIST

VALERIE JORGENSEN, M.D.

Throughout the Women's Liberation Movement literature, the women's magazines, the women's public forums, and the gynecology waiting rooms are heard complaints about medical care. Women in increasing numbers are voicing dissatisfaction with the quality of their medical care. Obstetricians and gynecologists are the focal point of this discontent. As a woman and a gynecologist, I sit on both sides of the fence and hear both points of view. I can only conclude that it is time to listen to one another, time to learn from one another, time to give up meaningless generalizations, and time to work on compromises to improve gynecologic care. It is time for change!

HUMAN RIGHTS-PATIENT RIGHTS

The women's movement in medicine is not an issue of women's rights versus men's rights, but rather it is an issue of human rights for all patients within the medical care system.[1,2] It is a movement for equal rights in medicine for both the patient and physician.[1] Well over one hundred books and articles have been written in the last decade criticizing the medical care system. The majority of these writings express criticism of obstetric and gynecologic care given women. Generally, most women authors reflect tremendous anger and frustration over what they feel are physicians' lack of respect and dignity for their female patients.[1-7]

RESPECTFUL CARE

The early models for medical care were structured around the physician (parent)-patient (child) relationship.[8] Women were taught to respect the knowledge and skills of their gynecologists and to trust these professionals with their bodies, their reproductive lives, and their physical and emotional health. Today, women generally find this type of "blind faith medicine" dehumanizing, disrespectful, and irrelevant. Women want mutual respect in a medical partnership!

Has medical care been "authoritarian, paternalistic, sexist and degrading"? Has medicine guarded medical facts as "privileged information," failed to gain "informed consent," failed to include women in medical care decisions, and failed to treat women as whole human beings? The majority of female authors writing about medical care answer in the affirmative.[1-7, 9-11] This is a searing condemnation of medical care. Is there any truth to these charges?

Let us briefly take a look at how physicians act when they are patients. When a physician-patient enters medical care, he or she expects the answers to the following questions:

1. What is my diagnosis?
2. What tests are you going to do and why?
3. How are you planning to treat my illness?
4. What is my prognosis?
5. What does this mean to my life style and career?

Physicians feel that they have a "right to know" because they are part of the medical profession. Doctors feel they have a right to answers "because they can live with the truth" and because this information is necessary for "putting their lives together." Yet these are the very answers we often deny our female patients. We fear "telling the truth for fear of harming her." We fear discussing her disease because "she won't understand and will only worry." We fear discussing the realities of her illness because "she will give up hope." Yet, if we listen to our female patients, these are our fears and not their fears. Women are seeking answers. They are asking to be educated about their bodies, asking to be informed about their medical care, asking to discuss medical care options, and asking for help to live and help to die. Women want humane, relevant medical care.

A POINT OF VIEW: WOMEN'S VIEWS

We would be hiding our heads in the sand if we did not acknowledge that women are reading, writing, and listening to one another about their common medical concerns. For the last decade, women have been demystifying medicine through many articles and books. They have started to translate medical care into a language that any person can comprehend.

Ellen Frankfort in *Vaginal Politics*[2] writes that authoritarianism in medicine belongs in the past. She goes on to state that women are dissatisfied with their medical care because "they are not treated as rational, responsible allies in health care matters." Women want to be treated as unique individuals with a mind and a body that the physician respects.[8]

Dependency is a big issue. A woman is often made to feel very dependent upon her gynecologist because she is not informed. For instance, she often does not know the medication she is taking or why. Prescriptions are written in ways that are not understood by the patient, and often no reasonable explanation is given. She fears verbal reprisal if she questions and is not totally submissive to her doctor's orders. Physicians often keep their patients submissive by professing that "she really doesn't want to know," "she shouldn't worry her pretty little head about it," or "she wouldn't understand the technical terms." Ms. Frankfort stresses that women do want to know and can comprehend the truth.

Frankfort goes on to state that gynecologists often reflect their own puritanic attitudes toward women when giving sexual and contraceptive information. A patient may often get the favorite advice or care of the doctor depending on his or her own sexual and moral values, rather than a frank medical discussion of contraceptive methods and sexual practices.

Barbara Seaman in *Free and Female*[7] writes a chapter entitled, "How to Liberate Yourself from Your Gynecologists." She feels that gynecologists do not respect their patients and impose authoritarian medical ritual on them. She concludes that prenatal care, labor and delivery, gynecologic examinations, and operations are done for and at the convenience of doctors and not for patients. Women have major concerns about the rigid "standard routines" that they are forced to accept.

Ms. Seaman feels that the doctrine of "reasonable informed consent" is completely ignored. Generations of women have been taught to worship their gynecologists' opinions. Those who dare to raise questions are quickly labeled eccentric or neurotic and are sharply reminded of the "physicians' long years of training and his expertise." She feels that women must question and seek second opinions because, "the removal of normal, healthy organs is carried out all too frequently." The medical consumer should not feel intimidated when she is inquiring about her own body and her own care. Medicine is far from an exact science, and physicians should stop pretending that it is absolute. A good gynecologist like any other good doctor is human first and not any all-purpose authority. Physicians should be willing to listen to their patients and should not pretend that they have all the easy answers. The doctor and patient are partners in the patient's health and welfare, not master and serf.[7]

A similar point of view is illustrated in an article written by Mary Lynn M. Luy entitled, "What's Behind Women's Wrath Towards Gynecologists."[5] She notes that women from all age groups are voicing complaints. Perhaps the outrage is best expressed by militant women's groups, but it is felt by all. Women are complaining that their gynecologists are "specialists in insensitivity." In general, the complaints are focused on the doctor's:

   1. patronizing, dictatorial attitudes,
   2. lack of sensitivity,
   3. sexist attitudes and sexual biases,
   4. demeaning, humiliating pelvic examination.

Women interviewed felt that doctors regarded them as inferior and incapable of understanding explanations. Accordingly, they were treated as children who could not make decisions and should be guarded from harsh medical realities. Women object that gynecologists are "more interested in treating patients than in treating people."[5] When women have asked for explanations doctors have bristled, regarding such questions as challenges to their medical competence and judgment. Patients do not want to be excluded from deciding important matters, especially those involving health care options and alternatives. When the doctor is annoyed at his patient's independence, he may retort with statements such as, "so you think you are the doctor," or "why don't you find another doctor?" Can we begin to understand that women ask questions *only* to understand their care? Women want to be able to give informed consent, and they can accomplish this only through a meaningful dialogue with the medical profession.

Ms. Luy elaborates that gynecology textbooks are often purveyors of "sexist myths." From Novak's *Textbook of Gynecology* (1970) she quotes, "The frequency of intercourse depends entirely on the male sex drive. The bride should be advised to allow her husband's sex drives to set their pace and she should attempt to gear hers satisfactorily to his." From Green's *Gynecology* (1971) she quotes, "Although the instinctive sexual drive of the male is greater than hers, it is nevertheless of fundamental importance for the woman to make herself available for the fulfillment of this drive, and perfectly natural and normal that she will do it willingly and derive satisfaction and pleasure from the union." Such generalizations are meaningless, as documented in *The Pleasure Bond* by Masters and Johnson.[12]

Some textbooks encourage young doctors to think that they have an obligation and right to be the moral guardians of their women patients. The great irony lies in the fact that gynecologists are socially sanctioned as sexual advisors and yet are "astoundingly ignorant of female sexuality."[1] *Our Bodies Ourselves*[1] serves as a widely used medical reference for women of all age groups. The book states that "every woman should realize that just because a physician is certified in OB-GYN, doesn't mean that he or she is qualified, trained or prepared in any way to give advice or counsel in any human relations area of a woman's life."Gynecologists have been given the role, but have not fully assumed the responsibility or the training. "The image and myth that physicians are all knowing and humanitarian is now very far out of date."[1] These women authors caution patients not to let themselves be stampeded into any sudden medical decisions or be forced to accept any medications or procedures that they do not understand or want. "You have a right to know the meanings of the tests and your diagnosis and treatment from your gynecologists."[1] "You have a right to know the indications for treatment, the varieties of treatment, and pros and cons of the treatment chosen."[1]

CHANGING ATTITUDES

Women are becoming increasingly vocal and demonstrative over their medical needs, their medical demands, and their medical ideals. Their criticisms are harsh and of course are not entirely valid. We cannot ignore that American medicine has been good to women. We cannot ignore that gynecologists have provided one of the highest standards of medical care. This has been well documented. However, women's needs are changing and the way in which we care for them must change also. Women are asking to be educated about their bodies and their medical care. They are seeking honest discussions of medical options and the opportunity to participate in health decisions. Women are seeking contraceptive and sexual information without sensual slurs or judgmental platitudes. Good preventive medicine is a major concern. The issue in gynecology is how to care effectively. It is time to shift gears, to listen, to change old ways, and to make medical care meaningful for today's and tomorrow's women.

GYN CARE: MY VIEW

New ideas, new treatments, new techniques, and new ways of caring keep the practice of medicine alive and well. Both patients and physicians have the same goals. How do we meet them effectively?

Respect for the individual patient is generated out of the physician's ability to listen. A history should be taken without prejudging the patient's symptoms. We should be historians, not judge and jury. Each physician should be listening to the patient as a total person, not as a pregnancy, a pelvis, or a pain. We should acutely respect that her body has a head, and that her life style and life stresses may have a great deal to do with her diseases and her complaints.

The gynecologist should be technically competent, but not a medical machine. He or she should be able to relate to each patient first as a human being, then as a doctor. Physicians are people treating other people!

A gynecologic examination should educate the patient about herself. One reasonable approach to doing a respectful examination is as follows:

1. Begin by asking the patient what she expects and what would make her comfortable.

2. Allow her some control over the examination. If the routines of disrobing and using an office gown or draping her during the pelvic examination are objectionable, offer her the alternatives of remaining in her own slip and not using the drape. Office routines should be flexible enough to preserve each woman's dignity and respect.

3. Proceed with the pelvic examination when the patient indicates she is ready. Explain your every move as you are doing it.

4. Start with the *internal* examination. Choose the smallest warm speculum necessary to visualize the cervix and vagina adequately and to take the appropriate tests. A large speculum is used far too often and only traumatizes her. Never do a procedure without telling her what you are doing and why. Describe what you see and interpret the findings. Tell her when you are removing the speculum.

5. Explain the bimanual examination as you are doing it. Women relax much better when they concentrate on what you are doing. Discuss her physical findings and their meaning. Translate scientific terms into meaningful language.

6. Continue with the rectal or rectovaginal examination, explaining that there will probably be some discomfort.

7. Examine her external genitalia last. Acknowledge that examination of the erogenous zones may make her uncomfortable. Palpation should be brief and informative.

8. Complete the pelvic examination and allow her a few moments before the breast exam. Educate the patient about her breast during your examination and then teach her how to examine herself.

Good crisis care is important, but prevention is still our best cure. Gynecologists should take every opportunity to teach each woman about her body and how to do a meaningful self-examination. It should be made very clear that self-examinations complement but do not substitute for regular gynecologic examinations.

Speak about her body in anatomical, nonsexual, noncosmetic terms, avoiding value judgments or flattering terms.

9. Allow her to dress and return to a consultation room to discuss her examination. The gynecologist should explain the meaning of the physical findings, the tests that were done, and the diagnostic tests or procedures that should be done. Honestly discuss pathology, using nonscare tactics. Explore and explain her medical options.

There are very few medical or surgical emergencies. Allow each woman reasonable time to make rational decisions. Encourage her to discuss her problems with her family. Support her right to seek another opinion. Women have a grave responsibility to themselves and their families to understand any treatment and its sequelae and to participate actively in medical care decisions.

Every gynecologist should know how and when to make an appropriate referral. Physicians should not imply that they are angry or that the patient is "wrong" or "bad" because another specialist is needed. One should simply state that one has reached the limit of his expertise in dealing with the problem and that another physician may have more information and help to give her. A kind referral could save her life.

CONCLUSION

Change has come. Gynecology must change also. Good obstetrics and gynecology is more than health maintenance and the prevention and treatment of disease. It has become the full time shared responsibility of both the physician and patient in the total care of the whole human being. Women need their gynecologists more than ever before. They have told us that and continue to tell us. What could be more of a challenge?

REFERENCES

1. Boston Women's Health Book Collective, *Our Bodies Ourselves*, Simon and Schuster, New York, 1976.
2. Frankfort, E, *Vaginal Politics*, Quandrangle Books, 1972.
3. Greer, G, *The Female Eunuch*, McGraw-Hill, New York, 1971.
4. Janeway, E, *Man's World Woman's Place*, Dell, 1971.
5. Luy, MLM, What's Behind Women's Wrath Towards Gynecologists, Mod Med *42*:17, 1974.
6. Morgan, R, (editor), *Sisterhood is Powerful—An Anthology of Writings from the Women's Liberation Movement*, Random House, 1970.
7. Seaman, B, *Free and Female*, Fawcett Inc., 1973.
8. Eckstein, G, *The Body Has a Head*, Harper and Row, New York, 1969.
9. Hayes, HR, *The Dangerous Sex*, G. P. Putnam's Sons, 1972.
10. Horney, K, *Feminine Psychology*, W. W. Norton, 1967.
11. Morgan, E, *The Descent of Woman*, Stein and Day, 1972.
12. Masters, WH, and Johnson, VE, *The Pleasure Bond*, Little, Brown, 1974.

11

RAPE

JAMES L. BREEN, M.D.

EARL GREENWALD, M.D.

Few crimes create as great an impact on the victim and perpetrator as does the act of rape. The derivation of the word "rape" is from the Latin word, "rapere," meaning "to seize."[1]

All violent crimes, including robbery, assault, rape, and murder, have increased since 1960. The rate of increase in the incidence of rape is noted in Table 11.1. This rise is part of a general increase in the frequency of violent behavior in the United States, as reflected by the corresponding increase in the incidence of other felonies.

The number of reported rapes increased 146% between 1960 and 1971, and an additional 11% between 1971 and 1972.[2] Criminologists estimate that 4 to 10 times as many rapes are committed as are reported, that fewer than 50% of reported rapes are brought to trial, and that very few such trials end in a conviction of the alleged assailant.

Rape is one of the least reported crimes,[3] for victims fail to report the event for fear of physical harm or because of parental or peer rejection. There is also a general belief that any legal action by the victim will engender considerable humiliation, psychological trauma, and expense, with little probability of retribution or of separating the rapist from society.

In 1933, the frequency of rape was 2/100,000 in the United States. This increased to 9.2 in 1960 and 11.6 in 1965.[4] An interview-survey revealed that forcible rape occurred at a frequency 3½ times the rate reported, or, using the 1965 statistics, at the rate of 40.6/100,000 population.[5] These statistics suggest that the likelihood of a serious personal attack on the females of America, each year, is approximately 1 in 12,000, with the greatest risk occurring in the lower socioeconomic groups.[5]

A comparison with other countries, including Luxembourg, France, Holland, and Belgium, shows a dramatically lower incidence of rape, i.e. approximately 2 to 3 women/100,000.[6] The difference is impressive and difficult to explain on the basis of legal considerations. Indeed, the penalty for rape is much less severe in countries other than the United States. The reasons for this disparity are probably related to complex factors dealing with attitudes toward sexual expression and to the legality and, therefore, availability of acceptable forms of sexual release, such as prostitution.

The physician is one of the first professionals to enter into the evaluation and management of rape victims. He must be thoroughly cognizant of the techniques

TABLE 11.1
Rape, Reported Annual Incidence in the United States

Year	Number of rapes
1965	22,460
1966	25,330
1967	27,100
1968	31,060
1969	36,470
1970	37,270
1971	41,890
1972	46,430

utilized in evaluating a physically and emotionally traumatized person. He must effectively elicit relevant information, perform a careful and complete examination, and record all observations pertinent to the legal and medical needs of the patient.

DEFINITIONS

The precise meaning of the various terms used in describing sexual offenses should be understood. "Sexual assault" is a general term used to describe manual, oral, or genital contact by an offender with the genitalia of a victim without the victim's consent.

"Molestation" is a noncoital form of sexual assault. Coital forms of sexual assault include "incest" and "rape." "Incest" is coital contact between blood relatives. Force is not a necessary element for allegation and conviction. It is interesting to note that voluntary incest is included in the definition of, and penalized in the same manner as, forcible rape with a nonrelative in some states.

"Rape" has three basic components. The perpetrator's genitalia must contact the genitals of the victim ("carnal knowledge"), this must be accomplished "against the victim's will," and there must be an element of "compulsion."

Definitions of these various components vary widely from state to state, although some consistency is evident. Table 11.2 shows, for all states, the District of Columbia, and Puerto Rico, the ages of consent and peculiarities relating to definitions of rape and to the sentences prescribed.

It should be noted that rape is not an offense invariably committed by a male against a female. A female can rape a male, and this is explicitly specified in some state laws.

The first factor requiring consideration in the definition of rape is to determine the extent of sexual contact necessary for the event to be considered rape. Many states require evidence of penetration only, explicitly excluding the necessity for the male to ejaculate.

It is not uncommon for a state law to indicate that the "penetration" however slight, be "adequate." Introduction of the penis between the labia majora, but not into the vagina, represents a case of rape in many or most states.

It should be noted that actual laceration of the hymen may not be a prerequisite for the charge of rape, although many states require that victims, beyond a

TABLE 11.2
State Laws

State	Age of consent	Sentence	Peculiarities of definition
Alabama	16	Death or Prison	Penetration adequate
Alaska	16	Prison	Includes incest
Arizona	18	Prison	Corroboration by witness not needed; not wife
Arkansas	16	Death or Prison	Penetration adequate
California	18	Prison	Corroboration required unless victim is 18 years or less; perpetrator 14 years or older, unless prove ability
Colorado	18	Prison	Female can rape male younger than 18 years of age
Connecticut	16	Prison	—
Delaware	7	Death or Prison	—
Florida	10	Death or Prison	Ejaculation not necessary
Georgia	7	Death or Prison	Penetration adequate; must corroborate by witness
Hawaii	None	Life imprisonment at hard labor	No corroboration by witness needed
Idaho	18	Prison	Perpetrator must be 14 years or older, or must prove ability
Illinois	14	Prison	Penetration only; perpetrator must be 14 years or older, or must prove ability
Indiana	16	Prison	Not wife; perpetrator must be 14 years older, or must prove ability
Iowa	16	Prison	Penetration only; must corroborate by witness
Kansas	18	Prison at hard labor	Female can rape male younger than 18 years of age
Kentucky	18	Death or Prison	Not wife or husband; penetration only
Louisiana	Common law	Death or Prison	Not wife; penetration only, however slight
Maine	14	Prison	Penetration only
Maryland	14	Death or Prison	Penetration only; female older than 18 years can rape male younger than 14, misdemeanor
Massachusetts	16	Prison; if victim is sexually delinquent, 1 day to life	—
Michigan	16	Prison	Penetration, however slight
Minnesota	18	Prison	Not wife
Mississippi	18	$500.00 fine or prison	Victim must be previously chaste
Missouri	16	Death or Prison	Penetration adequate
Montana	18	Prison	Incest considered rape
Nebraska	18	Prison	Victim must be previously chaste if older than 15
Nevada	16	Death or Prison	Penetration, however slight; not wife
New Hampshire	16	Prison	"Copulation" defined as a form of rape
New Jersey	16	$5,000.00 and/or Prison	Perpetrator must be 16 years or older, or must prove ability
New Mexico	16	Prison	Not wife
New York	17	Prison	Corroboration necessary; includes bestiality and sex with a dead human body, consensual sodomy
North Carolina	12	Life imprisonment	—
North Dakota	18	Prison	Not wife; perpetrator must be 14 years or older, or must prove ability; penetration only, however slight
Ohio	18	Prison	Incest considered rape

TABLE 11.2—*Continued*

State	Age of consent	Sentence	Peculiarities of definition
Oklahoma	16	Death or Prison	—
Oregon	16	Prison	Incest and sex with wife's daughter considered rape
Pennsylvania	16	$2,000.00 or Prison at hard labor in solitary confinement	Perpetrator must be 15 years or older, or must prove ability
Rhode Island	16	Prison	—
South Carolina	14	Death or Prison at hard labor	—
South Dakota	18	Prison	Perpetrator must be 14 years or older, or must prove ability
Tennessee	12	Death by electrocution or Prison	"Commencement of sexual connection" adequate; penetration not necessary
Texas	18	Prison	Victim 15 years or older must be previously chaste; perpetrator must be 14 years or older, or must prove ability
Utah	13	Prison	—
Vermont	16	$2,000.00 or Prison	Perpetrator must be 16 years or older, or must prove ability; if perpetrator and victim are less than 16, misdemeanor
Virginia	16	Death or Prison	—
Washington	18	Prison	Not wife or husband; penetration however slight; female can rape male younger than 18 years of age
West Virginia	16	Prison	Not wife or husband; victim older than 10 must be previously chaste
Wisconsin	None	Prison	—
Wyoming	18	Prison	—
District of Columbia	16	Death by electrocution or Prison	—
Puerto Rico	14	Prison	Not wife; perpetrator must be 14 years or older, or must prove ability; penetration, however slight

specified age, be "previously chaste." Other common restrictions in the definition of rape include that the victim is not the spouse of the perpetrator; in several states, the event must be corroborated by an eyewitness.

The fallacies in these requirements are obvious. The marital status of a woman and the integrity of her hymen are in no way related to the physical and psychologic trauma experienced by coercion to perform a sexual act. Most rapes are not spontaneous but are premeditated, and it is unlikely that an assailant will commit this crime without carefully excluding witnesses.

The second important component in rape is the lack of consent of the victim, equivalent to "against the victim's will."[7] This includes sexual contact by force, fear, or fraud, or under circumstances in which the female is unable, by law, to consent to sexual activity.

The word "force" is difficult to define. English law requires that the victim must resist until overcome by unconsciousness, exhaustion, brute force, or fear of death.[8] American law requires only that force consist of physical harm, or that the fear of physical harm be transmitted to the mind of the victim in the form of intimidation by threat.[8]

"Force," therefore, includes physical violence or threat with a weapon which may injure, mutilate, or kill. Threat of future harm to the victim or to her family or acquaintances constitutes that use of "fear." "Fraud" includes the promise of marriage or the victim's belief that he or she is already validly married to the perpetrator.

Under certain circumstances a person is considered unable, by law, to consent, and sexual activity with such persons, even without coercion, is considered "statutory rape." This includes individuals below the age of consent, which is defined by individual state laws (Table 11.2), and individuals whose state of consciousness has been altered by illness, sleep, drugs, or alcohol.[7]

Legally, "consent" implies "intelligent will," or a capacity of the participants, in sexual intercourse, to understand the nature and consequences of their activity.[7] The lack of consent, therefore, implies that one participant is deprived of the power to entertain an intelligent opinion or to understand the implications of the sexual contact in which they are involved. This would be true for individuals institutionalized for psychiatric problems, and for persons with mental retardation and psychologic disabilities. The fact that a noninstitutionalized individual is incapable of exercising judgment in terms of sexual contact may not be evident. A reasonable defense, therefore, for a perpetrator is that he was unaware of the fact that, or had no reasonable opportunity to know that, the victim was incapable of an intelligent decision and, therefore, of consent.

Several states provide that a male below a specific age, usually 14, cannot be convicted for rape unless his physical ability to accomplish intromission is unequivocably proven. This and many other restrictions create a situation in which proof of the allegation is difficult or impossible. These restrictions exist, obviously, for the protection of improperly accused assailants, but they also prevent valid prosecution because of their highly restrictive nature.

It is not the responsibility of the physician, in the course of his evaluation of the victim, to reach a conclusion or to offer an opinion, whether in a written report or under courtroom interrogation, concerning the validity of the charge of rape or the identity of the perpetrator. The examining physician must always be cautious of the necessity to remain objective and to use the phrases "suspected" or "alleged" in reference to the event. He must not create an impression that he has reached a conclusion and/or is expressing an opinion.

PENALTY FOR RAPE

The sentences rendered after a conviction of rape differ considerably among the various states. The most severe penalty is death, but since capital punishment is, at the time of this writing, unconstitutional, individuals so sentenced are serving life terms. Monetary fines vary widely (from $500.00 in Mississippi to $5,000.00 in New Jersey), as do prison sentences (from 1 day to 1,500 years).

The penalties in some states are more severe for younger victims, and less severe for younger perpetrators. Indeed, in Vermont, if both the victim and assailant are less than 16 years of age, the offense is considered a misdemeanor.

The statute in Massachusetts specifies that, if the victim can be proven "sexually delinquent," the sentence can be imprisonment for as little as 1 day to as much as life. The penalty for incest, when defined and described under the rape law for the individual state, tends to be more severe than for forcible rape of a nonrelated individual of the same age.

EVALUATION AND MANAGEMENT OF THE ALLEGED VICTIM OF RAPE

The major objectives during the physician's examination of the victim of an alleged rape are the following: (1) administer any treatment necessary because of life-threatening injuries, (2) obtain an informed consent for examination, (3) notify the authorities, if they are not already present, (4) obtain and carefully record a thorough history, (5) perform a complete physical examination, and in so doing, collect relevant specimens and photographs, accurately recording all examination findings, (6) effect legal transfer of specimens to laboratory personnel to complete evaluations, (7) protect the patient against venereal disease, pregnancy, and phychologic sequelae, and (8) release information and data to proper authorities.

Administration of First Aid

The first concern of the attending physician is to evaluate the patient for the presence of life-threatening injuries and to treat them immediately. It is obvious that further steps in evaluation or management should not be approached until the patient's condition is stable.

Rape is a crime of violence, and it is generally met by the victim with resistance, unless she is threatened with a lethal weapon. A considerable proportion of women suffer injuries, ranging from minor lacerations and abrasions to death. Approximately ½ of 1% of rapes terminate in the death of the victim, 8.7% of patients sustain major genital or nongenital injury, and one-third of all patients sustain minor genital or nongenital injuries.[9]

A preliminary physical examination is performed in order to determine the extent of physical trauma and the presence or absence of active bleeding from genital or extragenital injuries. Hemostasis is achieved, and suspected fractures are splinted. Repair of nonthreatening injuries may be deferred until a thorough examination and collection of necessary specimens are completed.

Informed Consent

Prior to proceeding with a more thorough evaluation, a third party should be called to witness the proceedings. This individual should be a registered nurse or a police officer. If the victim is a child, the parent or legal guardian should be present. It should be understood by the third party that he or she may, at a later date, be asked to corroborate the physician's recorded findings. In addition, the third party serves the vital function of eliminating the possibility that charges of rape will be leveled against the examining physician himself.

A suggested consent form is illustrated in Figure 11.1. Permission is granted for complete examination of the victim, for collection of specimens for laboratory evaluation, and for photography of physical injuries.

This must be signed by the patient, a witness, and the legal guardian of a patient who is below the age of consent or who is not mentally competent. If an appropriate consenting guardian cannot be reached, permission may be granted by

Case No._____ Name_____
Date_____ Address_____
Time_____ City_____
Witness_____ Guardian _____

Consent for Examination

I hereby authorize Dr._____ and Dr._____
_____to perform a complete medical examination, including pelvic (internal) examination, on my person and record for the proper law enforcement agency their findings as related to the prosecution of my assailant(s).

I further authorize the collection of necessary specimens for laboratory tests and the taking of necessary photographs by a competent photographer on the condition my identity is not revealed in said photographs.

Witness_____ Signed_____
                                        Parent (Guardian)_____

FIG. 11.1 Rape: recommended consent form

a court order, either in writing or by telephone. If such is not readily available, many state laws provide that any law enforcement officer can order an examination if a crime has allegedly been committed.[10] If the patient is a minor or if the examiner is acting on a court order, the wishes of an uncooperative victim may be totally disregarded.

Obtaining and Recording a History[3, 11]

A statement is obtained from the victim or, if the victim is incapable of response, from an accompanying individual, including full particulars, such as date, time, place, and circumstances of the alleged attack. A complete description of and/or the identity of the perpetrator should be ascertained, and the names, addresses, and telephone numbers of witnesses should be accurately recorded.

A thorough description of resistance offered should be recorded, and all areas of physical or sexual contact described. This assists the physician in focusing close attention on areas of the body which might otherwise be superficially examined. Sodomy, oral-genital contact, and other forms of sexual activity may be forced upon the victim during or after the initial insult, particularly during gang rapes.

During the history-taking process complete notations should be made, and the notes should be transcribed into a final form immediately on conclusion of the examination. The history should be recorded in the victim's precise words, enclosing the statement in quotation marks and using the first person.

The examining physician should not, and the courts will not, rely on the physician's memory. Months, and occasionally years, may elapse between the event and the court hearing. The form which has been most useful is illustrated in Figure 11.2.

The presence of a female third party is of value during the interview and examination, particularly if conducted by a male physician. The female assistant, with whom the victim may more closely identify, offers the elements of reassurance and support.

If not already present, the police should be notified. The primary reason for police presence is that they can institute necessary medicolegal procedures for the

MEDICAL REPORT Suspected Rape		Date
	(Hospital Name) Receiving Ward	Brought by
Name of Patient		Birthdate
Address		Age

AUTHORIZATION FOR RELEASE OF INFORMATION

I hereby authorize_____ to supply copies of ALL medical reports,
(Hospital Name)
including any laboratory reports, immediately upon completion, to the Police Department and the
Office of the District Attorney having jurisdiction.

Person
Examined _____

Address _____

Parent or
Date_____   Guardian_____

Witness_____   Address_____

MEDICAL REPORT	Time arrived	Date & Time of Alleged Rape

History (as related to physician)

EXAMINATION	Date	Time

General Examination (include ALL signs of external evidence of trauma)

Laboratory Specimens Collected	Pelvic Examination (include ALL signs of trauma, size, and development of female sex organs)
Yes No (Mandatory, or explain absence)	Vulva
	Hymen
Date _____ Time _____	Vagina
Smears _____ Vulva	
_____ Vagina _____ Cervix	Cervix
	Fundus
Saline Washings _____ Vulva	Adnexa (right)
_____ Vagina	Adnexa (left)
	Rectal
(Laboratory Reports Attached)	Examining Physician

I hereby certify that this is a true and correct copy of the official _____
(Hospital Name)

records concerning the examination of the above named patient.

Date _____   Title _____

FIG. 11.2. Recommended record form

assistance and protection of the victim. They can make an initial determination of the likelihood of the event's having occurred, assist in the identification and apprehension of the assailant, and, at a later date, assist in the prosecution of the perpetrator.

The physician must constantly remain objective in his or her investigational capacity, yet he or she should attempt to offer understanding and emotional support. There is a tendency on the part of the examining male physicians, who are repeatedly involved in evaluation of rape victims, to have one of two emotional responses. The first, because of the relative frequency of unjustifiable complaints, is to feel and convey to the patient the feeling that she in some way encouraged the rape. This may be reflected in an attitude of disbelief. Another undesirable reaction occurs in the clinical situation of forcible rape, with physical trauma. Disgust and anger may be elicited from the examining physician and be reflected directly to the patient and witnesses. Objectivity of all persons involved is thereby lost.

The examiner must be sensitive to the fact that victims of rape are suffering a bewildering spectrum of emotional responses, ranging from rage to humiliation. The physician's anxiety and horror in dealing with victims of bona fide rape may be conveyed by an unwillingness to talk clearly and freely about the event.

The feeling of shame is frequently intensified by family members, who attempt to protect the patient from the publicity involved in seeking medical evaluation and prosecution. Frequently the family conveys to the victim some question about her role in encouraging the rape experience. This severely exacerbates the patient's feeling of shame, rather than encouraging the more favorable feeling that she is a victim of the crime, not a perpetrator, and that she has the right and the responsibility to pursue prosecution.

An important component in the recorded history is the description of the patient's attitude and general status. The patient must, among other things, specifically be asked whether she bathed, showered, douched, urinated, or defecated since the assault, for these activities may alter the physical and laboratory findings.

The date and type of last voluntary sexual experience should be ascertained as well as the date and normalcy of the last menses and a thorough description of the patient's contraceptive habits. These assist the physician in evaluating her risk of pregnancy resulting from "forced" sexual intercourse.

The phase of the menstrual cycle is an important factor in the patient's history, for it determines the degree of concern about ensuing pregnancy and assists in the selection of an interceptive method. In addition, many victims are raped during menses, with tampon in situ. In this situation, the physician must be careful to search for and remove a tampon that may have been pushed into the cul de sac, and particular attention must be directed toward vaginal injury, the possibility of which appears to be increased by the presence of a tampon in the vagina at time of sexual assault.[12]

Attention should be directed toward signs by the patient's general appearance or behavior, of the use of alcohol or drugs, despite a verbal denial. If the use of alcohol or drugs is suspected, appropriate specimens should be obtained for toxicologic evaluation. Sexual intercourse with a patient whose consciousness or rationality is altered by intoxication may be grounds for a charge of statutory rape, as noted above.

Physical Examination

The record of the physical examination should include a description of the type and style of clothing worn and any disturbances of attire. If a change of clothing is available, garments worn by the victim should be preserved for examination by the authorities, particularly in cases of rape with homicide.

Subsequent evaluation is directed toward detecting and describing, in written form, the following: (1) the presence or absence of stigmata of trauma to all areas involved in the sexual assault, (2) a precise description of evidence of recent sexual intercourse, including a description of the status of the hymen, (3) collection of specimens to support or deny an episode of sexual intercourse, (4) institution of surveillance for sequelae of the sexual experience, including venereal disease, pregnancy, and adverse psychological reactions.

A complete physical examination of all areas of the body must be performed. Particular attention should be directed toward all extragenital areas. Frequently the mouth and rectum are allegedly involved in the sexual assault. All positive findings and pertinent negative observations must be included in the final report.

Written descriptions of the genital examination should begin with a description of the external genitalia, noting the presence or absence of blood, moist or dry secretions on the mons pubis, vulva, perineum, rectum, buttocks, or thighs. All evidence of trauma should be described in detail.

The labia majora should be separated, and the status of the hymen observed. There are four basic descriptions which may be used: (1) the hymen is present, intact, and demonstrates no evidence of recent trauma, (2) the hymen is present, intact, and demonstrates evidence of recent trauma, (3) the hymen is present, intact, and demonstrates evidence of old scarring, or (4) the hymen is absent. The precise meaning of hymenal integrity is unclear, but it may be of great legal significance, since the definition of rape in some states includes the necessity that the victim be "previously chaste" (see Table 11.2).

Penetration of the vagina by any object, including the erect penis, may occur through a fimbriated, highly elastic hymen without laceration. On the other hand, the hymen may be ruptured by trauma other than sexual intercourse. A variety of noncoital sexual activities may destroy the hymen, including various forms of autostimulation, such as digital or mechanical masturbation or the introduction of foreign bodies into the vagina. In addition, children occasionally rupture their hymens by falling on objects such as bicycle handles or rocks. In such patients the absence of hymenal integrity has no relevance whatsoever to their prior sexual behavior, and cannot, or should not, be used as a factor in judging their prior chastity.

Hymenal laceration is not a prerequisite for diagnosis in many states, in which mere introduction of the glans penis between the labia majora of the victim, without entry beyond the introitus, is sufficient to warrant the allegation of rape. In all practicality the physician can only determine, from examination of the introitus and determination of the state of hymenal integrity, whether coitus was "anatomically possible." Signs of recent laceration of the hymen, the presence of other genital trauma, or the identification of semen within the vagina utilizing the tests described below are supportive evidence for recent sexual intercourse.

During examination of the external genitalia, pubic hair in which secretions of semen adhere or on which such secretions have dried should be trimmed with a scissor and submitted separately to the laboratory for evaluation. The pubic hair should then be combed and loose hairs preserved for evaluation. Police laboratory facilities can differentiate between male and female hair. As noted above, all clothing, if damaged or stained with blood or secretions, should be submitted for hospital and police laboratory evaluations. Dried secretions are scraped from the skin into vials for analysis.

A speculum of appropriate size is moistened with water and gently introduced into the vagina. The mucosa is carefully inspected for abrasions and lacerations. If there is active bleeding but the source is not apparent, attention must be directed toward the fornices, which are frequently difficult to inspect adequately. Significant bleeding from cervical trauma is uncommon; therefore, vaginal lacerations should not be ruled out until these areas have been thoroughly visualized, even if general anesthesia is required to do so. With a speculum in place the necessary specimens, as described below, should be obtained.

This part of the examination may be difficult or impossible to perform when dealing with a child. It is particularly important that the genitalia of the child be inspected, for they are predisposed to significant trauma because of their incomplete physical development. General anesthesia is frequently desirable in order to avoid the physical and psychological trauma involved. A vaginoscope may be useful in the examination of the vagina.

The laboratory investigations which should be carried out are outlined in Table 11.3. The tests are directed toward the identification of spermatozoa, determination of the presence of acid phosphatase, and identification of ABH factors in the collected fluid.

Identification of Spermatozoa. A wet mount of vaginal fluid should be examined to determine the presence or absence of spermatozoa and , if present, their motility. Sperm may maintain motility for a period ranging from 30 minutes to 28 hours.

The presence of motile sperm implies recent sexual contact, although not necessarily with the alleged offender, within the previous 28 hours. The presence of nonmotile sperm has little significance, since the duration of motility may be variable in the spermatozoa of some males while others produce ejaculates with no motile spermatozoa. Nonmotile sperm may be found in a favorable, moist environment, such as the vagina, for as long as 48 hours. Spermatozoa dried on the surface of the body, pubic hair, or clothing lose their motility immediately, although they may be identified many hours after deposition.

The absence of spermatozoa in the vaginal fluid does not prove that the observed fluid is not seminal in origin. Some men are azospermic or oligospermic because of congenital testicular malfunction or testicular injury, as from mumps orchitis. In addition, approximately 450,000 vasectomies are performed annually in the United States.[13] All such ejaculates do, however, contain acid phosphatase.

The extremely uncommon and improbable possibility that the assailant used a condom must be considered. Coitus also may have been interrupted prior to ejaculation because of the victim's efforts, discovery by a third party, or the use of coitus interruptus.

Specimens for examination for sperm should be obtained from the introitus, in the presence of an intact hymen, or from the vaginal pool when accessible. Aspirated fluid should be placed on a slide, covered with a cover slip, and examined immediately for motility by the evaluating physician. A smear should be made of the aspirate, fixed by using a spray fixative of 95% alcohol, and sent for cytologic evaluation, specifically requesting an examination for sperm. The specimen should also be evaluated for cellular atypia. Another smear is made of the aspirate, air dried, and sent to the laboratory with a request for hematoxylin and eosin, gram, or fluorochrome staining for the presence of spermatozoa.

An endocervical specimen is obtained, by cotton-tipped applicator, and innoculated into an appropriate medium, such as a Thayer-Martin medium, for culture for *Neisseria gonorrhea*. Cultures for gonorrhea should also be obtained from the rectum.

Acid Phosphatase Determination. An aspirate from the vagina, of at least 1 ml of fluid, is submitted for evaluation of acid phosphatase. This enzyme is not unique to semen, for it has been found in blood, urine, normal vaginal fluid, all tissues of the human body, meat gravy, beet juice, mayonnaise, and a variety of other food products. The most relevant factor is not the presence of acid phosphatase, but its quantity. A fresh ejaculate contains between 400 and 8,000 King-Armstrong units per ml. This is measurable for at least 12 hours, but probably less than 24 hours after ejaculation. Determination of deposition of semen, using the acid phosphatase tests, has been performed with success on the victim's clothing as long as 6

TABLE 11.3
Rape, Summary of Suggested Laboratory Evaluations

Blood
    Complete blood count
    Serology, repeated in 4 weeks if negative
    Beta subunit human chorionic gonadotropin until positive or menstruation begins; if negative, weekly
Urine
    Urinalysis
    Pregnancy test; if negative, weekly
Vaginal aspirate
    Air-dried smear for hematoxylin and eosin, gram, or fluorochrome stain for sperm
    Fixed smear for cytology and sperm
    Wet mount for sperm and motility
    Acid phosphatase
    ABH antigen
    Culture for *Neisseria gonorrhea*, repeated in 4 weeks if negative
Other
    Appropriate color photographs
    Hair combed from perineal and pubic areas, all clothing, debris from beneath fingernails to police
    Dried secretions on hair and scraped from skin for acid phosphatase and ABH antigen
    Segments of stained clothing for acid phosphatase and ABH antigen

months after the assault. Activity of 20 or more King-Armstrong units per ml is considered positive for semen.

Hair apparently encrusted with dried semen and dried secretions scraped from skin and clothing should also be submitted to the laboratory, without fixation or alteration. Acid phosphatase can be eluted and identified from these encrustations.

ABH Secretion Detection. Some individuals, called "secretors," have detectable levels of A, B, or H agglutinogen in their seminal and other body fluids. Any material suspected of representing dried semen and an aspirate of vaginal fluid or fluid obtained by lavaging the vagina with 1 ml of normal saline are sent for laboratory evaluation. Only 0.25 square inch of cloth or 1 square mm of encrusted material is required to perform this test. All clothing should be submitted for police evaluation after representative sections have been removed for analysis for sperm and ABH typing.

These specimens are evaluated against the victim and suitable positive controls whose sputa are tested on clean white paper toweling. The procedure is an absorption-inhibition test and readily detects the blood type in approximately 80% of secretory specimens, such as semen, urine, saliva, and sweat.[14] The reaction weakens as specimens become older, and the validity of this test may be lost with time.

The form illustrated in Figure 11.2 is completed in its entirety, in triplicate. One copy is submitted to police authorities, one copy enters the patient's hospital file, and the original is retained by the physician for future reference.

Photography. Obtaining relevant color photographs of physical findings may be essential. All clothing disarray, injuries, and encrusted secretions should be photographed. This serves as a reminder to the physician of critical findings and is more explicit than the written report when the necessity arises to present this information in court. Photographs are retained in the patient's file and transferred, on request, to appropriate authorities.

Transfer of Evidence

It is mandatory that the physician personally transfer all laboratory specimens and clothing obtained to a responsible technician, obtaining signed receipts for all material submitted. If the chain of transfer is not documented and completed by responsible individuals, the prosecuting attorney may find difficulty in presenting any information as evidence.

Preventive Therapy

Having stabilized the patient, performed the examination and recorded the results, the physician directs his or her efforts toward preventive therapy. Basically three problems are encountered: (1) venereal disease, (2) pregnancy, and (3) psychologic sequelae.

Venereal Disease. Initial tests should include cervical and rectal cultures for gonorrhea and a serologic test for syphilis. The test for syphilis should be repeated on appearance of a genital lesion or 4 weeks later. In a recent study of 2,190 alleged female victims of rape, 82 patients were found to have contracted a venereal disease. This included 76 cases of gonorrhea, 5 cases of syphilis, and 1 case of lymphogranuloma venereum.

It is generally recommended that prophylaxis against venereal disease be administered. Probenecid, 1 g, is taken orally and simultaneously 2.4 million units of benzathine penicillin G or an appropriate age-adjusted dose are administered. In a penicillin-sensitive patient, tetracycline, 500 mg orally, 4 times daily for 15 days is an appropriate alternative.

Pregnancy. In the study of 2,190 patients evaluated for rape noted above, 13 conceived as a result of the sexual assault. It is particularly important to obtain a pregnancy test at the time of initial evaluation, because the differentiation between pregnancy resulting from and not resulting from the rape is of critical importance. Therapeutic abortion can be used to terminate a pregnancy resulting from rape, but it is preferable to prevent a pregnancy. Effective regimens for postcoital contraception (interception) have included stilbestrol, 5 mg orally, daily for 25 days if the sexual assault occurred in the follicular phase of the menstrual cycle, or stilbestrol, 25 mg orally, daily for 5 days if the rape occurred near the time of ovulation. Medroxyprogesterone acetate, 100 mg intramuscularly as a single dose, and conjugated equine estrogenic substances, 40 mg intravenously as a single dose, have proved effective.

Considerable nausea is experienced with the use of stilbestrol. There are fewer side effects with the injection of medroxyprogesterone acetate or conjugated equine estrogens. A single parenteral dose of medication eliminates the major factor which causes failure of postcoital contraception, namely, lack of patient reliability. Failure to complete a course of oral interception is usually related to the various side effects, such as anorexia, nausea, and vomiting; or it may occur because of forgetfulness or because of the advice of a third party.

Because of the correlation between in utero exposure to nonsteroidal estrogenic substances and adenosis and mesonephric adenocarcinoma of the vagina, some physicians have hesitated to use stilbestrol. If pregnancy is not prevented and the patient refuses abortion, there may be concern for the female offspring. No nonsteroidal estrogen-exposed females have developed vaginal adenocarcinoma if exposure occurred in the first 4 weeks of pregnancy, so this factor should be of little relevance in choosing the form of postcoital contraception.

The most sensitive mean of following a patient for pregnancy is the determination of plasma or serum Beta subunit human chorionic gonadotropin (BS-HCG) level. This gonadotropin can be detected 9 to 10 days after fertilization of the ovum. Accordingly, if uterine bleeding does not occur within 1 week of completion of postcoital contraception, a plasma or serum BS-HCG should be performed. If this is negative, it should be performed on a weekly basis until it becomes positive or until menstrual bleeding occurs. Menstrual extraction or dilatation and evacuation should be performed if the BS-HCG determination becomes positive.

Postcoital contraception should be instituted as soon after sexual exposure as possible, preferably within 72 hours. If a patient presents more than 3 days after the assault, a suitable form of post coital contraception can be offered, even though its value is questionable at that time.

It should be emphasized to all patients that postcoital contraception is not effective in all women and that pregnancy may ensue. This encourages the patient to submit to close followup, so that a pregnancy may be detected and terminated as soon as possible.

Successful interception has been obtained with the immediate insertion, at the time of physical examination, of an intrauterine device. Relatively few patients have been evaluated with this form of postcoital contraception, but it may be an appropriate approach in certain situations, particularly if the use of estrogens is contraindicated.

Psychologic Sequelae. A description of the psychologic reactions of the rape victim to the sexual assault is beyond the scope and intent of this article. It should be noted, however, that such complications may arise at any time, from the moment of the experience to years later. The psychologic sequelae manifest themselves in many phases of the patient's behavior.

Many victims have sought expert assistance, prior to medical evaluation, from professional or paraprofessional organizations, such as Women Organized Against Rape (WOAR) and rape crisis centers (RCC). These specialists generally accompany the patient and are of great assistance to her during medical examinations and police interrogation. They lend emotional support at this time, when most needed, and can serve as a single individual continuously available throughout the emotionally and physically exhausting evaluative process.

They perform immediate postevaluation counseling and initiate an ongoing relationship with the victim, consisting of telephone calls and visits over the succeeding months. These meetings provide opportunities for the patient to re-enact the traumatic episode with an understanding, objective individual who will not reflect anxiety or a judgmental attitude. The objectives are to assist the patient in converting feelings of guilt and shame to "healthy anger," to convey empathy (not sympathy), and to assist the patient in understanding, correctly interpreting, and dealing with the numerous extreme emotional responses which she is experiencing.[2]

For an indefinite period after the rape experience, victims benefit from organized group discussions in which they can share their ongoing feelings and responses with others who have had similar experiences. This opportunity is provided by several organizations and rape crisis centers.

Basically, there are three phases of reaction to rape. The first, lasting several days or weeks, is the acute reaction, in which the patient has difficulty expressing her feelings about or describing the assault. Any reminder of the event may result in a great emotional outpouring. Shock and dismay are usually replaced by marked anxiety.

Recollection of the experience may create such extremes in affect and behavior that the patient may become totally nonfunctional in everyday activities. She suffers from feelings of shame and self-recrimination and from fear of the reactions of others toward her. She is also fearful of the physical sequelae, such as venereal disease and pregnancy.

The second phase, in which the acute anxiety reactions have been resolved and the patient returns to normal daily function, represents one of "pseudo-adjustment." Anxiety in this phase, is managed by denial, repression, and rationalization.[2] The victim becomes able to deal with the event by displacing blame to fate or to the psychopathology of the perpetrator. The patient frequently withdraws from group sessions and therapeutic efforts.

In the third phase, patients become depressed by recollections of the rape event. At this time, the patient is attempting to resolve her feelings about the assault, and may require extensive counseling in order to achieve this.

Psychologic problems are more complex and intense in victims in the pediatric age range. During the initial evaluation and interview, attempts to obtain relevant information may be difficult because of the patient's severe anxiety and her inability to communicate in clear, understandable terminology. It is essential that the physician display a respect for the patient and a sincere interest in her feelings. In addition, the examiner must communicate in a manner which she understands and, in turn, attempt to understand the meaning of the words which she uses in describing the event.

Parents of assaulted children generally display considerable anxiety about the psychologic and physical well-being of the child. They express this in a forceful, demanding behavior toward attending personnel and other forms of behavior often somewhat detrimental to the well-being of the assaulted child.[15] Basically, the parents' reaction is one of anger, guilt, and helplessness.

SUMMARY

The physician plays an important part in the evaluation and management of alleged victims of rape. It is his or her responsibility to treat life-threatening injuries, accurately record data required for conviction or acquittal of the suspected sexual assailant, protect the patient from disease and pregnancy, establish contact with and transfer relevant data to authorities and attorneys, provide contact for the patient with counseling organizations for continued psychologic evaluation and therapy, and, on occasion, testify in court as to his or her findings on interview and examination.

An organized approach to the procurement of laboratory specimens, to the examination of the assault victim, and to the completion of an accurate written documentation of findings are mandatory. Above all, the examining physician must remain objective and supportive in his evaluation and dealings with the alleged victims of rape.

REFERENCES

1. Webster's New Collegiate Dictionary, 1973 Edition, G & C Merriam, Springfield, Mass.
2. Wasserman, M, Rape: Breaking the Silence, Progressive, 37:19, 1973.
3. Zussman, S, Treatment of the Victim of Rape. B. Psychological and Legal Aspects: The Woman's Point of View, Abstract, In Wilson, RA, and Craver, BN, eds, Clinical Uses of the Female Sex Hormones and Early Diagnosis of Treatment of Mammary Cancer, Int Cong Ser, Excerpta Medica, Amsterdam, 1971.
4. Sutherland, S, and Scherl, DJ, Patterns of Response Among Victims of Rape, Am J Orthopsychiat, 40:503, 1970.
5. Jungblut, JJ, The Challenge of Crimes in a Free Society, President's Commission on Law Enforcement and Administration of Justice, U.S. Government Printing Office, Washington, 1967.
6. Schiff, AF, Rape in Other Countries, Med Sci Law 11:139, 1971.
7. Perr, IN, Statutory Rape of an Insane Person, J Forensic Sci 13:433, 1968.
8. Schiff, A. F.: Statistical Features of Rape, J Forensic Sci 14:102, 1969.
9. Hayman, CR, Lanza, C, Fuentes, R and Algor, K, Rape in the District of Columbia, Am J Obstet Gynecol 113:91, 1972.
10. Schiff, AF, Examining the Sexual Assault Victim, J Florida Med Assoc 56:731, 1969.
11. Breen, JL, Greenwald, E, and Gregori, CA, The Molested Young Female—Evaluation & Therapy of Alleged Rape, Ped Clin North Am 19:717, 1972.

12. Burgess, AW, Holmstrom, LL, The Rape Victim in the Emergency Ward, Am J Nurs *73:*1741, 1973.

13. Schiff, AF, Modification of the Berg Acid Phosphatase Test, J Forensic Sci *14:*538, 1969.

14. Procedure for Handling and Obtaining of Specimens for Alleged Rape Cases, Department of Pathology, St. Barnabas Medical Center, Livingston, NJ.

15. Lipton, GL, and Roth, EL, Rape: A Complex Management Problem in the Pediatric Emergency Room, J Ped *75:*859, 1969.

12

DYSPAREUNIA

MICHAEL J. DALY, M.D.

More frequently today than in the past, physicians are confronted by patients with the problem of painful intercourse or dyspareunia. More open discussion of sexual problems in our culture and greater expectation for sexual fulfillment have brought about this change. Unfortunately, many practicing clinicians have difficulty in managing the patient whose chief complaint is dyspareunia. It is also unfortunate that many physicians have received inadequate training in the medical aspects of human sexuality.[1]

Dyspareunia is a disruptive symptom to most women and their partners. It can totally destroy their relationships, as well as their ability to achieve fulfillment in their sexual lives.[2] It is, therefore, a symptom that the physician should not pass over lightly. By recognizing its importance, the doctor will be in a position to ascertain its etiology and to find appropriate measures for its management. The importance of taking an adequate sexual history cannot be overemphasized.[3] Not only is this important for patients who openly express their symptoms, but also for those patients who are more reserved in expressing their problems.

By one estimate, dyspareunia occurs in approximately 10% of women patients.[4] Townsend[5] found that it occurred in 20% of his patients, while Masters and Johnson[6] state that 8% of women who are sexually dysfunctional report painful intercourse. In practice, dyspareunia often coexists with vaginismus, and the two have similar causative origins. Vaginismus is an involuntary spasm of the pelvic musculature and lower third of the vagina. This spasm makes penile entry difficult, if not impossible, and there are cases in which it has prevented a marriage from being consummated. It often eventuates in the husband's impotence.

ETIOLOGY

When dyspareunia and vaginismus are psychogenic, the background factors are similar to those for frigidity. Pain in coitus and subsequent spasm are often a result of lack of vaginal lubrication. This lubrication should occur on initial sexual stimulation of the woman, and its absence is to be expected when there is a total inhibition of erotic activity as a consequence of intense guilt, anxiety, or fear associated with the sexual act. When symptoms have been manifested from the first attempt at intercourse, one is dealing with psychodynamic factors identical to those in primary orgasmic dysfunction, although they are often more intense in these disorders. On the other hand, if these symptoms appear in women who were previously orgasmic in coitus, one must consider the situational factors in the present milieu. Obviously, organic disease can produce similar symptoms in both of these problems. In the absence of any obvious traumatic experiences such as rape or beating by a male, there would be a strong presumption that a somatic problem has intervened and is accounting for the painful intercourse. A thorough gynecologic examination is always indicated.

The types of somatic pathology that may be involved in cases of dyspareunia and vaginismus are manifold. They include: disorders of the vaginal outlet, such as (1) an intact hymen or irritated hymeneal remnants, (2) painful scars, either traumatic or postepisiotomy, (3) infections of the Bartholin glands, (4) clitoral disorders, or (5) irritations or trauma; disorders of the vagina, such as (1) infectious vaginitis, (2) allergic reactions to douches, creams, jellies, or the latex in condoms or diaphragms, (3) senile vaginitis, (4) radiation vaginitis, (5) painful scarring of the roof of the vagina after a hysterectomy; and disorders of the pelvis, such as infections, endometriosis, tumors, or cysts. Occasionally after hysterectomy or genital tract surgery a transitory vaginismus can occur. This is not due to any somatic factor, but to the woman's anxiety that she may be hurt by coitus. A physician's reassurance to these patients concerning their sexuality usually overcomes this problem.

Etiologic factors, therefore, can be organic, psychosomatic, or a combination of both.

Organic Factors

Green-Armytage[7] found imperforate hymens in 5% of women who were unable to consummate their marriages. Patients with testicular feminization syndrome or other congenital abnormalities may not have a vagina or may have only a vaginal pouch. Obviously these conditions lead to mechanical obstruction and can produce severe dyspareunia. Other abnormalities, such as double vagina, can also produce dyspareunia and these can be treated surgically.

Another possible cause of dyspareunia is retroversion of the uterus. On deep penetration the penis can dislodge the uterus by pulling on the uterosacral ligaments, thus producing pain. The pain occurs on deep penetration or during coitus with the woman's legs elevated. This can usually be treated by simply instructing the male not to penetrate too deeply and by changing coital positions.

Vaginitis due to trichomonas or *Candida albicans* and local infections secondary to herpes and nonspecific vaginitis can produce a great deal of discomfort during coitus. Acute genital tract gonorrhea will also produce the same symptom, as will the presence of venereal warts in the vagina. Lymphopathia venereum and granuloma inguinale are rare, chronic types of venereal disease that can produce dyspareunia secondary to scar tissue. Obviously, examination will lead the physician to the appropriate diagnosis. Endometriosis is not an uncommon factor in producing dyspareunia. The history will reveal that the pain is noted usually on deep penetration and is worse just prior to the onset of menstruation. Pelvic examination will reveal nodules in the cul-de-sac or on the uterosacral ligaments. This diagnosis can be confirmed by laparoscopy, and therapy with progestins instituted. Occasionally surgical removal of the implants will be required. Pregnancy in these patients often alleviates the pain of endometriosis.

Atrophic vaginitis is becoming an increasing problem as women live longer and develop new expectations for sexual fulfillment in the later years.[8] Diagnosis can be made by inspection of the vagina and examination of a vaginal smear. Therapy can be instituted either with oral estrogen or estrogens applied locally in a vaginal cream.[9]

Post-operative Dyspareunia. Occasionally inappropriate scarring, secondary to episiotomy or an episiotomy that became infected, will produce pain during intercourse. This is usually present during initial penetration. Careful history and physical examination will confirm the diagnosis. One must be careful in prescribing operative removal of scars in these patients. The scar tissue may not be the true source of the symptom, particularly in a patient who has strong emotional problems.[10, 11] Rectal operations also can produce scar tissue that may cause dyspareunia. Occasionally a patient who has undergone radical pelvic surgery for malignancy in which a large portion of the vagina has been removed will develop coital pain. It should be remembered that even when most of the vagina is removed, patients may be able to have normal coitus as a new vagina will develop. Occasionally estrogens may be needed in these patients as well as vaginal dilations during their postoperative management.

Abitbol and Davenport[12] have demonstrated that dyspareunia is less apt to develop after radical surgery for pelvic cancer than when radiation is the mode of therapy. Patients who have had exenterations performed for advanced cancer of the pelvis may develop coital pain because of the presence of scar tissue. Reconstruction of a vaginal barrel may be helpful.

Radiation. Patients who have received radiation for pelvic malignancy, usually for carcinoma of the cervix, not infrequently develop dyspareunia. This may be prevented or alleviated in most patients. Our management has been to first allay the woman's fears that intercourse will bring about a recurrence of her cancer or subject her sexual partner to malignancy. This reassurance includes a discussion of her sexuality and her image of herself as a sexual person. She needs to feel that she is capable of performing in a normal sexual way, that she is still sexually attractive, and that normal sexual function is still attainable. Many of these women avoid sexual activity out of fear or shame. This inhibition of sexual behavior accounts for the development of vaginal constriction so that when coitus is attempted pain is experienced. We place these patients on estrogen, either 1.25 or 0.625 mg of Premarin, for 25 days per month. And, finally, we encourage coitus in a frank discussion with the partner when this is feasible.

Tumors of the pelvis may produce pain on intercourse as an early symptom. These usually are ovarian cysts caught deep in the cul-de-sac or myomata. An adequate pelvic examination should reveal these tumors. If normal pelvic structures are palpated and if there are no abnormal masses, needless surgery, such as exploratory laparotomy, should not be recommended. Rather, the etiological alternatives should be explored. If these prove to be negative, diagnostic laparoscopy may be warranted to uncover pelvic pathology.

Occasionally urethritis or cystitis will cause coital discomfort. These conditions are often associated with other genitourinary complaints such as frequency or burning on urination. Examination of the urine, including culture, will usually confirm the diagnosis. If these symptoms recur the patient warrants a complete urological evaluation including an intravenous pyelogram, cystoscopy, and urethroscopy.

Psychosomatic Factors

Pain on intercourse may be primarily a somatic response to an emotional state as well as being secondary to organic disease. These emotional states are usually related to fear, anxiety, guilt, and even, on occasion, hostility. It has also been suggested that this emotional response could very well be secondary to, or in concert with, organic disease. But it must be recognized that dyspareunia may be primarily psychological in origin.[13]

A number of women who complain of dyspareunia will be found to have inadequate preparation for coitus. The work of Masters and Johnson,[14] in describing the normal physiologic response of the vagina as well as other body changes, has been an immeasurable help in our understanding of human sexuality. If the proper milieu, both emotional and physical, is not present for a woman prior to intercourse, pain may result. The initial response of the normal vagina to adequate sexual stimulation, without emotional roadblocks such as fear, anxiety, guilt, or hostility, is wetness of the vaginal barrel. This lubrication of the vagina is the result of a diaphoresis from the blood vessels surrounding the vagina. If this initial response to sexual stimulation does not occur penetration by the penis will produce discomfort. This can result further in the woman's responding with contractions of the levator muscles, thus producing vaginismus. One can readily understand how this can become a vicious cycle, producing more pain, not only because of lack of lubrication, but also because of the contractions of the pelvic floor muscles. Often the sexual partner either is inept in his approach or lacks understanding of the emotional component of human sexuality.

Commonly there is a breakdown in communication between the male and the female on both a verbal and a feeling level, especially as these feelings relate to their sexuality. The misconception that many males have concerning their total responsibility for the female's sexual pleasure still exists in our society. A more appropriate concept is that the woman must learn to take her sexual pleasure and teach the male what pleases her.

TREATMENT OF PSYCHOGENIC DYSPAREUNIA AND RELATED VAGINISMUS

The treatment of dyspareunia of psychogenic origin requires an appropriate doctor-patient relationship which will allow for free communication between therapist and patient. In this way an adequate history can be obtained to uncover the underlying emotional conflict, so that an appropriate strategy of therapy can be developed.

The Doctor-Patient Relationship

The relationship between physicians and their patients depends on a number of factors, including the attitudes, the behavior patterns, and priorities of the physician as well as his or her personality. The patient's needs will reflect her cultural, social, and psychological background. The patient's emotional stability and learned responses will influence attitudes and behavior towards the physician.

It is important for the therapist to adopt a nonjudgmental attitude toward the patient. This does not require that the physician change his or her own moral beliefs relative to sexual attitudes, but rather that the doctor be noncommittal concerning those sexual practices of the patient's that may differ from his or her own, as long as they are not destructive to the patient. Within this milieu, the patient can develop the necessary trust in the therapist. The patient's early experiences with authority figures, such as parents and teachers, can act as a negative or positive influence on the degree of trust. It is of prime importance that the physician never tarnish this response. The establishment of an adequate history can require a number of visits while this transference is developing. The history should not only uncover the physical symptoms, but also how the patient feels about her symptoms, about her partner, and about other significant people. The quality of the sexual relationship as well as the expectations of both partners should be learned. This requires the involvement of the male partner. It is almost always helpful to see the couple together, so that interaction between the two can be observed. An overdependent relationship should be noted, and any hostility, anxiety, or guilt feelings between the two partners should be identified and dealt with. Each partner may be seen separately at a subsequent visit, so that the physician can deal with underlying fears that are painful to express in the presence of the partner. Naturally, the history of frequency of sexual desire and experiences should be obtained, but this is of far less importance than the degree of fulfillment, pleasure, or needs. Alternate sexual outlets, such as masturbation or homosexual experiences, also need to be discussed.

The diagnosis of a psychosomatic disorder is made on positive findings, not on exclusion of organic disease. Positive findings include the uncovering of a conflict, such as a wish for sexual fulfillment versus a fear of sexual injury, or anxiety or guilt relative to sexual behavior. The patient who does not wish sexual expression or fulfillment will not ordinarily complain of dyspareunia. It is the uncovering of this anxiety, fear, guilt, or hostility toward the sexual partner or the projection of emotional problems related to previous sexual traumas onto the present sexual partner that may be at the root of psychosomatic elements of dyspareunia. The primary principle involved in the psychotherapy of patients with dyspareunia is that this is a symptom of underlying emotional conflicts concerning sexuality. Many strategies of treatment have been successful,[15-19] including behavioral therapy, psychotherapy, and psychoanalysis, and each is effective when the proper patient choice is made. Psychoanalysis, which is a long term intensive therapy, should be used only for individuals attracted to the idea of gaining insight and understanding of their total psychic life. O'Connor and Stern[20] found a 77% improvement rate in 96 cases of functional sexual disorders treated by psychoanalysis. Behavioral therapists have reported higher cure rates using relaxation and desensitization techniques. Sufficient data in a large group of patients treated by behavioral therapy are not yet available. A combination of therapy methods—-behavioral therapy, psychotherapy, and psychoanalysis—can be used flexibly in the same case. Many of these techniques have been combined in the development of a so-called new sex therapy.

This combined sex therapy concept of treating sexual dysfunction by focusing on altering behavior is not new. This is really a combination of behavioral therapy, psychotherapy, conjoint therapy, and marriage counseling. This can be effective using a single therapist or (in conjunction with) co-therapists. When co-therapists are used, one should ordinarily be a man and the other a woman. The sexual unit, in which both partners are involved in the therapy sessions and responsible for the outcome, is an important concept even though the sexual problem may be present as a symptom of only one partner. It is difficult to treat a sexual problem, whether it be in a woman or a man, without also getting the involvement and the commitment of the other partner.

The principle of sensate focus promulgated by Masters and Johnson is also of prime importance. This allows the patient to become aware of his or her sexuality. This is accomplished by increasing the awareness of body image and touch. The couple is placed in a nondemanding situation in which they learn to appreciate the pleasure of the sensations of touch, vision, smell, and sound. They learn to communicate what pleases and displeases them. Intercourse is prohibited at this time to help in focusing attention on the body's total sexual response and to remove the pressure for performance. In addition, communication is encouraged. The principles of communication, both verbal and nonverbal, are developed by each partner so that there is a realization of the erotic body areas, including the skin, mouth, ears, breasts, and, finally, the genitals. At different times one partner may be the recipient and the other the giver, with roles being reversed when appropriate. And, finally, the removal of stress is essential. It is important that neither partner be placed in a stressful position. The couple are reassured that their bodies are functioning properly and that the pleasure of coital union is a natural process that can be blocked by the processes of the mind. Too much thought about performance, and the injury to self-esteem which occurs when there is failure, is presented as a major problem. Partners are alerted to be aware of the anxiety and worry that act as blocking agents to the pleasure of their sexual experience. These feelings must be dispelled before the problem is solved.

A more simplified approach to the treatment of dyspareunia, in which the woman learns from the therapist about her genital function, has also been successful. She develops an awareness of her vagina by being instructed first to touch herself externally and then by using vaginal bougies of increasing size. She learns to insert the bougies up to a size equivalent to the size of the male penis. This is a behavioral approach in which desensitization takes place as she becomes aware of lack of vaginal pain on insertion, primarily because of her ability to control the situation. There is also an intellectual learning experience in this process. For some women, without deep-seated emotional problems relative to their dyspareunia, this may be a helpful form of therapy.

In those women who have a great deal of hostility toward the male, or in those women who have undue amounts of guilt or anxiety, more frequent sessions dealing with the emotional component of sexual feelings are required. The physician who feels comfortable in dealing with these problems can be quite successful in the management of such a woman and her partner. Frequently, however, these patients will require referral to a psychiatrist or psychologist. On the other hand, only a small percentage of women whose chief complaint is dyspareunia will require psychiatric referral. The interested physician who undertakes the care of these patients in a comprehensive manner will usually be rewarded with successful results and a well cared for patient.

REFERENCES

1. Daly, MJ, The Physician's Role in Human Sexuality of the Future, South Med J *65:*1475, 1972.
2. Weiner, MF, Wives Who Refuse Their Husbands, Psychosomatics *XIV:*277, 1973.
3. Chez, R, Obtaining the Sexual History in the Female Patient, Am Acad Gen Pract *30:*123, 1964.
4. Jeffcoate, TNA, *Principles of Gynecology*, 2nd ed, Butterworth, London, 1962.
5. Townsend, L, *Gynecology for Students*, 2nd ed, Melbourne University Press, Carleton, p. 172, 1966.
6. Masters, WH, and Johnson, VE, *Human Sexual Inadequacy*, Little, Brown, Boston, 1970.
7. Green-Armytage, VB, Dyspareunia, Brit Med J *1:*1238, 1956.
8. Daly, MJ, and Winn, H, The Change of Life in Women, Geriatrics *26:*104, 1971.
9. Waxenberg, SE, Drellich, M, and Sutherland, H, The Role of Hormones in Human Behavior, J Clin Endocrinol *19:*193, 1959.
10. Rankin, J, The Use of Z-plasty in Gynecologic Operations, Am J Obstet Gynecol *117:*231, 1973.
11. Daly, MJ, Psychological Impact of Surgical Procedures on Women, in Freedman, AM, and Kaplan, HI, eds., *Comprehensive Textbook of Psychiatry*, 2nd ed., Williams & Wilkins, Baltimore, 1974.
12. Abitbol, MM, and Davenport, JN, Sexual Dysfunction after Therapy for Cervical Carcinoma, Am J Obstet Gynecol *119:*181, 1974.
13. Daly, MJ, Emotional Aspects of Obstetrics and Gynecology, J Mich State Med Soc *61:*1495, 1962.
14. Masters, WH, and Johnson, VE, *Human Sexual Inadequacy*, Little, Brown, Boston, 1970.
15. Kaplan, HS, *The New Sex Therapy*, Brunner/Mozel, New York, 1974.
16. Bandura, A, *Principles of Behavior Modification*, Holt, Rinehart and Winston, New York, 1969.
17. Ullman, LP, and Krasner, L, *A Psychological Approach to Abnormal Behavior*, 2nd ed, Prentice-Hall, Englewood Cliffs, NJ, 1975.
18. Hoch, KF, et al., Hypo-desensitization Therapy of Vaginismus, Int J Clin Exp Hypnosis *XXI:*144, 1973.
19. Annau, JS, The Therapeutic Use of Masturbation in the Treatment of Sexual Disorders, Adv Behav Ther *4:*199, 1973.
20. O'Connor, JF, and Stern, LO, Results of Treatment in Functional Sexual Disorders, NY State J Med *72:*1927, 1972.

13

HIRSUTISM AND DYSFUNCTIONAL UTERINE BLEEDING

WILLIAM R. KEYE, JR., M.D.

ROBERT B. JAFFE, M.D.

HIRSUTISM

Because abnormal endocrine function occurs in only a small number of individuals with excessive hair growth,[1] hirsutism is often primarily of cosmetic concern. The problems associated with excessive hair growth are often not medical but psychological, and result from personal, familial, and cultural attitudes.

However, excessive hair growth in a woman who has signs of defeminization or virilism may be a clue to a serious underlying medical disorder. Therefore, it is important in this group of patients to ascertain the cause of the excessive hair growth and to institute therapy when appropriate.

In this chapter we will present our approach to the differential diagnosis of hirsutism and the physiologic and clinical basis for this approach. In addition, we will describe the medical treatment of hirsutism.

Definition

There is a large degree of individual variation in hair growth in normal women, which is influenced by racial and familial factors. Thus it often may be difficult to determine whether, in fact, a woman has excessive hair growth. This situation is reflected by the varying definitions of hirsutism in recent reviews.

Muller[1] uses the term hirsutism interchangeably with hypertrichosis, which is defined as an abnormally excessive growth of hair. Leng and Greenblatt[2] use the term hirsutism to denote a condition of excessive growth of sexual hair, i.e. pubic, axillary, abdominal, chest, and facial hair. Finally, Karp and Herrmann[3] define the hirsute patient as any woman who complains of "too much hair."

While the differences in these definitions may be a source of confusion, each definition focuses on a different aspect of hirsutism, and each aspect should be considered when the physician is confronted with a hirsute patient.

Normal Hair Growth

While most hair growth is either dependent upon or influenced by androgens, the relation between hair growth and androgens is complex. Some hair (trunk, limb, upper pubis, beard, ears, and nasal tip) is dependent upon the high levels of circulating androgens which occur in adult males. The initiation of hair growth of the axilla and lower pubis, which typically appears at puberty in both sexes, requires androgens but can occur at lower levels. And, finally, lanugo hair and the hair of the eyebrows and eyelashes appear to be independent of androgens.[4]

Recent studies of androgen metabolism by isolated hairs have demonstrated that differential androgen responsiveness of different hair roots is not determined by differences in androgen metabolism.[5, 6] This suggests that differences must exist in the ability of the hair follicles to bind the androgens to intracellular receptors or to respond to the androgen-receptor complex.[5]

Although most reviews speak of hirsutism as an easily definable and clearly distinguishable state, there is no clear dividing line between normal and hirsute females. Most reviewers provide a conceptual definition of hirsutism as "excessive hair growth," without providing an operational definition, i.e. a set of criteria by which to judge whether or not an individual woman is hirsute.

The inability to provide an operational definition of hirsutism is the result of several factors. First, body hair growth is a graded characteristic. Second, the amount and distribution of hair growth is partially determined by racial factors. For example, Chinese women rarely have facial or body hair except in the pubic and axillary regions, while East Asian, Arctic, and Mongol women frequently have little or no pubic hair. Japanese women have much less axillary hair than American women. A great diversity exists even among Caucasians. Nordic groups have relatively less hair than descendants of Irish, English, Welsh, and Russian Jewish immigrants. Third, familial patterns of hair growth are not uncommon. A recent study by Lorenzo[7] demonstrated that the amount and distribution of hair was more similar among family members than between unrelated controls. And, finally, the amount and distribution of hair normally changes in the female from childhood until well after the menopause. An extensive study of 430 women from ages 15 to 74 demonstrated that adolescence is a period of increasing hair growth and that after age 45–54 hair tends to increase on the face and to disappear on the trunk and limbs.[8]

Androgen Metabolism

Only three of the naturally occurring androgens have been shown to have sufficient potency to stimulate and regulate hair growth in man. These are testosterone, androstenedione, and dehydroepiandrosterone.

Testosterone is produced in women by the ovaries, by the adrenal glands, and in peripheral tissues from precursor hormones. Peripheral conversion is the major source of testosterone.

While testosterone is the most potent androgenic hormone, it appears that the conversion of testosterone to dihydrotestosterone is an important event in its androgenic action. Dihydrotestosterone is 1½ to 3 times more potent than testosterone in some test systems.[11]

In women, 20% of circulating dihydrotestosterone is derived from the peripheral conversion of testosterone,[12] while most of the remainder is derived from androstenedione.[13] There is little evidence of secretion of dihydrotestosterone in normal women. It is further metabolized and excreted as androstanediol. The manner in which dihydrotestosterone acts at the cellular level to influence hair growth is currently under study.

Determining Excessive Hair Growth

In determining whether, in fact, a patient has hirsutism, the physician should determine first whether she is abnormal with respect to the amount and distribution of hair. If no abnormality exists (in the doctor's opinion), then the patient should be reassured and offered symptomatic (cosmetic) treatment to allow her to achieve a "normal" amount of hair (in the patient's opinion).

If the patient does have excessive hair growth the physician should determine whether this involves sexual (pubic, axillary, abdominal, chest, or facial) or nonsexual hair. The excessive growth of nonsexual hair may reflect congenital anomalies, side effects of medications, or underlying systemic disease. Obviously, these conditions should be diagnosed and treated.

Finally, investigations should be undertaken to determine the nature of abnormal endocrine function in women with excessive growth of sexual hair. Establishing the exact nature of the underlying endocrinopathy makes it possible to institute specific therapy.

Differential Diagnosis of Excessive Nonsexual Hair

As most women who present with the complaint of hirsutism will not have an underlying endocrinopathy, it is important for the clinician to be familiar with, and recognize, nonendocrine causes of hirsutism.

Hair growth which is viewed as excessive by the patient but which is of no medical significance may result from the racial or familial heritage of the individual. In addition, some women may be alarmed by the increase in body or facial hair which may accompany adolescence or the menopause. Some of these women may be satisfied with the explanation that their particular pattern of hair growth is normal for them. However, others will request advice regarding the removal of what they consider excessive amounts of hair, even though such hair is of no medical significance.

Extrinsic Factors. Repeated, prolonged, and severe trauma to the skin may result in localized areas of hirsutism. Common examples are the increased hair on an extremity seen after the removal of a cast[2] or in an area of skin of some mentally retarded patients who chew and bite their skin repeatedly.

Drug-induced hirsutism may develop as a side effect of either steroid or nonsteroid drugs. Reversible hirsutism may occur after several months of administration of diphenylhydantoin (Dilantin).[9] The excessive hair growth involves the extensor surfaces of the extremities and usually disappears within 1 year of the withdrawal of treatment. Increased hair growth on the face, trunk, and extremities occurs in some children who receive the antihypertensive hyperglycemic agent diazoxide. Hirsutism has also been reported following the ingestion of the fungicide hexachlorobenzene.[10] Steroidal drugs such as androgens, anabolic agents, and some C-19 progestogens may cause hirsutism and virilism by virtue of their androgenic properties.

Localized hirsutism has been reported in large nevi. While such localized hirsutism is not of itself medically significant, it may provide a clue to the presence of underlying conditions such as neurofibromatosis or abnormalities of the spinal column.

Differential Diagnosis of Excessive Sexual Hair

Hirsutism can reflect increased production of androgens by the ovaries and/or adrenal glands. The less frequent causes will be mentioned briefly.

Congenital Adrenal Hyperplasia. The virilizing forms of congenital adrenal hyperplasia represent mainly diseases of infancy and childhood, although a few such individuals remain undiagnosed until adulthood. Congenital adrenal hyperplasia results from an autosomal recessive inherited disorder in which there are specific deficits in steroid-hydroxylating enzyme activities. In the most common form, the 21-hydroxylase deficiency, there is reduced conversion of 17-hydroxyprogesterone to 11-deoxycortisol (compound S), and thus reduced formation of cortisol (Compound F) from 11-deoxycortisol. As a result, there is an accumulation of 17-hydroxyprogesterone which in turn is converted to Δ^4-androstenedione. Androstenedione may then be metabolized to testosterone. Excessive amounts of androstenedione and testosterone can virilize a female fetus, resulting in clitoral hypertrophy with or without ambiguous genitalia in the form of labial fusion and a urogenital sinus.

Adrenal Tumors. Hirsutism which results from adrenal adenomas or carcinomas is generally rapidly progressive and associated with virilization in the form of frontal balding, clitoromegaly, increased muscle size, and deepening of the voice.

Adrenal vein catheterization in patients with adrenal tumors has shown marked elevation of testosterone, androstenedione, and dehydroepiandrosterone.[11, 14, 15] Dehydroepiandrosterone sulfate is secreted in large amounts by these tumors, resulting in extremely high 17-ketosteroid excretion. A given tumor may produce normal amounts of one androgen and greatly increased amounts of others.

Recently, several patients have been reported who have testosterone-secreting adrenal tumors, at least one of which was felt to be under gonadotropin control.[16, 17]

Cushing's Syndrome. Hirsutism may also be seen in Cushing's syndrome secondary to adrenal hyperplasia when there is elevation of both 17-ketosteroids and 17-hydroxycorticosteroids. Excessive adrenocorticotropic hormone (ACTH), originating from either pituitary or nonpituitary tumors (carcinoma of the bronchus, thymus, pancreas, or thyroid) results in hypersecretion of both corticoids and androgens. The clinical picture reflects the increase in both of these groups of hormones, as hirsutism coexists with the classical features of Cushing's syndrome (truncal obesity, muscle wasting, moon facies, purple striae, hypertension, and weakness). Menstrual disorders appear late in the course of the disease, suggesting an adrenal rather than an ovarian source of the increased androgens.[3]

Ovarian Tumors. The presence of a virilizing ovarian tumor should be suspected in women who rapidly develop a marked degree of hirsutism associated with signs of virilization (deepening of the voice, clitoromegaly, temporal balding, and a masculine body configuration). There may or may not be a readily palpable adnexal mass.

Arrhenoblastoma. The most common of these rare tumors is the arrhenoblastoma, thought to arise either from undifferentiated hilus cells in the rete ovarii or as a teratomatous change. It occurs most often during the third and fourth decades, but is also found in adolescent women in association with either primary or secondary amenorrhea. Only two cases have been reported in women younger than 13 years.[18] Virilization rapidly disappears and normal menses return in most cases after surgical removal of the tumor.

Most women with arrhenoblastomas have serum testosterone levels in the male range, with normal or slightly increased urinary 17-ketosteroids. Analysis of ovarian vein blood in patients with arrhenoblastomas has shown testosterone to be the chief secretory product of the tumor,[19] although large amounts of dehydroepiandrosterone and androstenedione may occasionally be secreted. Arrhenoblastomas have been reported coexisting with adrenal androgenic hyperfunction, polycystic changes of the ovary, and a mucinous cystadenoma. The coexistence of these lesions can make the diagnosis of the tumor difficult if too much reliance is placed on suppression and stimulation studies of the adrenal gland.

A small number of arrhenoblastomas have been reported to have components of a granulosa cell carcinoma and are referred to as gynadroblastomas. While the clinical features are primarily those of masculinization, the presence of endometrial hyperplasia with excessive uterine bleeding reflects increased estrogen production, perhaps by peripheral conversion of androgens to estrogens.

Lipoid Cell Tumor. Slightly more than 100 lipoid cell tumors of the ovary have been reported. These tumors have also been referred to as hypernephroma, luteoma, masculinovoblastoma, adrenal rest tumor, or any of the 19 other synonyms. They are thought to arise either from adrenal rests or ovarian stroma. These tumors may produce androgens, both androgens and estrogens, or they may be nonfunctioning.[20] In addition to virilizing features, women with this tumor frequently display clinical features of Cushing's syndrome, although plasma and urinary cortisol levels are normal.

Hilus Cell Tumor. This rare tumor is thought to originate from cells that are homologous to the interstitial or Leydig cells of the testes. These tumors are usually small (less than 5 cm), unilateral, virilizing, and benign, although at least two cases with metastatic disease have been reported. They also have been reported in association with pure gonadal dysgenesis.

Polycystic Ovary Syndrome. Although much of the preceding discussion, and much of the diagnostic workup of the hirsute patient, is concerned with relatively rare syndromes and tumors, the greatest number of hirsute patients who have a demonstrable cause of their hirsutism will suffer from a variant of the polycystic ovary syndrome.

The classical form, the Stein-Leventhal syndrome, is characterized by infertility, oligo- or amenorrhea, obesity, and hirsutism, associated with bilateral ovarian enlargement. Essential to the diagnosis is the presence of a thickened ovarian capsule, often pearly gray or oyster white in color, below which are numerous follicles in various stages of development, but an absence of corpora lutea. Since the description by Stein and Leventhal in 1935,[21] a similar histologic appearance has been seen in hirsute women whose ovaries are not enlarged or in association with other ovarian or adrenal disorders (Cushing's syndrome, hilus cell tumor, arrhenoblastoma, adrenal rest tumors, granulosa cell tumors, and benign cystic teratoma).[22]

Patients with polycystic ovary syndrome usually present with slowly progressive hirsutism which begins soon after menarche. These patients frequently do not establish regular menstrual cycles, but experience progressive oligomenorrhea or amenorrhea. While they are hirsute, and may be obese, they are also well feminized and do not appear virilized. There appears to be a familial occurrence of polycystic ovary syndrome, which may be inherited in a pattern consistent with autosomal dominance.

Although the pathogenesis of this syndrome is not clear, most patients have a recognizable profile of pituitary, adrenal, and ovarian hormones. A recent study by DeVane et al.[23] has shown significant elevations in circulating luteinizing hormone (LH), estrone, testosterone, androstenedione, and dehydroepiandrosterone sulfate in these patients. Serum follicle-stimulating hormone (FSH), estradiol, and dehydroepiandrosterone concentrations were not significantly elevated when compared to early follicular phase controls.

On the basis of sampling of the adrenal and ovarian vein blood, it appears that increased androgens may be the result of increased secretion by the adrenals or ovaries or the result of increased peripheral conversion.[24, 25]

In contrast to the detailed description of the histologic and hormonal alterations in the polycystic ovary syndrome is the relative lack of information regarding the etiology of this disorder. While it is clear that there are alterations in hypothalamic, pituitary, ovarian, and adrenal function, the site(s) at which the primary endocrine defect originates is yet to be determined.

Recent studies of gonadotropin responses to synthetic gonadotropin-releasing hormone (GnRH) have demonstrated that the pattern of elevated LH secretion and diminished FSH secretion is due to an alteration in pituitary response to hypothalamic stimulation.[26] However, it is unclear whether this is a primary defect in pituitary gonadotropin synthesis, storage, or secretion, whether it is secondary to a primary disorder of hypothalamic GnRH, or whether it merely reflects altered sex steroid secretion and the modulating effects of these steroids upon a normal hypothalamic-pituitary axis.

In vitro studies of androgen metabolism by ovarian wedges have suggested that the primary defect in polycystic ovary syndrome is a failure of ovarian enzymes. These enzymatic defects result in a decreased formation of estrogen from androgens and the accumulation of the androgens dehydroepiandrosterone and androstenedione. Greenblatt[27] has suggested that this failure in ovarian enzymes results when there is a depletion of enzymes secondary to chronic overstimulation by the persistently elevated levels of LH.

Finally, the adrenal cortex has been implicated as a source of excess androgen production in women with polycystic ovaries. This has been suggested by combined ovarian and adrenal vein catheterization in women with polycystic ovary syndrome.[25] A recent study by Polansky[28] has demonstrated that adrenal androgen production is probably not responsive to LH. This suggests that increased adrenal androgen secretion may be due to a primary biochemical lesion of the adrenal and not secondary to the chronically altered gonadotropin secretion by the pituitary.

In summary, the basic lesion in the polycystic ovary syndrome may be a specific biosynthetic abnormality in androgen metabolism and/or a dysfunction in the hypothalamic-pituitary-ovarian axis.

Hyperthecosis. Hyperthecosis is a pathologic process which produces a clinical picture similar to that seen in the polycystic ovary syndrome. It is characterized by obesity, hypertension, and an abnormal glucose tolerance. Clinically it overlaps with the polycystic ovary syndrome, although most subjects display virilism in addition to hirsutism. Histologically it is identified by the presence of nests of lutein cells within the ovarian stroma but apart from the walls of follicles. These features may coexist with those of the polycystic ovary syndrome,[29] although Givens et al.[30] have described a paucity of primordial, developing, and Graafian follicles which is in contradistinction to the normal population of primordial follicles in the polycystic ovary.[31]

The biochemical features of ovarian hyperthecosis also are similar to those of the polycystic ovary syndrome; normal or elevated serum LH, testosterone, and androstenedione; normal or slightly elevated urinary 17-ketosteroids (17-KS) and 17-hydroxycorticosteroids (17-OHCS); normal or low serum FSH; and elevated production rates of testosterone and androstenedione. The administration of dexamethasone results in the suppression of urinary 17-KS and 17-OHCS and the partial suppression of serum testosterone.[30] Ovarian vein catheterization studies have shown the ovaries to be the source of the increased amounts of testosterone in the peripheral plasma.[32]

While this syndrome has been considered by most to be a variation of the polycystic ovary syndrome, Farber et al. have urged its separation from the polycystic ovary syndrome, for these women do not respond to clomiphene citrate and only on occasion respond to ovarian wedge resection.[33] Unfortunately, the diagnosis is only suggested by clinical features (abnormal glucose tolerance, hypertension, and signs of virilism: clitoromegaly or frontal alopecia). Diagnosis can be made only by ovarian biopsy.

Wedge resection is the most effective form of therapy for anovulation, while bilateral oophorectomy may be necessary to remedy the progressive virilism.[32]

Genetic Disorders of Sexual Development. Hirsutism may also occur in phenotypic females with gonadal dysgenesis (streak ovaries), mixed gonadal dysgenesis (testes plus steak ovary), true hermaphroditism (ovary plus testes), or male pseudohermaphroditism (testes).

The term idiopathic hirsutism has been applied to women with hirsutism, some of whom may have oligomenorrhea and elevated serum testosterone concentrations of either adrenal or ovarian origin, but no demonstrable abnormality of these organs. Shuster has proposed that the primary defect in this disorder is an increase in the capacity of the skin to metabolize androgens, which results in secondary adrenal androgen overproduction.[34] He suggests that this syndrome be referred to as primary cutaneous virilism and defines it as a genetically determined condition of enhanced cutaneous metabolism of androgens.

Diagnostic Workup

A review of the literature reveals many elaborate, expensive, and time-consuming approaches to the diagnostic evaluation of patients with hirsutism. While these studies may be appropriate and necessary in some hirsute women, they are not necessary in most. The initial evaluation of these women can be simple, quick, and relatively inexpensive.

Fortunately, the polycystic ovary syndrome and idiopathic hirsutism account for most of the hirsutism seen by the gynecologist. The natural history of these disorders is quite characteristic: slowly progressive hirsutism beginning between the ages of 15 and 20 associated with oligomenorrhea or dysfunctional uterine bleeding. Therefore, when interviewing a hirsute patient, the physician should look for variations from this familiar history.

First, the age of the patient at the onset of hirsutism should be determined. The onset of hirsutism prior to definite signs of feminization at puberty suggests one of the disorders of sexual development, congenital adrenal hyperplasia, or an adrenal or ovarian tumor. On the other hand, the onset of hirsutism after the age of 30 is more consistent with an ovarian or adrenal tumor or Cushing's syndrome.

Next, the presence or absence of menses and the relationship between the development of hirsutism and the onset of menstrual irregularity should be determined. As Karp and Herrmann[3] have pointed out, menstrual difficultues occur late in the course of hirsutism due to adrenal causes (adrenal tumors or Cushing's syndrome) and earlier in the case of ovarian disorders. Hirsutism is associated with primary amenorrhea in true hermaphroditism, male pseudohermaphroditism, and in some cases of congenital adrenal hyperplasia or adrenal and ovarian tumors.

Third, the rate of development of hirsutism should be determined. It develops slowly in the polycystic ovary syndrome, but may be rapid in patients with ovarian or adrenal tumors.

During the physical examination, one should first determine the somatotype of the woman, looking for signs that reflect the amount of estrogen (female body contours and adult breast development) and androgen (increased muscle size, frontal balding, and increased laryngeal size) stimulation. Hirsute women with polycystic ovary syndrome rarely have signs of excessive androgen production other than hirsutism and acne. Therefore, hirsute women with frontal or occipital balding, clitoromegaly, masculine body habitus, or increased laryngeal size and deepening of the voice should make the physician very suspicious of an androgen-secreting tumor, hyperthecosis, or congenital adrenal hyperplasia.

Examination of the skin may reveal acne in any of these conditions, but thin skin and abdominal striae are typical in Cushing's syndrome.

The patient's height may also be a clue to the etiology of the hirsutism. Patients with congenital adrenal hyperplasia are often short (under 5 feet) because of premature epiphyseal closure resulting from exposure to increased amounts of androgens prior to puberty. Patients with mixed gonadal dysgenesis may also be short.

Clitoromegaly is rare in polycystic ovary syndrome; its presence suggests either an androgen-secreting tumor or one of the intersex disorders such as female pseudohermaphroditism (congenital adrenal hyperplasia), true hermaphroditism, mixed gonadal dysgenesis, or male pseudohermaphroditism. In the case of androgen-secreting tumors, the clitoromegaly develops after menarche, while clitoromegaly associated with an intersex disorder is present at birth and may be associated with other signs of external genital ambiguity (perineal urethra, labioscrotal fusion, or a urogenital sinus). Other findings, such as the absence of a uterus or the presence of a testis in an inguinal hernia, are diagnostic of male pseudohermaphroditism. Bilateral enlargement of the ovaries is most often seen with polycystic ovary syndrome or hyperthecosis, while unilateral ovarian enlargement may be the result of an ovarian androgen-secreting tumor.

Laboratory Evaluation

Laboratory evaluation of the hirsute female may take one of several forms, depending upon the results of the history and physical examination.

If the patient has an increase in growth of nonsexual hair without disordered menstruation, *no* studies of androgen metabolism are necessary. Likewise, patients with disorders of menstruation who do not have hirsutism or other signs of androgen excess do not need laboratory studies of androgen metabolism.

Since obesity is frequently associated with hirsutism, and patients with polycystic ovary syndrome, hyperthecosis ovarii, or a lipoid cell tumor may appear Cushingoid, it is often necessary to perform appropriate laboratory tests to rule out Cushing's syndrome.

A simple screening test for Cushing's syndrome is the overnight dexamethasone suppression test. The patient receives 1.0 mg of dexamethasone orally at 11 p.m. together with a sedative (e.g. 200 mg of secobarbital orally). A sample of venous blood is drawn at 8 a.m. the following morning for determination of plasma cortisol. A plasma cortisol of less than 5 μg/100 ml excludes Cushing's syndrome. A concentration greater than 10 μg/100 ml establishes the diagnosis. If the value is between 5 and 10, the test should be repeated. If the plasma cortisol concentration is greater than 10 μg/100 ml the patient should be hospitalized for additional tests to differentiate adrenal hyperplasia from a tumor.

Hirsute patients who have physical findings suggesting an intersex disorder should have cytogenetic studies.

In the remaining hirsute women, laboratory studies are done to distinguish the benign conditions of idiopathic hirsutism, polycystic ovary syndrome, or hyperthecosis from the more serious androgen-secreting tumors or congenital adrenal hyperplasia.

Therefore, following the initial history and physical examination of the patient, a 24-hour urine collection for measurement of 17-ketosteroids and 17-hydroxycorticosteroids and a plasma sample for testosterone are obtained. Once these samples have been collected, the patient is placed on one of the commercially available oral contraceptives containing norethindrone, 2 mg, and mestranol, 0.10 mg. This is done for two reasons: to initiate what may be the appropriate hormonal therapy of hirsutism and to determine the ability of exogenously administered hormones to suppress endogenous androgen production. If either 17-ketosteroid or testosterone values are above normal, 0.5 mg of dexamethasone can be administered orally every 6 hours during the last 5 days of the 21-day cycle of oral contraceptives. Urine and blood samples are collected on the 21st day of oral contraceptives (5th day of dexamethasone), and the determinations of 24-hour urinary 17-ketosteroids or plasma testosterone are repeated. A second month of oral contraceptives is begun 1 week later. During the second month of oral contraceptives, the results of these studies are reviewed.

If the initial 17-OHCS and 17-KS values are elevated, Cushing's syndrome should be suspected and the patient screened with the dexamethasone suppression test described above.

An elevated 17-ketosteroid value ($>$ 20 mg/24 hours) with a normal or low 17-hydroxycorticosteroid level and normal plasma testosterone is consistent with adrenal hyperplasia of the congenital or postpubertal types. This diagnosis can be confirmed by an elevated 24-hour urinary pregnanetriol value ($>$ 2.0 mg) and the reduction of the 17-ketosteroid value to $<$3 mg/24 hours by the combined oral contraceptive and dexamethasone therapy. Some endocrinologists feel that the postpubertal development of adrenal hyperplasia is rare.

Normal basal values for urinary 17-ketosteroid and plasma testosterone are consistent with either the polycystic ovary syndrome or idiopathic hirsutism. However, the basal values for 17-ketosteroids or testosterone may be elevated in the presence of either of these functional disorders as well as with an androgen-secreting tumor of either the adrenal or the ovary. The ability of combined estrogen-progestin and adrenal corticoid therapy to suppress elevated androgens may be useful in distinguishing the functional from the neoplastic disorders. In a study reported by Benjamin et al.[35] the combined use of an oral contraceptive and dexamethasone suppressed the urinary 17-ketosteroids to $<$3 mg in normal women, in women with polycystic ovary syndrome or idiopathic hirsutism, and in women with congenital adrenal hyperplasia. On the other hand, 17-ketosteroid values remained at $>$ 3 mg/24 hours in patients with adrenal adenomas and in one patient with an arrhenoblastoma. The inability of this combined regimen to reduce the plasma testosterone concentration to normal female levels is also presumptive evidence for a tumor of either the adrenal or the ovary. Therefore, hirsute women whose androgens are not suppressed by combined estrogen-progestin-dexamethasone therapy should be hospitalized for additional diagnostic studies. Other patients who should be hospitalized for more elaborate testing are those with elevated cortisol levels after dexamethasone suppression, an ovarian mass, or sexual ambiguity. Patients admitted for evaluation of a possible androgen-secreting tumor should have direct tests of adrenal and ovarian androgen secretion. The best technique appears to be retrograde venous catheterization of the ovarian and adrenal veins with selective samples and the subsequent determination of androgen secretion of each of these glands.[36] Using this technique, the excessive androgen production may be localized to the specific ovary or adrenal, thereby simplifying the surgical removal of the tumor.

Treatment

Modes of therapy may be either specific or nonspecific. Specific forms of treatment are directed at reducing the amount of circulating androgens or interfering with their effect on the hair follicle. These specific forms of treatment vary with the nature of the underlying disorder. Nonspecific forms of therapy may be effective regardless of the underlying disorder and are directed at reducing either the number of hairs or their undesirable cosmetic effect.

Specific Therapy. Specific therapy for hirsutism associated with adrenal or ovarian tumors or intersex disorders consists of adrenalectomy, oophorectomy, or removal of gonadal tissue bearing a Y-cell line. Appropriate therapy for Cushing's syndrome may be bilateral adrenalectomy.

The use of synthetic glucocorticoids to suppress ACTH overproduction and thus the excessive androgen production of congenital adrenal hyperplasia not only prevents progressive virilization in women but may also correct menstrual abnormalities and restore potential fertility. Laboratory guidelines to adequate therapy are reduction of urinary 17-ketosteroids, urinary pregnanetriol, and blood testosterone to normal levels.

Specific treatment of hirsutism in patients with the polycystic ovary syndrome consists of combined estrogen-progestin therapy. The estrogen and progestin act to reduce androgen production by suppressing gonadotropin stimulation of ovarian steroidogenesis. They also cause increased protein binding of circulating testosterone and may reduce the effect of testosterone on the hair follicle by preventing its binding to the follicle.

Many patients with the polycystic ovary syndrome will respond to any of the combination oral contraceptives. However, the improvement may be slight and may not occur for six months or more after the institution of such therapy. An occasional patient will be so sensitive to androgen stimulation that hirsutism or acne is actually made worse by the oral contraceptive preparation. These patients may respond best when given an oral contraceptive which has as its progestin a compound which is not androgenic, such as Enovid. Unfortunately, the improvement is usually not permanent and hirsutism may worsen when therapy is discontinued.

Wedge resection may restore ovulation in these women, but it seldom has a beneficial effect on hirsutism. Another form of therapy not yet available in the United States involves the use of the anti-androgens cyproterone acetate or 17α-methyl-β-nortestosterone. Additional experience must be gained with these drugs to define their role in therapy. Patients with hyperthecosis may require oophorectomy to control their hirsutism.

Nonspecific Therapy. In some women, improvement in hirsutism can be achieved by nonspecific means designed to make the excessive hair less noticeable. The best of these is electrolysis to remove the offending hair. Unfortunately, the cost of these treatments may be prohibitive, and, unless some means of inhibiting new hair growth is also employed, improvement may be short lived. Therapy with oral contraceptives is useful in accomplishing this goal.

Other less effective means of reducing the excessive hair include (1) pumice, wax, or chemical depilatories, (2) bleaching, and (3) shaving.

DYSFUNCTIONAL UTERINE BLEEDING

Introduction

Menarche, the menstrual cycle, and the menopause are three of the four major reproductive events in women, pregnancy being the fourth. Abnormalities of uterine bleeding associated with these events are among the most common, and perhaps the most confusing, of the problems facing the gynecologist. The application of radioimmune assay techniques for hormone determinations and the use of purified and synthetic hypothalamic and pituitary hormones, coupled with an understanding of the normal physiology of the menstrual cycle, have led to a description of the pathophysiologic mechanisms underlying abnormal uterine bleeding. This, in turn, has made possible specific, rational, and effective therapy of abnormal uterine bleeding.[37]

In this section we will review the recent studies which shed light on the hormonal causes of abnormal uterine bleeding and offer a diagnostic and therapeutic approach to these abnormalities based on this understanding.

Definition

Dysfunctional uterine bleeding (DUB) refers to excessive uterine bleeding which is due to persistent anovulation in a woman of reproductive age who has ovaries capable of producing estrogen.[38] It does not include abnormal uterine bleeding due to gross uterine lesions (polyps, leiomyomata, or malignancy), pregnancy, or disorders of blood coagulation. Bleeding may be excessive in frequency (more often than every 20 days), duration (greater than 8 days), or amount (greater than 150 cc per episode).

In contrast to the predictable, self-limited nature of menstrual flow in ovulatory cycles, DUB is characterized by its unpredictability. Thus, women with DUB may present with either a very heavy and prolonged episode of bleeding which follows an interval of amenorrhea or a pattern of completely irregular and frequent bleeding. The final common denominator in both forms of bleeding is the persistent stimulation of the endometrium by estrogen unopposed by the periodic influence of progesterone.

While the final common denominator in DUB is the same in all age groups, the discussion of this disorder will be divided into DUB in the adolescent, the postmenarcheal, and the perimenopausal women, since the differential diagnosis is different in each age group.

Dysfunctional Uterine Bleeding in the Adolescent

The initiation of gonadal function at puberty begins with an increasing secretion of pituitary gonadotropins, postulated to result from a decreasing sensitivity to the negative feedback effect of ovarian steroids on the hypothalamic pituitary unit. In response to the increased gonadotropins, there is increased production of estrogens by the ovary, which results in the development of pubertal changes in the woman. The secretion of gonadotropins by the pituitary is relatively constant in the pubertal but premenarcheal adolescent. With the onset of menarche, the cyclic patterns of gonadotropin and ovarian steroid secretion associated with ovulation occur. However, it appears that the initial menses are not associated with ovulation in most girls. A recent study of the hypothalamic-pituitary-ovarian axis in puberty suggests that ovulation begins within the first year after menarche. The development of ovulation at approximately monthly intervals does not occur for the next 2 to 5 years. It is during this interval between menarche and the establishment of regular ovulatory cycles that DUB most often occurs in the adolescent.

Dysfunctional uterine bleeding in most adolescents is due to "immaturity of the hypothalamic-pituitary unit" or the polycystic ovary syndrome. Detailed studies of pituitary and ovarian function in patients with an immature hypothalamic-pituitary axis have demonstrated that anovulation results from the absence of a cyclic surge of gonadotropins. In some cases, the absence of this gonadotropin surge is due to an inability of the hypothalamic-pituitary axis to respond to the positive feedback effect of increasing concentrations of estradiol.

Anovulation in women with Stein-Leventhal syndrome is associated with tonic elevation of pituitary luteinizing hormone (LH) and tonic secretion of ovarian estrogens and androgens. There is an absence of a cyclic surge of gonadotropins, which results from the elevated ovarian androgens and/or estrogens.

Evaluation. The evaluation of an adolescent patient with DUB should include determination of the extent of blood loss and a search to rule out other causes of abnormal vaginal bleeding.

The patient should first be questioned regarding the nature and extent of the bleeding and symptoms of acute or chronic blood loss. She should be asked questions about the frequency and duration of bleeding, the number of pads used, and the degree to which the pads are saturated.

In determining the extent of blood loss, signs of acute (postural hypotension) or chronic (pale skin and mucous membrane) blood loss should be looked for, as they influence the course of therapy. Initial evaluation should also include a hemoglobin and hematocrit.

Having determined the extent of blood loss, the diagnosis of DUB is made by ruling out other causes of excessive vaginal bleeding. A pelvic examination may reveal that, in fact, the bleeding is not uterine but vaginal in origin. Vaginal lacerations due to attempts at intercourse, the insertion of a foreign body, or trauma often result in episodes of sudden profuse bleeding and hypotension. Frequently the patient will deny intercourse or the insertion of a foreign object. Thus inspection of the vagina is mandatory regardless of history. Other vaginal lesions such as sarcoma botryoides, adenosis, or clear cell carcinoma may present as unpredictable episodes of spotting or mild bleeding, in contrast to the heavier bleeding often associated with vaginal laceration.

Cervical lesions rarely result in abnormal vaginal bleeding in this age group. Nonetheless, sarcoma botryoides, mixed mesodermal sarcoma, cervical polyps, and endocervical polyps should be ruled out. Cyanosis of the cervix or dilatation of the endocervical os suggest an intrauterine pregnancy.

Bimanual examination may demonstrate an enlarged uterus of an early pregnancy. Bilateral adnexal masses suggest the polycystic ovary syndrome, whereas a unilateral adnexal mass may be an ectopic pregnancy or an estrogen-secreting granulosa or theca cell tumor.

A history of regular but excessive menses resulting in anemia and repeated dilatation and curettage is typical of von Willebrand's disease. The diagnosis of this coagulopathy can be made by demonstrating a prolonged bleeding time and a decreased concentration of factor VIII (antihemophilic factor). Women with von

Willebrand's disease may also present with midcycle bleeding from the site of ovulation on the ovary.

Finally, when the diagnosis of DUB is made, the patient should be examined for the presence of thyroid dysfunction, liver disease, or renal disease which may cause anovulation. However, DUB in the adolescent is usually not associated with these systemic diseases.

Treatment. The therapeutic approach to DUB in the adolescent depends on the hemoglobin concentration, the degree of active bleeding, the pattern of bleeding, and the presence of associated nongynecologic disease.

In patients with symptomatic anemia or hypotension, transfusion with packed cells or whole blood is indicated.

The treatment of choice for active and heavy bleeding consists of oral estrogen-progestin preparations. A popular and effective protocol utilizes nore-thynodrel with mestranol. The administration of four 5-mg tablets (norethynodrel 5 mg and mestranol 75 μg) or two 10-mg tablets (norethynodrel 10 mg and mestranol 150 μg) will greatly decrease the bleeding within 1 to 2 days and usually stop it in 3 to 4 days. On day 5 the dose is reduced to 10 mg daily and maintained for 20 more days. Withdrawal bleeding will then occur within 2 to 3 days of the discontinuance of therapy. The tablets are then restarted on the fifth day for 21 days. After three more cycles, hormone therapy can be discontinued. Effective control can be maintained after the initial cycle with usual contraceptive dosages utilizing pills containing 50 μg of estrogen.

If bleeding is profuse on admission and rapid control is desired the tablets can be supplemented by Premarin, 20 mg intravenously. The dose can be repeated at 2-hour intervals for a total of 3 or 4 injections.

The important features of this or similar protocols are the administration of relatively high doses of progestin combined with a synthetic estrogen. In addition, the therapy is administered almost continuously for several months and the amount of medication is decreased after the first month of therapy.

A common problem with this therapy is nausea and vomiting. This annoying side effect can be reduced by administering the tablets at 4- to 6-hour intervals throughout the day and night.

Some patients will not (because of nausea) or cannot take progestins combined with estrogen (because of hypertension or a history of thrombophlebitis). Potent progestins can be administered to these patients with little or no nausea and little aggravation of pre-existing medical problems. Norethindrone, five 5-mg tablets, or norethindrone acetate, three 5-mg tablets, may be administered in place of the combination oral contraceptives.

If the pattern of bleeding is one of frequent episodes of mild bleeding or spotting, a combination of a progestin and estrogen is also administered, but in a lower dose. Bleeding can usually be controlled with standard doses of combination oral contraceptives which contain 1 mg of progestin and 80 to 100 μg of estrogen. These preparations are administered for 3 weeks out of every 4.

If bleeding continues in spite of hormonal therapy, the diagnosis of dysfunctional uterine bleeding may be incorrect and a dilatation and curettage (D and C) or hysterogram should be considered to rule out intrauterine lesions.

The long-range management of these patients depends upon several factors. Continued use of a low estrogen (50 μg) combination oral contraceptive may be indicated in sexually active adolescents in whom a pregnancy is not desired. It should be explained to the patient that continued use of oral contraceptives may interfere with the maturation of the hypothalamic-pituitary axis. Prolonged amenorrhea and primary infertility may follow the discontinuance of long term contraceptive therapy, although the therapy may not have been causative.

The recurrence of DUB in patients who do not resume ovulatory menstrual cycles after hormonal therapy can be prevented if necessary by medroxyprogesterone acetate, 10 mg a day for 5 days every 6 to 8 weeks. This will result in regular episodes of several days of withdrawal bleeding. When regular ovulatory menses begin, therapy is discontinued.

Postadolescent Dysfunctional Uterine Bleeding

Dysfunctional uterine bleeding is not as common in women between the ages of 20 and 35 as at the time of menarche or menopause. While the differential diagnosis of abnormal uterine bleeding is similar to that of the adolescent, the underlying pathologic processes responsible for anovulation may be different.

Pathophysiology. Some women may continue to have dysfunctional bleeding beyond adolescence because of dysfunction of the hypothalamic-pituitary axis, others because of the polycystic ovary syndrome, and still others because of premature ovarian failure.

Evaluation. Clues as to the origin of anovulation in women with dysfunctional uterine bleeding in this age group may be obtained when interviewing the patient. A history of irregular menses from menarche is seen in some women with hypothalamic-pituitary dysfunction, whereas irregular vaginal bleeding after several years of regular menses, with or without pregnancy, is typical of premature ovarian failure. Occasionally, the onset of DUB can be related to psychologic stress, excessive weight gain, the administration of drugs (e.g. phenothiazines, reserpine, or methyldopa), or other extrinsic factors.

The patient's physical features also may suggest the underlying cause of the failure to ovulate. Many of these patients are obese, for obesity may be part of the polycystic ovary syndrome or may be related to hypothalamic-pituitary dysfunction.

Signs of androgen excess of the polycystic ovary include hirsutism and acne. If there are also signs of virilism such as clitoromegaly, frontal balding, or masculine body build the patient should be evaluated for a more serious disorder of androgen production, such as an adrenal or ovarian tumor. However, amenorrhea is more frequently encountered with these disorders. Bilateral ovarian enlargement is also consistent with the diagnosis of the polycystic ovary syndrome.

In differentiating hypothalamic-pituitary dysfunction, the polycystic ovary syndrome, and premature ovarian failure, the measurement of circulating gonadotropin concentrations and the determination of adrenal and ovarian steroid hormone production can be helpful.

Typically, LH and follicle-stimulating hormone (FSH) concentrations in peripheral venous blood samples are in the low or low normal range in hypothalamic-pituitary dysfunction, LH values are elevated and FSH values low normal in the polycystic ovary syndrome, and FSH and LH values are elevated and in the postmenopausal range in women with premature ovarian failure. This rise may not occur, however, prior to the development of amenorrhea.

Serum testosterone concentrations may be elevated (greater than 0.8 ng/ml) in the polycystic ovary syndrome, but not in premature ovarian failure or hypothalamic-pituitary dysfunction.

Treatment. Control of the dysfunctional bleeding can be achieved by the same medication schedule suggested for the adolescent patient. However, because of the older age of some of these patients, pre-existing medical problems may contraindicate the use of high doses of estrogens. Therefore, patients should be evaluated for past or present thrombophlebitis, liver dysfunction, migraine headaches, breast masses, cervical abnormalities, seizure disorders, or hypertension. Lesions of the uterus such as polyps, cervicitis, and pregnancy occur frequently in this age group. For this reason, a dilatation and curettage, a hysterogram, or hysteroscopy may be helpful diagnostic aids in those patients who fail to respond to hormonal therapy.

The long term treatment of patients in this age group depends upon the nature of the underlying disorder. Clomiphene may be used to establish the competence of the hypothalamic-pituitary-ovarian axis and to induce ovulation in those women who wish to become pregnant. Clomiphene therapy is most successful in women with the polycystic ovary syndrome, less so in women with dysfunctional bleeding and hypothalamic-pituitary immaturity, and of no use in women with premature ovarian failure.

Women who do not wish to conceive can be treated with combination oral contraceptives. Such therapy will provide a method of contraception as well as correct the symptoms, but not the cause, of dysfunctional bleeding. Women with dysfunctional bleeding and the polycystic ovary syndrome may notice improvement in hirsutism and acne while taking the oral contraceptives.

Cyclic progestin therapy (medroxyprogesterone acetate, 10 mg/day for 5 days every 6 weeks) should be given to those women who remain anovulatory, cannot take estrogen, or are not desirous of pregnancy. This therapy will prevent the development of endometrial hyperplasia which may otherwise occur in response to prolonged exposure to unopposed estrogen stimulation.

Of course, specific therapy directed at associated medical problems, such as weight reduction and emotional support in the obese patient or thyroid replacement therapy in the hypothyroid patient, may result in the resumption of regular ovulatory cycles.

Dysfunctional Uterine Bleeding in the Perimenopausal Woman

Women in the perimenopausal period with DUB pose several problems to the gynecologist. First, the differential diagnosis of dysfunctional bleeding includes malignancies of the genital tract, which must be ruled out prior to therapy. Second, prolonged or heavy bleeding and moderate degrees of anemia may not be well tolerated because of the presence of pre-existing chronic conditions. And third, conditions which contraindicate high dose estrogen-progestin therapy are more prevalent in this age group.

Pathophysiology. Dysfunctional uterine bleeding is more frequent in this age group because anovulatory cycles are more frequent. The major cause of anovulation appears to be incipient ovarian failure. With the depletion of responsive follicles, estrogen production is diminished and unpredictable and there may be an absence of cyclic gonadotropin secretion and ovulation. As a result, the endometrium is stimulated by estrogen alone, without the cyclic increase in progesterone. Bleeding then occurs from a proliferative or hyperplastic endometrium and in an erratic and unpredictable fashion.

Uterine bleeding may also occur in some postmenopausal women who show signs of increased estrogen production and who have a proliferative or hyperplastic endometrium. As is true in the premenopausal woman, the uterine bleeding occurs in response to prolonged and unopposed stimulation of the endometrium by estrogens. However, unlike the premenopausal woman whose estrogens originate primarily from the ovary, the increased estrogens in the postmenopausal woman result from increased conversion of adrenal androgens (particularly androstenedione) to estrogens. This increased conversion is particularly apt to occur in postmenopausal women who are obese or who have liver disease. It has been proposed that prolonged exposure of the endometrium to estrogens formed in this manner not only leads to dysfunctional uterine bleeding but may predispose to endometrial carcinoma.[39]

Women who present with abnormal uterine bleeding after the age of 35 should have endometrial sampling (D and C or multiple endometrial and endocervical biopsies) to rule out endometrial adenocarcinoma or other uterine lesions. Once this has been done, hormonal therapy may be initiated.

Since the uterine bleeding occurs in response to excessive or prolonged estrogen stimulation, women in this age group with dysfunctional uterine bleeding secondary to ovarian failure frequently do not have symptoms or signs of vasomotor instability. Therefore it may be helpful to obtain a serum sample for determination of FSH and LH concentrations. A marked elevation of serum FSH (greater than 40 milli-International Units (mIU) per ml) and a moderate elevation of serum LH (greater than 30 mIU/ml) with a ratio of FSH:LH of greater than 1 is indicative of ovarian failure. Early in the course of ovarian failure, when dysfunctional uterine bleeding is most common, LH and FSH concentrations may be in the normal or upper normal range, but the ratio of FSH:LH is greater than 1.[40]

In addition to endometrial sampling to rule out endometrial carcinoma and serum FSH and LH concentrations to establish ovarian failure, a thorough history, physical examination, and gynecologic examination should be performed to rule out other local and systemic causes of abnormal vaginal bleeding, as discussed earlier.

Treatment. Treatment of dysfunctional bleeding in women over 35 years of age is made easier by the fact that pregnancy is seldom desired. Therefore, therapeutic measures can be directed toward regulation of the uterine bleeding with less concern for restoring ovulatory cycles.

The principles of therapy are the same as those for bleeding in the younger woman. Most women respond well to 1 to 3 months of therapy with a combination oral contraceptive. Patients should be carefully questioned regarding possible contraindications to this hormonal therapy. Because of the higher risk of coronary artery disease, combined pills should be used with caution in women age 40 or older. Periodic withdrawal with Provera may be preferable.

Summary

The symptoms of DUB in women from menarche to menopause can be successfully managed by the administration of combination progestin-estrogen medications. The success of this therapy depends upon the careful search for other causes of abnormal bleeding, for these disorders require specific or nonhormonal modes of therapy. This search will be facilitated by a thorough understanding of the differential diagnosis of DUB in the perimenarcheal, postmenarcheal, and perimenopausal woman. Obviously the ultimate goal, still not attainable in a significant number of patients, is elucidation of a specific cause of the anovulation and appropriate treatment so that ovulatory cycles may ensue.

REFERENCES

1. Muller, SA, Hirsutism: A Review of the Genetic and Experimental Aspects, J Invest Derm 60:457, 1973.
2. Leng, JJ, and Greenblatt, RB, Hirsutism in Adolescent Girls, Ped Clin North Am 19:681, 1972.
3. Karp, L, and Herrmann, WL, Diagnosis and Treatment of Hirsutism in Women, Obstet Gynecol 41:283, 1973.
4. Garn, SM, Types and Distribution of the Hair in Man. Ann NY Acad Sci 53:498, 1951.
5. Schweikert, HU, and Wilson, JD, Regulation of Human Hair Growth by Steroid Hormones. I. Testosterone Metabolism in Isolated Hairs, J Clin Endocrinol Metab 38:811, 1974.
6. Schweikert, HU, and Wilson, JD, Regulation of Human Hair Growth by Steroid Hormones. II. Androstenedione Metabolism in Isolated Hairs. J Clin Endocrinol Metab 39:1012, 1074.
7. Lorenzo, EM, Familial Study of Hirsutism, J Clin Endocrinol Metab 31:556, 1970.
8. Ferriman, D, and Gallway, JD, Clinical Assessment of Body Hair Growth in Women, J Clin Endocrinol Metab 21:1440, 1961.
9. Bray, PF, Diphenylhydantoin (Dilantin) after 20 Years, Pediatrics 23:151, 1959.
10. Cam, C, and Nigogosyan, G, Acquired Toxic Porphyria Cutanea Tarda due to Hexachlorobenzene, JAMA 183:88, 1963.
11. Kirschner, MA, and Bardin, CW, Androgen Production and Metabolism in Virilized Women, Metabolism 21:667, 1972.
12. Ito, T, and Horton, R, The Source of Plasma Dihydrotestosterone in Man, J Clin Invest 50:1621, 1971.
13. Mahoudeau, JA, Bardin, CW, and Lipsett, MB, The Metabolic Clearance Rate and Origin of Plasma Dihydrotestosterone in Man and its Conversion to the 5α-Androstanediols, J Clin Invest 50:1338, 1971.
14. Mahesh, VB, Greenblatt, RB, and Coniff, RF, Urinary Steroid Excretion before and after Dexamethasone Administration and Steroid Content of Adrenal Tissue and Venous Blood in Virilizing Adrenal Tumors, Am J Obstet Gynecol 100:1043, 1968.
15. Korenman, SG, Kirschner, MA, and Lipsett, MB, Testosterone Production in Normal and Virilized Women with the Stein-Leventhal Syndrome or Idiopathic Hirsutism, J Clin Endocrinol Metab 25:798, 1965.
16. Werk, EE, Sholiton, LJ, and Kalejs, L, Testosterone Secreting Adrenal Adenoma under Gonadotropin Control, New Eng J Med 289:767, 1973.
17. Burr, IM, Graham, T, Sullivan, J, Hartman, WH, and O'Neill, J, A Testosterone Secreting Tumor of the Adrenal Producing Virilization in a Female Infant, Lancet 2:643, 1973.
18. Novak, ER, and Lang, JH, Arrhenoblastoma of the Ovary, Am J Obstet Gynecol 92:1082, 1965.
19. Greenblatt, RB, Mahesh, VB, and Gambrell, RD, Jr, Arrhenoblastoma, Obstet Gynecol 39:567, 1972.
20. Wagner, VP, and Smale, LE, Androgen and Estrogen Production by a Lipid Ovarian Tumor, Obstet Gynecol 45:903, 1973.
21. Stein, IF, and Leventhal, ML, Amenorrhea Associated with Bilateral Polycystic Ovaries, Am J Obstet Gynecol 29:181, 1935.
22. Cooke, CW, McEvoy, D, and Wallach, EE, Polycystic Ovarian Syndrome with Unilateral Cystic Teratoma, Obstet Gynecol 39:789, 1972.

23. DeVane, GW, Czekala, NM, Judd, HL, and Yen, SSC, Circulating Gonadotropins, Estrogens, and Androgens in Polycystic Ovarian Disease, Am J Obstet Gynecol 121:496, 1975.

24. Stahl, NL, Teeslink, CR, Beauchamps, G, and Greenblatt, RB, Serum Testosterone Levels in Hirsute Women, Obstet Gynecol 41:651, 1973.

25. Kirschner, MA, and Jacobs, JB, Combined Ovarian and Adrenal Vein Catheterization to Determine the Site(s) of Androgen Overproduction in Hirsute Women, J Clin Endocrinol Metab 33:199, 1971.

26. Patton, WC, Berger, MJ, Thompson, IE, Chong, AP, Grimes, EM, and Taymor, ML, Pituitary Gonadotropin Responses to Synthetic Luteinizing Hormone Releasing Hormone in Patients with Typical and Atypical Polycystic Ovary Disease, Am J Obstet Gynecol 121:382, 1975.

27. Greenblatt, RB, Diagnosis and Treatment of Hirsutism, Hosp Pract 8:91, 1973.

28. Polansky, S, Luteinizing Hormone, Adrenal Androgenesis, and Polycystic Ovarian Syndrome, Obstet Gynecol 45:451, 1975.

29. Kliman, B, Case Records of the Massachusetts General Hospital: Hyperthecosis of Ovaries, New Eng J Med 287:1192, 1972.

30. Givens, JR, Wiser, WL, Coleman, SA, Wilroy, RS, Andersen, RN, and Fish, SA, Familial Ovarian Hyperthecosis: A Study of Two Families, Am J Obstet Gynecol 110:959, 1971.

31. Goldzieher, JW, and Green, JA, The Polycystic Ovary. I. Clinical and Histologic Features, J Clin Endocrinol Metab 22:325, 1962.

32. Bardin, CW, Lipsett, MB, Edgcomb, JH, and Marshall, JR, Studies of Testosterone Metabolism in a Patient with Masculinization due to Stromal Hyperthecosis, New Eng J Med 277:399, 1967.

33. Farber, M, Daoust, PR, and Rogers, J, Hyperthecosis Syndrome, Obstet Gynecol 44:35, 1974.

34. Shuster, S, Primary Cutaneous Virilism or Idiopathic Hirsuties? Brit Med J 2:285, 1972.

35. Benjamin, F, Cohen, M, and Romney, S, Sequential Adrenal and Ovarian Suppression Tests in the Differential Diagnosis of the Polycystic Ovary (Stein-Leventhal) Syndrome, Fertil Steril 21:854, 1970.

36. Judd, HL, Spore, WW, Talner, LB, Rigg, LA, Yen, SSC, and Benirschke, K, Preoperative Localization of a Testosterone Secreting Ovarian Tumor by Retrograde Venous Catheterization and Selective Sampling, Am J Obstet Gynecol 120:91, 1974.

37. Keye, WB, Jr, Ho Yuen, B, and Jaffe, RB, New Concepts in the Physiology of the Menstrual Cycle, Clin Endocrinol Metab 2:451, 1973.

38. Altchek, A, Dysfunctional Menstrual Disorders in Adolescence, Clin Obstet Gynecol 14:975, 1971.

39. Grodin, JM, Siiteri, PK, and MacDonald, PC, Source of Estrogen Production in Postmenopausal Women, J Clin Endocrinol Metab 36:207, 1973.

40. Aksel, S, and Jones, GS, Etiology and Treatment of Dysfunctional Uterine Bleeding, Obstet Gynecol 44:1, 1974.

14

AMENORRHEA

LEON SPEROFF, M.D.

In terms of difficulty, the differential diagnosis and management of amenorrhea is one of the most overrated problems in clinical medicine. One reason most physicians regard the amenorrheic patient with apprehension is the standard treatment of the subject in books and lectures. What one usually remembers is a vast array of possible disorders underlying amenorrhea, frequently listed in page-filling tables. Actually, the majority of patients with amenorrhea have relatively simple problems which can be easily managed by the patient's primary care physician. Comfort and security in managing amenorrhea is derived from the utilization of a simple, but very effective, scheme for the differential diagnosis of amenorrhea of all types and chronology, requiring only routine procedures which are available to all physicians.

This "workup" is not new, but has been successfully applied by clinicians for many years. Careful adherence to the scheme of this workup will localize the disorder underlying the presenting symptom of amenorrhea. It will be seen that most of these disorders can be easily managed with the secure knowledge that one is not doing the patient a disservice by avoiding specialist referral. Indeed, the assistance of appropriate specialists can now be sought when indicated, bringing confidence to the referral for expert consultation.

Before presenting the diagnostic workup in detail, it is necessary to provide a definition of amenorrhea that will designate appropriate patients. In addition, a brief review of the physiologic mechanisms that produce a menstrual flow is included to clarify the logic of the various steps in the diagnostic procedure.

DEFINITION OF AMENORRHEA

Any patient fulfilling the following criteria should be evaluated as having the clinical problem of amenorrhea:

1. No bleeding by age 14 in the absence of growth or development of secondary sexual characteristics.

2. No periods by age 16, regardless of the presence of normal growth and development with the appearance of secondary sexual characteristics.

3. In a woman who has been menstruating, the absence of periods for a length of time equivalent to a total of at least three of the previous cycle intervals, or 6 months of amenorrhea.

Having affirmed the traditional criteria, let us now point out that strict adherence to these criteria may result in improper management of individual cases.

For example, there is no reason to defer the evaluation of a teen-age girl who presents with various characteristics of Turner's syndrome.

Experience has shown that categorization of amenorrhea as primary or secondary is unnecessary and only confusing. The workup to be detailed herein applies comprehensively to all amenorrheas, and the classic definitions of primary or secondary are only burdensome; hence, they are not retained.

Remember. the possibility of pregnancy should always be considered.

BASIC PRINCIPLES IN MENSTRUAL FUNCTION

The presence of menstrual function entails visible external evidence of the menstrual discharge. This requires an intact outflow tract which connects the internal genital source of flow with the outside. As such, the outflow tract requires patency and continuity of the vaginal orifice, the vaginal canal, and the endocervix with the uterine cavity. The presence of menstrual flow depends on the existence and development of the endometrium lining the uterine cavity. This tissue is stimulated and regulated by the proper quantity and sequence of the steroid hormones, estrogen and progesterone, and the gonadotropins, follicle-stimulating hormone (FSH) and luteinizing hormone (LH). Figure 14.1 depicts the blood levels of gonadotropins and gonadal steroids in a normal cycle as measured by saturation analysis methods. These hormonal changes can be best described by dividing the cycle into three phases: the follicular phase, ovulation, and the luteal phase.

The Follicular Phase

At 8 weeks of intrauterine life, rapid mitotic multiplication of oocytes begins, reaching a peak of 6 to 7 million by 20 weeks. Egg depletion by the process known as atresia begins at about 15 weeks of gestation, and by birth the total ovarian content of oogonia has fallen to 1 to 2 million. By the onset of puberty, the number of eggs has been reduced to 300,000 to 500,000. It is from this reservoir that the typical cycle of follicle maturation with ovulation and corpus luteum formation will arise. For every follicle which ovulates, close to 1,000 will pursue abortive growth periods of variable length and undergo atresia.

Until age 45 to 50, when the numbers of oogonia have been exhausted, primordial follicles are continuously undergoing an initial growth and development which in the vast majority of instances is rapidly followed by atresia. During the reproductive years this pattern is interrupted at the beginning of the menstrual cycle, when a group of follicles responds to a hormonal change and is propelled to further growth. The most important hormonal event at this time is a rise in FSH, leading to a direct stimulation of follicular growth. During this early period of FSH-stimulated follicular growth, there is little, if any, detectable change in the plasma levels of gonadal hormones. A rise in LH also occurs during menses, but this may simply reflect escape from luteal phase suppression, and no apparent function can be assigned to LH at the beginning of the cycle. The presence of LH is necessary, however, for estrogen production, and the period of initial follicular growth ends when a significant increase in plasma estrogen is detectable, 7 or 8 days before the preovulatory LH surge.

During the late follicular phase, estrogens rise slowly at first, then rapidly,

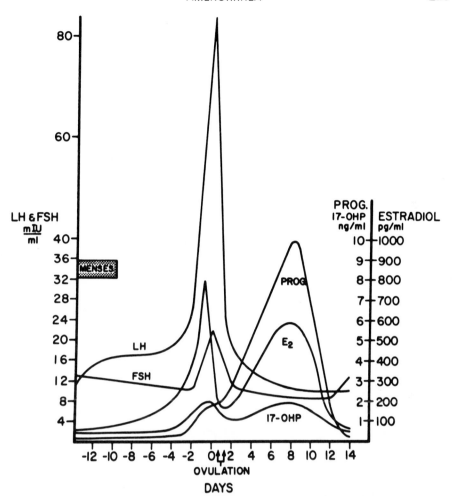

Fig. 14.1. Blood levels of gonadotropins and gonadal steroids in the normal menstrual cycle. E_2, estradiol; FSH, follicle-stimulating hormone; LH, luteinizing hormone; 17-OHP, 17-hydroxyprogesterone; PROG, progesterone. (From Speroff, L, and Vande Wiele, RL, Regulation of the Human Menstrual Cycle, Am J Obstet Gynecol *109*:234, 1971.)

reaching a peak just before ovulation. Concomitant with the rise in estrogens there is a decline in FSH, while in contrast LH increases steadily and then rapidly in a surge at midcycle.

The changes in hormonal levels are regulated by feedback mechanisms. In the case of FSH, there is a negative inhibitory feedback relationship with estrogen, while in the case of LH there is a negative inhibitory feedback at low levels of estrogen and a positive stimulatory feedback at high levels (see Fig 14.2). Thus, in the early part of the cycle as estrogens rise, FSH declines owing to a negative feedback effect. A concomitant decrease in LH does not occur since the negative feedback of estrogen on LH is already at a maximum. The rise in LH at midcycle

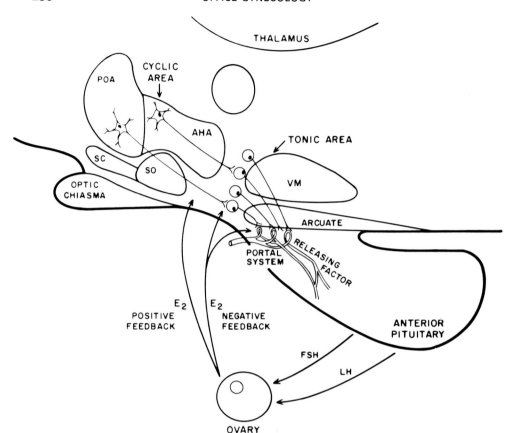

Fig. 14.2. Cyclic menstrual function is regulated to a large degree by feedback responses to estrogen. This diagram illustrates relationships established in experimental animals. The negative feedback action of estradiol (E_2) is responsible for tonic levels of gonadotropins and in particular for the level of follicle-stimulating hormone (FSH); this action is exerted in the medial area of the hypothalamus. The midcycle surge of luteinizing hormone (LH) represents a response to a positive feedback effect of estradiol, probably exerted in a more anterior area of the hypothalamus. POA, paraoptic area; SO, supraoptic nucleus; VM, ventromedial nucleus; SC, suprachiasmatic nucleus; AHA, anterior hypothalamic area.

is a response to the rising levels of estrogen stimulating a positive hypothalamic response. During the luteal phase LH secretion is suppressed by the negative feedback of progesterone in the presence of estrogen (the principle utilized in estrogen-progestin birth control pills).

The rapid growth of the follicle late in the follicular phase when FSH levels are actually decreasing indicates that as the follicle matures it becomes increasingly sensitive to FSH. With follicular growth the levels of estradiol rise and inhibit FSH secretion; however, the follicle destined to ovulate protects itself from atresia by its own hormone production. High local estradiol concentration increases follicular sensitivity to FSH, perhaps by promoting follicular binding of FSH. The decrease in FSH then would be significant in terms of a loss of growth stimulation to the smaller follicles which are producing less estrogen. A wave of atresia, therefore, is seen to parallel the rise in estrogen, reaching a maximum in the preovulatory period.

The tissue derived from the theca interna of atretic follicles is termed stromal tissue. This tissue is not truly atretic. It continues to secrete steroids but, rather than estrogen, the principal stromal products are androgens, androstenedione and testosterone. The increase in stromal tissue in the late follicular phase is associated with a rise in androgen levels in the peripheral blood. Abnormal accumulation of this tissue, such as in anovulation and polycystic ovaries, may give rise to increased androgen production and hirsutism.

Ovulation

The rise in estradiol during the late proliferative phase is the trigger that sets off the LH surge. This positive feedback stimulatory effect of estrogen requires centers in the hypothalamus which respond to rapidly increasing levels of estradiol with an outpouring of LH-releasing factor. The presence of elevated levels of androgens may inhibit this response. The simultaneous modest rise in FSH at midcycle does not appear to have functional importance.

The high levels of LH persist for approximately 24 hours, then decrease during the luteal phase to nadir values. The secretion of LH and of FSH is not smooth, but episodic with rhythmic release by the anterior pituitary. This pulse-like release may be important in the transmission of stimulatory and feedback messages.

An adequate LH surge does not ensure ovulation. The follicle must be at the appropriate stage of maturity in order for it to respond to the ovulating stimulus. In the normal cycle, LH release and final maturation of the follicle coincide because the timing of the LH surge is controlled by the level of estradiol. This in turn is a function of follicular growth and maturation.

Rupture of the follicle occurs approximately 24 hours after the LH peak.

The Luteal Phase

After rupture of the follicle and release of the ovum, the granulosa cells increase in size. They assume a characteristic vacuolated appearance associated with the accumulation of a yellow pigment, lutein, which lends its name to the process of luteinization and the new anatomical subunit, the corpus luteum. During the first 3 days after ovulation, the granulosa cells enlarge and capillaries penetrate into the granulosa layer. By day 8 or 9 after ovulation, a peak of vascularization, associated with peak levels of progesterone and estradiol in the blood, is reached. Steroidogenesis in the corpus luteum is dependent on the low but important quantities of LH available in the luteal phase. Beginning about 10 to 12 days after ovulation, the corpus luteum enters into a stage of regression, which is first marked by a gradual decrease of blood in the capillaries followed by decreasing steroid production.

It is well known that the variability in cycle length among women is due to the varying number of days required for follicular growth and maturation in the follicular phase.

In the normal cycle the time period from the LH surge to menses is consistently close to 14 days. The finite life span of the human corpus luteum may represent a response to the stimulation of the LH surge at midcycle. Degeneration and regression are inevitable unless pregnancy intervenes. With pregnancy, survival of the corpus luteum is prolonged by the emergence of a new stimulus of rapidly increasing intensity, human chorionic gonadotropin (HCG). This new stimulus first appears at the peak of corpus luteum development, just in time to prevent luteal regression. HCG serves to maintain the vital steroidogenesis of the corpus luteum until approximately the 9th or 10th week of gestation, by which time placental steroidogenesis is well established.

KEY EVENTS IN THE NORMAL MENSTRUAL CYCLE

There are several relationships in the regulation of the human menstrual cycle that are a key to understanding these events. The first is the rise in FSH which begins at the termination of the preceding cycle and is responsible for the stimulation of a new set of follicles, thus initiating a new cycle. The absence or blunting of this rise in FSH will prevent cycling.

Secondly, ovulation is due to a surge in LH which in turn is triggered by rapidly rising levels of estrogen. Inhibition of synchronous timing of the LH surge or inadequate follicular estrogen production will prevent ovulation and possibly create a set of circumstances which will not allow recycling.

Finally, a normal pregnancy will not occur without the concurrent normal lifespan of the corpus luteum, a lifespan which is dependent upon LH maintenance and perhaps upon the preovulatory adequacy of FSH to provide full follicular maturation.

The human cycle depends upon essential changes in estradiol levels at key moments. The initial rise in FSH occurs in response to the decline in estradiol in the preceding luteal phase. Successful follicular development without premature atresia depends upon adequate estradiol production by the growing follicle. Ovulation is triggered by estradiol at midcycle. The interplay among the follicle, the hypothalamus, and the anterior pituitary depends upon estradiol functioning as a classic hormone, to transmit the messages of negative and positive feedback, and also upon the local effect of estradiol within the follicle to ensure gonadotropin sensitivity. Events which prevent estrogen production, obtund the necessary fluctuations in circulating levels, or interfere with target organ estrogen action will result in abnormal or absent menstrual cycles.

THE DIAGNOSTIC WORKUP

The basic principles underlying the physiology of menstrual function permit formulation of several discrete compartmental systems on which proper menstruation depends. The diagnostic evaluation, therefore, segregates causes of amenorrhea into the following compartments:

   I.   Disorders of the outflow tract or the uterine target organ.
   II. Disorders of the ovary.
   III. Disorders of the anterior pituitary.
   IV. Disorders of the central nervous system (hypothalamic function).

A patient with amenorrhea is managed according to the flow diagram depicted in Figure 14.3. Amenorrhea is the sole pertinent initial item of information. Additional data available by history and physical examination will contribute, however, to the final diagnosis. There are three basic diagnostic steps to be followed. Adherence to this sequence of steps reliably avoids unnecessary laboratory procedures.

Step 1

The initial step is to assess the level of endogenous estrogen and the competence of the outflow tract and uterus. A course of a pure progestational agent totally devoid of estrogenic activity is administered. There are only two choices: parenteral progesterone in oil or orally active medroxyprogesterone acetate (Provera). The use of an orally active agent avoids an unpleasant intramuscular injection; the proper dosage of Provera is 10 mg daily for 5 days. Other progestins, such as those in birth control pills, are not appropriate since they are metabolized to estrogens within the body and, therefore, do not exert a purely progestational effect.

Within 2 to 7 days after the conclusion of progestational medication, the patient will either bleed or not bleed. If the patient bleeds, one has reliably and securely established a diagnosis of anovulation. The presence of a functional outflow tract and a uterus lined by reactive endometrium sufficiently prepared by endogenous estrogen are confirmed. With this demonstration of the presence of estrogen, at least minimal function of the ovary, pituitary, and central nervous system (CNS) is established. In the absence of galactorrhea, further evaluation for the presence of a pituitary tumor is unnecessary. Although a very rare patient may be found with a pituitary or nearby tumor presenting with anovulation (and hence with bleeding following progestational medication), it is a useful clinical rule of thumb that a positive withdrawal bleeding response to progestational medication effec-

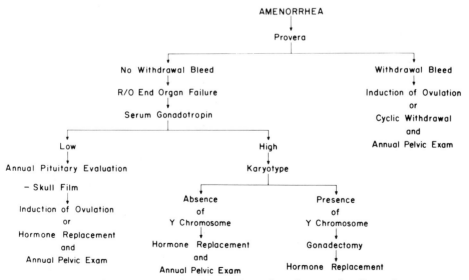

Fig. 14.3 The workup for amenorrhea. See the text for discussion.

tively rules out a pituitary tumor.[1] The presence of galactorrhea, regardless of the bleeding pattern, dictates pituitary evaluation.

Approximately 50% of patients with anovulation are amenorrheic. With the demonstration of a positive withdrawal bleed, therapy can be planned immediately. The patient who wants to become pregnant is a candidate for medical induction of ovulation (see Chapter 17). If the anovulation is associated with hirsutism or virilism, an adrenal cause must be ruled out. For the patient who is anovulatory and does not wish to become pregnant, therapy is directed toward interruption of the steady estrogenic effects on the endometrium. Certain potentially severe clinical consequences can be avoided. Estrogen breakthrough bleeding, which may at the least be inconvenient, can be irregular and very heavy. Endometrial cellular changes can progress to atypical hyperplasia and even to carcinoma. Appropriate management is considered essential for every anovulatory patient.

Provera (10 mg daily for 5 days every 2 months) is favored to ensure withdrawal bleeding and thus to prevent endometrial buildup, irregular bleeding, and hyperplasia. Spacing the medication every 2 months will allow the patient to be aware of spontaneous bleeding which could herald the onset of ovulatory cycles. If patients develop a failure to have withdrawal bleeding, they have moved to the negative category and the remainder of the workup must be pursued.

When reliable contraception is essential, the use of low estrogen oral combination pills in the usual cyclic fashion is appropriate. Recent information from the English prospective study indicates that the fertility rate upon discontinuing the birth control pill is normal;[2] thus, pill use and postpill amenorrhea and anovulation are probably not related as cause and effect. Anovulation with amenorrhea or oligomenorrhea should not be a contraindication to the use of oral contraception.

How much bleeding constitutes a positive withdrawal response? The appearance of only a few bloody spots following progestational medication implies marginal levels of endogenous estrogen. Such a patient should be followed closely and periodically reevaluated, since the marginally positive response may progress to a clearly negative response, placing the patient in a new diagnostic category. Bleeding in any amount beyond a few spots is considered a positive withdrawal response.

Step 2

If the course of progestational medication does not produce withdrawal flow, either the target organ outflow tract is inoperative or preliminary estrogen preparation of the endometrium has not occurred. Step 2 is designed to clarify this situation. Orally active estrogen is administered in quantity and duration certain to stimulate endometrial proliferation and withdrawal bleeding provided that a completely reactive uterus and patent outflow tract exists. An appropriate dose is 2.5 mg of Premarin daily for 21 days. The terminal addition of an orally active progestational agent (Provera, 10 mg daily for the last 5 days) is useful to achieve withdrawal, but not essential. In this way the capacity of Compartment I is challenged by exogenous estrogen. In the absence of withdrawal flow, a validating second course of estrogen is a wise precaution.

As a result of the pharmacologic test of Step 2, the patient with amenorrhea will either bleed or not bleed. If there is no withdrawal flow, the diagnosis of a defect in the Compartment I systems (endometrium, outflow tract) can be made with confidence. If withdrawal bleeding does occur, one can assume that Compartment I systems have normal functional abilities if properly stimulated by estrogen.

In a patient with normal external and internal genitalia by pelvic examination, and in the absence of a history of trauma (such as a dilatation and curettage) or infection, Step 2 can be safely omitted. Abnormalities in the systems of Compartments I are not commonly encountered.

Step 3

If Steps 1 and 2 have demonstrated the amenorrheic patient's inability to provide adequate stimulatory amounts of estrogen, the physiologic mechanisms responsible for the elaboration of estrogen must be tested. In order to produce estrogen, ovaries containing normal follicles and sufficient pituitary gonadotropins to stimulate the follicles are required. Step 3 is designed to determine which of these two crucial components (gonadotropins or follicular activity) is functioning improperly.

Step 3 involves an assay of the level of gonadotropins in the patient. Since Steps 1 and 2 involved administration of exogenous steroids, endogenous gonadotropin levels may be artificially but temporarily altered from their true baseline concentrations. Hence, a delay of at least two weeks following steroid administration must ensue before doing Step 3, the gonadotropin assay.

The bioassay of urinary gonadotropins is notoriously unreliable and should be abandoned. In its place, one should obtain the radioimmunoassay measurement of FSH and LH in a serum sample. The convenience of a single blood specimen is matched by the reliability of the method. In 2 weeks time the result can be obtained from various commercial or academic laboratories. Local standards may dictate different normal values, but most laboratories conform to the values presented in Table 14.1.

Step 3 is designated to determine whether the lack of estrogen is due to a fault in the follicle (Compartment II) or in the CNS-pituitary axis (Compartments III and IV). The result of the gonadotropin assay in the amenorrheic woman who does not

TABLE 14.1
Radioimmunoassay Levels of Gonadotropins

Clinical state	Serum FSH	Serum LH
	mIU/ml	*mIU/ml*
Normal adult	5–30, with ovulatory midcycle peak about 2 × base level	5–20, with ovulatory midcycle peak about 3 × base level
Hypogonadotropic state: prepubertal, hypothalamic, and pituitary dysfunction	<5	<5
Hypergonadotropic state: postmenopausal, gonadal failure, castrate	>40	>25

bleed following a progestational agent will be abnormally high, abnormally low, or in the normal range.

If the FSH is over 40 mIU per ml, the cause of the amenorrhea is gonadal failure. If gonadotropins are abnormally low or in the normal range, pituitary failure or inactivity is diagnosed.

The clinical utility of Step 3 is based on the absolute reliability of the negative homeostatic feedback relationship between estrogen and gonadotropins. In practice, a low LH (less than 5 mIU/ml) has been found to be a more reliable indicator of hypogonadotropism, while a high FSH (over 40 mIU/ml) has proved to be a reliable indicator of ovarian failure. FSH values within the normal range (5 to 30 mIU/ml) indicate the presence of ovarian follicles, whereas values over 40 mIU/ml are found only when the supply of ovarian follicles has been exhausted.[3] These patients will not respond to ovulatory drugs and should be considered sterile. The association between a high FSH and ovarian failure is so reliable that further attempts to document the state of the ovaries are unnecessary and unwarranted. Specifically, laparoscopy in order to visualize the ovaries and attempts to demonstrate the presence of follicles by biopsy only expose the patient to unessential surgical and anesthetic risks. Because the result of a high FSH has such an immense bearing on the future fertility of the patient, repeat sampling is a wise precaution.

Be aware that high levels of LH do not reliably establish ovarian failure. Occasional high peaks of LH may be found in the presence of adequate ovarian follicles. This can be partly explained by the pulsatile secretion pattern associated with LH, producing a marked variation in single measurements taken at random.[4] However, serial determinations of LH and FSH do not yield any additional information and are not worthwhile.[1]

All patients under the age of 35 who have been assigned a diagnosis of ovarian failure on the basis of a FSH level over 40 mIU/ml must have a karyotype evaluation. The presence of mosaicism with a Y chromosome requires laparotomy and excision of the gonadal areas because the presence of any testicular component within the gonad carries with it a 25–30% chance of tumor formation. Approximately 30% of patients with a Y chromosome will not develop signs of virilization. Therefore, even the normal appearing adult with an elevated serum level of FSH must be karyotyped. Over the age of 35, and perhaps over 30, amenorrhea with a high FSH is best labeled premature menopause and genetic evaluation is unnecessary.

Why is it that hypoestrogenic (negative progestational withdrawal) patients will frequently have normal circulating levels of FSH and LH as measured by the radioimmunoassay? The answer to this question is not known. However, it is probable that the radioimmunoassay recognizes (immunologically) FSH and LH molecules that are not biologically active. The significant clinical point is the following: FSH and LH levels in the normal range, just as extremely low gonadotropins, can indicate pituitary-CNS failure.

If the gonadotropin assay is abnormally low or in the normal range, one final localization is required to distinguish between a pituitary (Compartment III) or CNS-hypothalamic (Compartment IV) cause for the amenorrhea. Skull films (preferably tomograms) should be obtained to examine the sella turcica for signs of abnormal change. A very high serum prolactin level may be associated with a pituitary tumor even in the absence of galactorrhea.

If amenorrhea is the only presenting symptom in an otherwise normal individual, sella turcica evaluation and prolactin assay should be obtained annually as a precaution to rule out an emerging central tumor. Expectations for the utilization of gonadotropin-releasing hormone to discriminate between disorders of the hypothalamus and the anterior pituitary have not been realized. Tremendous variability in response is the rule, even to the degree that the patient with a pituitary tumor may or may not respond to releasing hormone stimulation.

The patient with an insidiously evolving pituitary tumor may present with amenorrhea years before the tumor becomes evident by sella turcica x-rays. A spectrum beginning with a mildly compromised ovulatory capacity and extending to panhypopituitarism can be encountered. Usually, over the course of time, deterioration in tropic activity is seen, with withdrawal of activity following a fairly predictable pattern: first growth hormone, then FSH and LH, and finally adrenocorticotropic hormone and thyroid-stimulating hormone. Less commonly, peculiar isolated loss of specific tropic hormones may be found.

If the x-ray of the sella, prolactin level, and neurologic scrutiny raise the suspicion of tumor, further evaluation now requires consultation with expert endocrine or neurosurgical resources.

HYPOTHALAMIC AMENORRHEA

Compartment IV (hypothalamic) problems are usually diagnosed by exclusion of pituitary lesions, and are the most common category of hypogonadotropic amenorrhea. Frequently there is an association with a stressful situation. In a study of the total female population aged 18–35 years of Uppsala, Sweden, pronounced psychologic stress was more frequent in women with secondary amenorrhea than in their age-matched controls.[5] There was also a higher proportion of underweight women and a higher occurrence of previous menstrual irregularity. Nevertheless, the physician is obliged to go through the process of exclusion prior to prescribing hormone replacement therapy or attempting induction of ovulation in order to achieve pregnancy. A good practice is to evaluate such patients annually after a 2-month period without hormone medication. Returning function will thus be detected by rising gonadotropins and the demonstration of a positive withdrawal response to a progestational agent. Even though a patient may not be currently interested in pursuing pregnancy, it is important to assure these patients that at the appropriate time treatment for induction of ovulation will be available and that fertility can be achieved. Concern with potential fertility is often an unspoken fear, especially in the younger patients. On the other hand, induction of ovulation (with clomiphene or Pergonal) should be carried out only for the purpose of producing a pregnancy. There is no evidence that cyclic hormone administration or induction of ovulation will stimulate the return of normal function.

A special example of hypothalamic amenorrhea is that associated with weight loss. Again the physician must exclude the presence of a tumor. Clinically a spectrum is encountered, from a limited period of amenorrhea associated with a crash diet to the severely ill patient with the life-threatening attrition of anorexia nervosa. It is a common experience for the gynecologist to be the first to recognize anorexia nervosa in a patient presenting with the complaint of amenorrhea. It is also not infrequent that a gynecologist will evaluate and manage an infertility problem due to hypogonadotropism and not be aware of a developing case of anorexia nervosa. In an adult weighing less than 100 pounds, continued weight loss requires psychiatric consultation.

It has been assumed that amenorrhea may reflect persistent suppressive effects of oral contraceptive medication or the use of the intramuscular depot form of medroxyprogesterone acetate. Recently it has been appreciated that the fertility rate is normal following discontinuance of either of these forms of contraception. Hence this amenorrhea must be investigated as described in order to avoid missing a serious problem.

HORMONE REPLACEMENT THERAPY

The patient who is hypoestrogenic and is not a candidate for induction of ovulation deserves hormone replacement therapy. This includes patients appropriately evaluated and diagnosed as gonadal failure, patients with hypothalamic amenorrhea, and postgonadectomy patients. A good schedule is the following: on days 1 through 24 of each month, take 1.25 mg of Premarin; on days 20 through 24, add 10 mg of Provera. Beginning medication on the first of every month establishes an easily remembered routine. Menstruation generally occurs 3 days after the last medication, the 27th of each month. In a few individuals the estrogen dosage must be reduced because of bothersome estrogenic effects such as fluid retention. In individuals who have not developed secondary sexual characteristics, it is best to start with higher doses of estrogen (5 and 10 mg of Premarin) in an effort to achieve breast development and a more feminine appearance.

Since many of these patients are in school, it is useful to adopt the academic year schedule for the annual re-evaluation process. Hormone replacement therapy can be discontinued in June and re-evaluation scheduled for August. If there is no change in status, hormone replacement therapy can begin again in September.

The importance of monthly menstruation to a young girl cannot be overemphasized. Regular and visible menstrual bleeding is often a gratifying experience in the young patient with gonadal dysgenesis and serves to reinforce her identification with a feminine gender role.

Patients with hypothalamic amenorrhea must be cautioned that replacement therapy will not protect against pregnancy in the event that normal function unknowingly returns. In the occasional patient who must have the most effective contraception possible, it is reasonable to utilize a low dose oral contraceptive to provide the missing estrogen.

REFERENCES

1. Kletzky, OA, Davajan, V, Nakamura, RM, Thorneycroft, IH, and Mishell, DR, Jr, Clinical Categorization of Patients with Secondary Amenorrhea using Progesterone-Induced Uterine Bleeding and Measurement of Serum Gonadotropin Levels, Am J Obstet Gynecol *121*:695, 1975.

2. Royal College of General Practitioners, *Oral Contraceptives and Health*, Pitman Publishing, New York, 1974.

3. Goldenberg, RL, Grodin, JM, Rodbard, D, and Ross, GT, Gonadotropins in Women With Amenorrhea: The Use of Plasma Follicle-Stimulating Hormone to Differentiate Women with and without Ovarian Follicles, Am J Obstet Gynecol *116:*1003, 1973.

4. Santen, RJ, and Bardin, CW, Episodic Luteinizing Hormone Secretion in Man, J Clin Invest *52:*2617, 1973.

5. Fries, H, Nillius, SJ, and Pettersson, F, Epidemiology of Secondary Amenorrhea, Am J Obstet Gynecol *118:*473, 1974.

15

THE MANAGEMENT OF THE POSTMENOPAUSAL WOMAN

NATHAN G. KASE, M.D.

INTRODUCTION

According to the 1970 U.S. census, of the 104,000,000 women in this country, 27,000,000 are 50 years of age or older. Most of these women have had, or shortly will sustain, their last menstrual period and have become postmenopausal. Statistics indicate that at age 50 a woman can expect an additional 28 years of life; therefore, something like one-third of a woman's life will be associated with the waning endogenous estrogen production of the postmenopausal period. The important political, social, and economic implications of these data are evident. The health maintenance responsibilities the physician must meet when dealing with this population are also obvious. However, the central issue for gynecologists, and indeed for all physicians offering care to women, is whether the decrease in estrogen their patients are experiencing is a sufficient liability to necessitate estrogen replacement therapy.

There is no simple answer to this question. The diversity of opinion ranges from the more conservative view that the menopause is an annoying but otherwise normal occurrence not worthy of therapy, to the most activist claim that the menopause and its attendant reduction in endogenous estrogen accelerate the aging process if left untreated. In this polarized situation, some women receive reassurance and support while others are given prompt and continuous high dose estrogen replacement therapy. In this chapter, the physiology of the menopause will be reviewed from the point of view of establishing the risk/benefit analysis for estrogen replacement therapy. Following this review, my own judgments and attitudes developed in clinical practice will be offered as suggested guidelines for physicians facing this challenge.

THE FEMALE CLIMACTERIC

The clinical manifestations of the female climacteric are the result of the impact of three categories of factors: estrogen depletion, the tendency to age, and the woman's perception of menopause as a "change of life."

Amount and Rate of Estrogen Depletion

Although attention is focused on the menopause, ovarian function has begun to wane years before the last menstrual period. Women in their late thirties experience decreasing frequency of ovulation which is accompanied by secondary infertility and irregular menstrual cycles. Follicle-stimulating hormone (FSH) levels in serum begin to rise during this time, and some women may even display vasomotor flushes during this premenopausal estrogen decline. At some point (usually around age 51–52 years), the estrogen produced is not adequate to proliferate an endometrium sufficient to cause menstrual flow. Estrogen production continues in lesser amounts, which are nevertheless sufficient to sustain secondary sexual characteristics for many years. Vaginal and vulvar atrophy may not appear until the 7th or 8th decade.

The ovary is not the source of the estrogen produced menopausally. The work of MacDonald and his associates[1] has shown the adrenal cortex to be the origin of the prehormone Δ^4-androstenedione, which is converted to estrone at peripheral nonendocrine metabolic sites, the most important of which is fat. This estrogen production is not under the control of the usual factors modifying pituitary-ovarian interactions which ordinarily maintain physiologically appropriate quantities of estradiol during the reproductive years. In the absence of this feedback mechanism aging, stress, and obesity become important elements that lead to variable, sometimes clinically important levels of estrone production in the latter third of a woman's life. As a result, from the point of view of estrogen depletion, there are not only *early and late stages of estrogen production*, in which estrogen declines from relatively high, biologically effective levels to the low levels of late life when dependent tissues atrophy, but also *variations in the rate of decline*, in which depletion is muted by factors which increase estrone production by either increasing prehormone production or increasing the efficiency of conversion of prehormone to estrone.

Tendency to Age

Although the operative mechanisms are obscure, there is a clinically observable propensity for some individuals to resist the impositions and manifestations of the overall aging process, while others succumb all too obviously to physical deterioration.

"Change of Life"

Just as the physical reaction to the aging process is variable, so is the psychologic impact of the change of life variable in women. In some, accommodation to the psychosocial and physical implications of aging is simple and nontraumatic. Others mistakenly assume their last menstrual period to be a signal of their entry into a period of life characterized by relentless physical disability on an ever-increasing scale, conflicts with and estrangement from family members, a dwindling sexual adequacy and interest—in short, inevitable loneliness, despair, and disability.

The clinical implications of the female climacteric can be viewed from a symptomatic point of view. In this postmenopausal period of life there will be (1) disturbances of menstrual pattern, with accompanying concerns with regard to neoplasia, (2) the sometimes troublesome but rarely disabling vasomotor disability seen early in the postmenopause, (3) the psychologic symptoms of anxiety, tension, depression, irritability, and presumptive changes in libido, (4) atrophy of specific organ systems leading to dyspareunia, pruritis, urinary urgency and frequency, osteoporosis, and vascular incompetence, and finally (5) the atrophy of personality and self.

ADVANTAGES OF ESTROGEN REPLACEMENT THERAPY

Advocates of estrogen replacement therapy claim that the superimposition of estrogen loss on aging, even if it does not accelerate aging, nevertheless places an unnecessary additional burden on the woman. On this basis, the following advantages are claimed for estrogen replacement therapy; control of vasomotor reactions, reduction of emotional reactions to the climacteric, provision of opportunities for the physician to practice preventive medicine, control and prevention of osteoporosis, and prevention of atherosclerosis.

Control of Vasomotor Reactions

From clinical experience, there is no question that the one clear therapeutic gain easily achievable by estrogen replacement therapy is control of the hot flash of the early postmenopausal period. The extent to which the vasomotor symptoms appear and become troublesome will depend upon the rapidity with which estrogen depletion occurs. Perhaps 20% of patients will experience sufficient difficulty as a result of this symptom to seek therapeutic relief. This can be achieved easily with low dose intermittent estrogen replacement therapy.

Reduction of Emotional Reactions to the Climacteric

Although there is little biophysical evidence to support the contention that depletion of estrogen alters brain function to yield psychologic disturbances, empiric observations abound which suggest that estrogen replacement therapy is associated with alleviation of these difficulties. Whether by a direct biologic replacement phenomenon or by the indirect gain of "having something done" for these reactions, this therapy does have a beneficial influence, an influence which should be acknowledged but not overemphasized.

Preventive Medicine

All too frequently the postmenopausal patient assigns a variety of symptoms to a mystical change of life mechanism. As a result, major disease entities may not be brought to physician care and management until serious consequences have occurred or until irreversible changes obtain. Advocates of estrogen replacement contend that the surveillance required on this therapy places the patient in closer relationship with her primary physician, enabling that physician to evaluate symptom complexes periodically. Semiannual examinations are helpful in disclosing the common inroads of atherosclerosis, colonic disease, and pulmonary problems in this age group.

Osteoporosis[2]

There is an age-related bone loss seen with increased frequency in females as opposed to males. In humans, bone mass reaches its peak at age 35, plateaus for several years, and finally declines beginning sometime within the 6th, and surely by the 7th, decade. The reduction in the mass and density of bone occurs in both cortical and cancellous bone. This reduction in overall bone density results in fragility of the bones and subsequent disabilities. In females, as opposed to males, there is increased frequency of spinal compression, hip fracture risk, and distal forearm fracture risk. Statistically, 25% of all females over 60 have evidence of spinal compression by x-ray. This is a rate 4 times greater than seen in males. The risk of hip fracture increases, in females, to 20% by the 9th decade. The seriousness of this problem is displayed in the fact that one-sixth of the women who suffer hip fracture will die within 3 months. The rate of hip fracture is 2 to 3 times greater than that seen in males. Finally, the frequency of distal forearm fracture is 10 times greater in females than in males.

Unquestionably, various exercise programs and dietary plans have a beneficial effect on osteoporosis. But the fact that osteoporosis is age related and pronounced in females gives rise to the questions, Is it related to estrogen depletion? Can estrogen replacement be beneficial? The long bone density loss is at least temporally related to estrogen loss. There is preliminary evidence that estrogen replacement therapy can retard the density loss in specific bones, such as the phalanges,[3] as well as the symptoms and x-ray appearance of postmenopausal osteoporosis.[4] Plasma calcium and phosphate are elevated in the menopause, and this can be reversed by estrogen. Tubal reabsorption of phosphate decreases when estrogen replacement therapy is given to postmenopausal females. As a result, a positive calcium balance can usually be seen. Finally, estrogens appear to suppress bone resorption, as measured by calcium tracer techniques, to an extent sufficient to explain the positive calcium balance. This can be displayed even in disuse osteoporotic states such as poliomyelitis. To the extent that the literature contains evidence in this regard, it appears that estrogen administration does have a beneficial effect on osteoporosis, via its effect on positive calcium balance and reduction of bone resorption. Estrogen therapy retards the otherwise relentless decrease in bone density in these women. Unfortunately, there is also an associated *decrease in bone formation* within 3 to 9 months of the initiation of estrogen replacement therapy. The result is a stabilized, lower rate of bone turnover. The obvious clinical implication of this fact is that if estrogen therapy is to be beneficial in prevention of osteoporosis it must be instituted early, before serious bone density has been lost. *No new bone formation results from estrogen replacement therapy.*

Atherosclerosis

Traditionally, three groups of observations are cited to support the use of estrogen replacement therapy to retard atherogenesis in the aging woman. These include retrospective autopsy data which indicated that women receiving estrogen replacement therapy have less atherosclerotic change in their large vessels than seen in control groups.[5] In addition, there was early evidence that serum lipoprotein constituents were beneficially converted by estrogen replacement therapy to those seen in younger women. Finally, the evidence that males had a significantly higher risk of death from coronary vascular disease than women was attributed to women's being protected in some way by estrogen. As will be seen below, additional information and controlled studies no longer substantiate the contention that estrogen replacement therapy has a beneficial influence on this process.

DISADVANTAGES OF ESTROGEN REPLACEMENT THERAPY

The disadvantages of estrogen replacement therapy can be considered in three general categories: the metabolic effects of estrogen, the side effects of estrogen therapy, and its impact on the development of cancer in estrogen-dependent tissues, such as the endometrium and the breast.

The Metabolic Effects of Estrogen

The evidence that the birth control pills containing combined progestin-estrogen have disadvantageous effects on both the venous and the arterial portions of the vascular tree led to a re-examination of the previously prevailing view that estrogen replacement therapy had some beneficial effect on the evolution of atherogenesis.

The statistical interpretations that once were considered to support the benefit of estrogen replacement therapy in coronary vascular heart disease are now considered to have been based on poorly controlled studies and the conclusions are deemed, at best, uncertain.[6] In fact, there is statistical evidence *against* a benefit in this problem. The ratio of male to female deaths from coronary artery disease is high up to the 5th decade but becomes unity by the 9th decade. There is no inflection in the steady increase in coronary artery disease mortality in females through the menopausal period. Furthermore, coronary artery disease has a curious demographic variability. The ratio of male to female coronary deaths at age 45 in the United States is 5:1, whereas in Italy it is 2:1, and in Japan, 1:1. Finally, while white healthy females in North America seem not to succumb to coronary artery occlusion, this advantage does not extend to black women of the same age group. These changing sex ratios lead to the conclusion that there are probably two populations of males in North America: a population which is very susceptible to fatal occlusion or arrhythmia early in life, and a second population experiencing coronary artery disease roughly similar to that of their female counterparts.

Despite this statistical evidence, there was sufficient feeling in the 1960's that estrogen replacement might have beneficial effects on arterial integrity to cause major nationwide studies to be initiated. In the coronary drug project,[7] daily high dose conjugated estrogens (5 to 10 mg) were given to prevent recurrent heart attacks in men. This therapy was associated with an excess of nonfatal myocardial infarcts over controls, which was not evident at lower doses. Indeed, there was a high incidence of early vascular accidents of all types at high dose levels, leading to withdrawal of a significant portion of the study group. Similarly, in a stroke study undertaken at V.A. hospitals,[8] estrogen was associated with an increased recurrence of cerebral accidents and myocardial infarcts rather than protection. A prospective study in males with prostatic disease[9] revealed that diethylstilbestrol, 5 to 10 mg, produced increased incidence of myocardial infarction, thromboembolic disease, and strokes over controls or lower dose recipients. These studies were compatible with the findings in British and American studies with respect to the influence of birth control pills on vascular complications.

Finally, review of the lipoprotein patterns subsequent to estrogen administration revealed that such therapy does *not* convert the patterns to those of younger women. All lipid fractions in females increase with age. On estrogen therapy there is further *increase* in triglycerides.[10] There is no decrease or, at best, a modest decrease in cholesterol, and there is an increase in phospholipids. Therefore, evidence is strong that estrogen replacement therapy at high doses can contribute to the risk of thromboembolic disease, cerebrovascular accident, and coronary artery disease. These effects are dose related, and the risks increase with age.[11]

At this moment, it can be said that estrogen replacement therapy does not appear to confer the protection that the premenopausal white woman possesses against arteriosclerotic vascular disease.

Other metabolic effects of estrogen can also be considered disadvantageous to the aging woman. The increased incidence of hypertension as a result of progestin-estrogen therapy, the peripheral decrease in insulin activity with the subsequent stress on insulin reserves, the alteration in bilirubin transport and the increase in gall bladder disease are distinct disadvantages to administration of therapy to aging females.

Side Effects of Estrogen

Given the psychologic disposition of the postmenopausal woman and her concerns over body image and function, it is obvious that the side effects of estrogen, such as bloating and edema, can be considered additional burdens affecting already disabled individuals.

Cancer Risk

The risk of cancer must be considered to be the major disadvantage of estrogen replacement therapy if it can be proven that there is a causal rather than casual relationship between this therapy and the incidence of breast and endometrial carcinoma.

Breast Carcinoma. Breast carcinoma increases in frequency in men given estrogen therapy for prostatic carcinoma or in the treatment and support of trans-sexual conversion, and in Bantu men with gynecomastia. Although there is a postmenopausal secondary peak in the incidence of breast carcinoma, generally it is known to rise to peak incidence at or just before the menopause. At the moment, there is no evidence to support a cause and effect relationship. Indeed, prospective studies of the effect of birth control pills on the incidence of benign and malignant breast disease showed that a relationship was proven *not* to exist thus far.

Endometrial Carcinoma. Although there is no causal relationship between breast carcinoma and estrogen, there is a very suggestive relationship between elevated endogenous estrogen and estrogen therapy and the incidence of endometrial hyperplasia and carcinoma. In general, there are certain constitutional stigmata displayed in patients with a high frequency of atypical adenomatous hyperplasia and endometrial carcinoma.[1] They appear with progressive aging, obesity, and with an inappropriately early incidence of polycystic ovarian disease and functioning ovarian tumors. They are rarely seen, however, in individuals with senile vaginitis or those complaining of vasomtor symptoms. The relationship between the presence of endogenous estrogen and endometrial hyperplasia and atypia is notable in the clinical observations of Gusberg. There are two mechanisms by which endogenous estrogen production could be increased in the postmenopausal individual. Because the prehormone androstenedione is converted to estrone, factors which increase the production of androstenedione or factors which increase its conversion to estrogen would lead to increased estrone, with consequent effects on the endometrium. Both have been noted in women who developed postmenopausal bleeding, adenomatous hyperplasia, and endometrial carcinoma. In patients with excess production of androstenedione, stress, various tumors, and, less frequently, obesity are seen. Increased conversion of androstenedione to estrone was associated predominantly with obesity, with a less frequent association with simple aging and, in some cases, liver disease. The contention, then, is that the constitutional stigmata yield endometrial hyperplasia and carcinoma by increasing the endogenous production of estrone. Furthermore, those physicians who consider estrogen replacement therapy with estrone sulfate to be disadvantageous because of the factor of endometrial neoplasia argue that this therapy can reproduce the picture of endometrial stimulation seen in the patients described above. Support for this view has recently been presented,[12, 13] in that a statistically increased incidence of endometrial carcinoma was noted in association with estrogen replacement therapy. In view of this finding, it is now our policy to include an orally active progestin (e.g. Provera, 10 mg) for each day of the terminal week of cyclic estrogen therapy. As further data appears, our position may change. For the moment, the advantages of judicious estrogen therapy continue to offset this new concern.

In conclusion, estrogen replacement therapy given continually or in injudicious doses to improper recipients (those who have increased endogenous estrogen) can exaggerate the constitutional predilection and possibly uncover a hereditary predilection for neoplasia.

CONCLUSIONS AND SUMMARY

Only hot flashes and genital atrophy are unique features of the menopause and are proven to be responsive to low dose estrogen replacement.

Estrogen can be produced after the menopause and can alter the clinical course of the climacteric as well as influence dosage and effectiveness of therapy.

While estrogen is not the sole factor in the incidence of osteoporosis, unfavorable ratios between females and males and its acceleration after menopause are noted. Estrogen replacement therapy probably retards the rate of osteoporotic change but cannot reverse it.

There is an increased incidence of myocardial infarction in males over females that is not understood. In prophylactic and therapeutic trials the results appear conflicting, but on the whole at higher doses there are worrisome increases in the incidence of a variety of thromboembolic disorders, cardiovascular accidents, and myocardial infarctions. Furthermore, there is evidence that the higher the dose of estrogen the more likely is the risk of thromboembolic disease, cerebrovascular accident, and possibly coronary disease.

Although there is a suggestion that breast disease may be related to either endogenous or administered estrogen, the data, in my view, are inconclusive. On the other hand, estrogen replacement therapy can be shown to influence progession of endometrial stimulation to hyperplasia and even carcinoma. This possibility must be considered in the cost/benefit analysis of estrogen replacement therapy in a particular patient.

At the present time, in my view, it is neither reasonable to deny relief of menopausal symptoms to patients by withholding moderate to low dose cyclic estrogen therapy, nor is it prudent to extoll estrogen as a panacea for aging, degenerative diseases, or psychic disturbances after the menopause. Estrogen obviously should not be used indiscriminately in the hope of correcting nonspecific ailments or complaints. Therefore, certain therapy decisions must be made in the female climacteric:

For the early menopause, in women over the age of 50 who have amenorrhea and are shown to have elevated gonadotropins (serum FSH >40 mIU per ml) but who are obese or stressed or who display cervical mucus or vaginal cornification, progestin along should be administered in anticipation that these patients will reveal slow estrogen loss. If no progestin-induced withdrawal bleeding occurs, then simple observation of endogenous estrogen decline by means of symptomatology, vaginal cornification, and cervical mucus should be pursued.

In women in the early menopause with rapid estrogen loss who are nonobese with little or no biological evidence of estrogen, low-dose equine urinary conjugated estrogens, 0.3 or 0.6 mg daily for 3 weeks, or ethinyl estradiol, 0.01–0.02 mg for 3 weeks, and off 1 week, can be utilized.

In the late menopause, when clear evidence of atrophy is seen, 0.625 but not higher than 1.25 mg of estrogen should be administered cyclically.

I cannot conceive of a circumstance where I would be required to administer estrogen parenterally; however, in certain situations local vaginal placement of estrogen may be useful.

Because of the increased concern over endometrial hyperplasia as a result of this therapy, periodic addition of progestin to determine whether withdrawal bleeding occurs should be instituted. If endometrial bleeds occur under these circumstances, then office aspiration biopsy should be performed.

The question of whether or not the addition of androgen is useful is often considered. In some patients the addition of methyltestosterone, 5 to 10 mg, does provoke a sense of well-being, but I have found no evidence to support any additional advantage of this therapy.

REFERENCES

1. Edman, CD, Hemsell, DL, Siiteri, P, and MacDonald, PL, Origin and Quantification of Estrone Production in Women with Endometrial Neoplasia, Gynecol Invest 6:23, 1975.
2. Heaney, RP, Menopausal Effects on Calcium Homeostasis and Skeletal Metabolism, in Ryan, KJ, and Gibson, DC, eds., *Menopause and Aging*, National Institutes of Health publication 73–319, Bethesda, Md, 1974, p. 59.
3. Aitken, JM, Hart, DM, and Lindsay, R, Oestrogen Replacement Therapy for Prevention of Osteoporosis after Oophorectomy, Brit Med J 3:515, 1973.
4. Gordon, G., Osteoporosis and Estrogens Ob-

Gyn Observer November 1973.

5. Rivin, AU, and Dimitroff, SP, The Incidence and Severity of Atherosclerosis in Estrogen-Treated Males, and in Females with a Hypoestrogenic or a Hyperestrogenic State, Circulation 9:533, 1954.

6. Furman RH, Coronary Heart Disease and the Menopause, in Ryan, KJ, and Gibson, DC, eds., *Menopause and Aging*, National Institutes of Health publication 73-319, Bethesda, Md, 1974, p. 39.

7. Coronary Drug Project Research Group, The Coronary Drug Project, Initial Findings Leading to Modifications of its Research Protocol, JAMA 214:1303, 1970.

8. Report of the Veterans Administration Cooperative Study of Atherosclerosis, Neurology Section, An Evaluation of Estrogenic Substances in the Treatment of Cerebral Vascular Disease, Circulation 33(SII):3, 1966.

9. Bailar, JC, Byar, DP, and The Veterans Administration Cooperative Urological Research Group, Estrogen Treatment for Cancer of the Prostate, Early Results with 3 doses of Diethylstilbestrol and Placebo, Cancer 26:257, 1970.

10. Hazzard, WR, Spiger, MJ, Bagdade, JD, and Bierman, EL, Studies on the Mechanism of Increased Plasma Triglyceride Levels Induced by Oral Contraceptives, New Engl J Med 280:471, 1969.

11. Shapiro, S, Oral Contraceptives and Myocardial Infarction: Editorial, New Engl J Med 293:195, 1975.

12. Smith, DC, Prentice, R, Thompson, DJ, and Herrmann, WL, Association of Exogenous Estrogen and Endometrial Carcinoma, New Engl J Med 293:1164, 1975.

13. Ziel, HK, and Finkle, WD, Increased Risk of Endometrial Carcinoma among Users of Conjugated Estrogens, New Engl J Med 293:1167, 1975.

16

INFERTILITY

ROBERT H. GLASS, M.D.

The diagnostic investigation of the infertile couple is straightforward, and the testing procedures are well known. The major problems faced by the practitioner are the proper interpretation of the tests and, if they are normal, the pressure exerted by many patients to "do something."

This chapter will discuss the various diagnostic tests and will also touch on some of the background work that has helped in the formulation of their interpretation. The practitioner must keep in mind that 15% of couples will have a problem that cannot be diagnosed by the currently known tests. Eventually, after a thorough investigation, it may be necessary to tell them that there is no known cause for their infertility and that further testing and treatment offer little chance for improving fertility. Provided a complete investigation has been made there is no disgrace in admitting our limitations. Well documented figures from large infertility clinics show that only 50% of couples seen will become pregnant.

The initial interview and physical examination will not be discussed here other than to stress the desirability of having the husband present and involved in the investigation from the onset. Early in the physician-couple interaction frequency of coitus and possible sexual problems should be ascertained.

Because the male factor is the largest single cause of infertility it is best to begin with a semen analysis. If the semen characteristics and the initial examination of the woman are normal, attention can then be directed to demonstrating the adequacy of cervical mucus, ovulation, and tubal patency. If the duration of infertility is one year or more there is no reason to delay the investigation by first requiring the woman to take 3 months of temperature charts.

SEMEN ANALYSIS

With 40 to 50% of infertility wholly or partially attributable to a male factor, it is important for the gynecologist to be able to interpret the results of a semen analysis. The specimen should be collected by masturbation into a clean glass jar, protected from cold, and brought to the laboratory within 2 hours of collection. Abstinence of 48 to 72 hours prior to ejaculation is recommended. The specimen should not be collected by withdrawal, because the sperm-rich fraction may be lost, nor should it be collected in a condom. The latter contain spermicidal agents. If the male cannot collect a specimen by masturbation he can be supplied with a special sheath, manufactured by the Milex Company, which does not contain a spermicide.

Interpretation of the semen analysis is often hampered by the erroneous "normal values" printed on data sheets supplied by many commercial laboratories. It is still common to see these laboratories quote the lower limits of normal as 60,000,000/ cc, 80,000,000/cc, or even 100,000,000/cc. The work of MacLeod has established that the percentage of pregnancies decreases when the sperm count drops below 20,000,000/cc, and this is the currently accepted lower limit of normal.[1] Because of the errors inherent in doing a sperm count we usually prefer the count to be 30,000,000/cc or higher. It should be pointed out that pregnancies do occur even with counts below 20,000,000/cc, and this has been emphasized by recent reports of sperm counts in fertile males prior to vasectomy.[2] Of 386 men undergoing elective vasectomy, all of whom had at least one child, 20% had sperm counts less than 20,000,000/cc.[3]

While the sperm count requires proper dilution of semen and placement of the diluted specimen on a hemocytometer chamber for counting, sperm motility determination is less rigorous and can be performed in any office equipped with a microscope and glass slides. A drop of semen is placed on the slide (or, ideally, on a coverslip which is then placed over a depression slide to make a hanging drop preparation) and looked at initially without a coverslip at 100x magnification. A rough estimate is made of both the percentage of motile sperm and the percentage of sperm that show *progressive* motility across the field. At least 50% of the sperm should show the latter quality, and this can be confirmed by placing a coverslip on the specimen and using 400x magnification. In order to compare specimens it should be standard procedure to evaluate motility 2 hours after ejaculation; there is no evidence that checking *in vitro* motility at more prolonged intervals (e.g. 24 hours) gives any useful information concerning the male's fertility potential.

There are simple staining methods which can be done in the office to evaluate sperm morphology but in general we rely on the clinical laboratory for this evaluation.[4] Over 60% of the sperm should have normal morphology.

The usual ejaculate volume is between 3 and 5 cc (range 1–7 cc) and it is influenced by the frequency of ejaculation. Low volumes in association with absence of sperm in the postcoital test suggest the possible need for artificial insemination with the husband's sperm. Higher than normal volumes associated with a lower concentration of sperm can be treated by the use of split ejaculate inseminations, a technique which will be discussed later in this chapter.

Other abnormalities in the semen which can contribute to infertility are:

   1. Infection, manifested by the presence of white blood cells. Almost all semen specimens contain some of these cells, and it is important for each laboratory to establish its own range for a normal reading.

   2. Failure of the semen to liquefy. Semen is ejaculated in liquid form; it quickly becomes a gel which again liquefies within 20 minutes. If a thick, viscid specimen is associated with a poor postcoital test, the semen can be liquefied by running it back and forth through a #19 hypodermic needle and then using it for insemination. Amelar has employed precoital douches with Alevaire, a mucolytic agent, to accomplish the same purpose.[5]

3. Agglutination of sperm. This occurs on occasion in most males, but if present in repeated specimens may represent an autoimmune reaction or may signal the presence of infection.

Our general approach, if the semen analysis is abnormal, is outlined in Figure 16.1. If the laboratory report on the initial semen analysis is abnormal we personally see a second specimen before forwarding it to the laboratory. If the semen characteristics are again abnormal inquiry is made concerning the presence of the following factors, any of which may produce abnormal sperm quality and quantity:

1. History of testicular injury, surgery, or mumps.

2. Heat. A small rise in scrotal temperature can adversely affect spermatogenesis, and a febrile illness may produce striking changes in sperm count and motility. The effect of the illness can still be reflected in the sperm count and motility 2 to 3 months later. This reflects the 70–74 days it requires for a spermatozoon to be generated from a primary germ cell. Environmental sources of heat—such as the use of jockey shorts

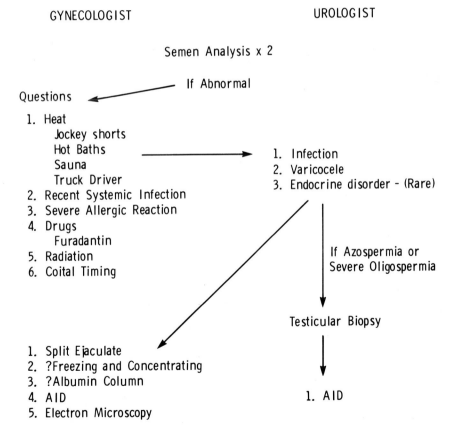

Fig. 16.1. A diagnostic and therapeutic approach to male infertility.

instead of boxer shorts, excessively hot baths, frequent use of a sauna or steam bath, or occupations that require long hours of sitting, such as long distance truck driving—may all diminish fertility potential.

3. Severe allergic reactions with systemic effects.[6]

4. Exposure to radiation.

5. Use of certain drugs such as Furadantin. The effect, if any, of marijuana on spermatogenesis is still uncertain, but there is some preliminary evidence that it can depress androgen levels.

6. Coital timing. Counts at the lower levels of the normal range may be depressed to below normal levels by ejaculations occurring daily or more frequently. Conversely, abstinence for 5–7 days or more "to save up sperm" is counterproductive because the minimal gain in numbers is offset by the lower motility produced by the increased proportion of older sperm. For most couples coitus every other day around the time of ovulation will give the optimal chance for pregnancy.

7. Cigarettes, alcohol, and hard work. While all three have been cited as causes of abnormal semen, there is very little evidence to either confirm or deny their connection. Working hours and alcohol are probably of more importance in infertility as a cause of impotence or decreased libido. A small proportion of alcoholics who are impotent will remain so even after discontinuing alcoholic intake.[7] The deleterious effects of nicotine on so many aspects of health certainly raises a suspicion that it can also depress semen quality.

If none of these problems pertains to the couple under investigation, then referral is made to a urologist in order to look for an anatomic abnormality, an infection, a varicocele, or an endocrine disorder.

Examination may reveal a physical impairment, such as a marked hypospadias which can cause sperm to be deposited outside the vagina. In rare cases of diabetes, in neurologic disease, or following prostatectomy there may be retrograde ejaculation into the bladder. Pregnancies have been reported after insemination of sperm obtained by catheterization of the bladder.[8] Emptying of the bladder and instillation of a buffer glucose solution prior to ejaculation will aid sperm survival. More recently therapy utilizing ephedrine or Ornade has been used with limited success in cases of retrograde ejaculation.[9, 10] Retrograde ejaculation may be only partial, and some men with this condition may have small amounts of ejaculate emitted from the urethra.

In a series of infertile males reported by Dubin and Amelar, 7.4% of the cases comprised some form of ductal obstruction.[11] The most common finding was epididymal obstruction due to gonorrhea or tuberculosis. A rarer finding was congenital absence of the duct system. If the ducts are congenitally absent, fructose will not be found in the semen because it is normally produced in the seminal vesicles. Charney mentions two cases in which rectal examination showed markedly dilated seminal vesicles.[12] Manual stripping through the rectal wall produced a gush of fluid and subsequently normal ejaculates. He suggests that mucus plugs may have occluded the excretory ducts.

Testicular damage may be found following mumps orchiditis and cryptorchidism. Finally, men with Klinefelter's syndrome usually have small testes and azospermia.

If the physical examination of the male does not uncover an abnormality, testicular biopsy may reveal the cause of the infertility. Azospermia associated with normal spermatogenesis indicates ductal obstruction. If the biopsy reveals complete hyalinization and fibrosis of the seminiferous tubules, there is almost no chance for fertility. Some who feel that hormonal therapy of male infertility is of value use testicular biopsy as a means of selecting those men who have the greatest chance of responding to drugs.[13, 14]

If the urologist finds infection in the genitourinary tract it can be cleared with antibiotics and possibly prostatic massage.

Endocrine disorders are a rare cause of male infertility and at the present time there seems to be no reason to use hormonal therapy unless there is evidence of deficiency. This viewpoint is contrary to current urologic practice. Cytomel is almost automatically prescribed, even when evidence of thyroid dysfunction is lacking. This treatment continues despite its condemnation by the urologists with the greatest experience in problems of male infertility.[12]

While treatment of males with low counts with clomiphene has on occasion raised sperm numbers, a recent double blind study using 100 mg daily for 3- to 10-day periods at monthly intervals revealed no consistent changes in sperm density.[15, 16] The same disappointing results have been found after therapy with human menopausal gonadotropins in men with normal levels of follicle-stimulating hormone and luteinizing hormone.[17] Injections of human chorionic gonadotropin (HCG) have been reported, in a few cases, to increase sperm motility. The usual dosage is 2,500 to 3,000 international units (IU) intramuscularly every 5 days. Substantial evidence is lacking for its clinical usefulness. In a study by Maddock and Nelson, injection of normal males with 5,000 IU of HCG three times a week for 1½ to 2 months resulted in severe damage to the seminiferous tubules.[18]

Testosterone rebound therapy has a long history and after years of disuse it has once again gained some adherents. Two to three months of testosterone, 30 mg daily, results in a marked depression of sperm count. In successful cases, 2 to 3 months after therapy is discontinued the sperm count is elevated above the pretreatment level. Urologic literature would suggest that these successes are a small minority. Two additional drawbacks are the often short duration of the improved sperm count and the occasional cases where the oligospermic male becomes permanently azospermic as a result of therapy.

Infusion of arginine or gonadotropin releasing factors can stimulate secretion of growth hormone or gonadotropins, respectively. There have been isolated reports of their usefulness in male infertility.[19] Because the evidence is, at the moment, equivocal, they should not be used except in investigational studies.

In a review of the management of male infertility de Kretser pointed out that many different medications have been claimed to exert an efficacious action on sperm, but that in the majority of cases claims have not been substantiated. He condemns empirical therapy with vitamins and thyroid.[20]

Varicocele

One of the most striking advances in the field of male infertility was the discovery of the importance of varicocele in influencing semen quality. Approximately 25% of infertile males will have a varicocele of the left internal spermatic vein. (It has also been noted in approximately 15% of men under age 20.) One study from Denmark showed that a number of males with improved spermatogenesis after surgery for varicocele had a small drop in left testicular temperature postoperatively, indicating that increased temperature could be the mechanism through which a varicocele exerts its deleterious effects.[21] Whatever the reason for the infertility associated with varicocele, ligation of the left internal spermatic vein in men with a varicocele results in a 40–50% pregnancy rate. The most striking improvement after operation is in sperm motility. MacLeod noted that 35% of the pregnancies occurred despite a sperm count remaining at 10,000,000/cc or under.[22] The stress pattern of sperm morphology, with tapering forms predominating, characteristic of varicoceles often remained after ligation.

Every infertile male requires a careful examination. Even small varicoceles may significantly affect semen quality. A varicocele may empty in the recumbent position, and the urologist must be alert to the need to examine the patient in the upright position. Dubin and Amelar also stress the importance of doing the examination while the patient performs a Valsalva maneuver.[11]

A recent European report stated that ligation of the left internal spermatic vein, even without a demonstrable varicocele, improved the pregnancy rate.

If the urologist is unable to find an anatomic abnormality, an infection, a varicocele, or an endocrine deficiency, we prefer to work on the ejaculate rather than subject the male to nonspecific endocrine therapy.

Two questions that often arise in cases where the male has poor sperm quality are the use of husband insemination and/or the possibility of freezing the husband's ejaculate and pooling a number of samples. While *a priori* it would seem logical to insert sperm with poor motility into the cervical os or uterus and save them part of their journey, this tactic has not been a successful one. Perhaps the poor sperm motility reflects only one aspect of a more profound deficiency in the sperm. While whole semen inseminations are seldom helpful in these cases, split ejaculate inseminations may be worthwhile. On the other hand, husband inseminations using whole ejaculates are of value in refractory premature ejaculation, retrograde ejaculation, and cases where the male cannot ejaculate in the vagina but can give a specimen by masturbation. Freezing and thawing depresses, to some extent, sperm motility. If a man has a low count with excellent motility there may be some rationale to freezing and pooling his specimens for later insemination. Unfortunately, poor counts are most often associated with poor motility. In these cases freezing is not feasible.

It is evident that in some males seminal fluid may be harmful to sperm. The first portion of the ejaculate contains the sperm-rich fraction and prostatic fluid. The remainder of the ejaculate originates in the seminal vesicles. Separating the two fractions by use of a split ejaculate can provide a specimen with a greater concentration of sperm and improved motility. In this technique the first few drops of the ejaculate are collected in one jar and the rest in a second jar. Collection can be facilitated by taping the two jars together. Both must be checked, for while the first jar contains the superior specimen in 90% of cases the second is better in 5%. (In 5% there is no difference between the two.) If one of the specimens is not substantially better than the whole ejaculate there is no reason for using it for inseminations. Amelar and Hotchkiss reported a series of couples in which split ejaculates were used and 22 of 39 (56%) achieved pregnancies.[23] However, males with very poor counts were largely excluded and some of the treated couples had counts and motilities in the whole ejaculates which now would be considered within the normal range. This should not detract from the usefulness of the technique, which can not only increase sperm concentration and motility but can also provide a specimen with less viscosity. In cases where split ejaculates are advisable the couple may also use an *in vivo* technique: the husband withdraws as soon as he feels that ejaculation is starting. Amelar and Dubin have reported 33 pregnancies in couples using this method.[24]

There have been a few reports of increased sperm motility following *in vitro* incubation with caffeine.[25, 26] Caffeine is mutagenic in bacteria, and therefore its use to treat sperm seems highly questionable.

Ericsson and coworkers have layered sperm on columns of liquid albumin as a means of separating out Y-bearing sperm.[27] While the success of the technique is still disputed, the albumin column does allow separation of the most vigorous sperm from the dead and poorly moving sperm.[27-29] Also removed are the debris and round cells often found in seminal plasma. The vigorously moving sperm suspended in physiologic solutions can be used for intrauterine inseminations. This technique is being studied in a number of clinics throughout the United States and Europe.

ARTIFICIAL INSEMINATION WITH DONOR SPERM (AID)

The combined problems of male infertility and decreased availability of adoptable babies has increased the interest and demand for AID. Thousands of babies are born each year in this country as a result of AID.

The procedure raises emotional, ethical, and legal questions. The husband may feel that he is devalued and his virility questioned. In a few cases a woman's ovulation may become abnormal in the cycle where inseminations have been planned. For obvious reasons the physician must never do inseminations without the consent of both husband and wife. Both must be strongly in favor of the procedure, and the stability of their marriage as well as their emotional maturity should be established by the physician. Cases where there is a suspicion that the wife is intimidating the husband into acquiescence should be avoided.

Three points are worth emphasizing to the couple:

1. Donor inseminations do not guarantee pregnancy. The success rate is about 70% (50% with frozen semen).

2. The couple should give some thought to their feelings should the child be born with a congenital anomaly. This will occur in perhaps 4–5% of all pregnancies, irrespective of whether they follow normal intercourse or artificial insemination.

3. It is a wise precaution to have both the man and the woman sign a

consent form. An example can be found in an article by Kleegman.[30] The procedure is covered by law in only a few states. In California, once the husband signs the consent form he is the legal father of the baby conceived through AID. In other areas it would be worthwhile for the physician to know the legal status of AID in his/her state so that correct information can be conveyed to patients. If the state has no law governing AID then the physician who does the inseminations should not be the obstetrician for that pregnancy. An obstetrician unaware of the inseminations can in clear conscience sign the birth certificate stating that the husband is the father of the child.

For obvious reasons, the donor should be unknown to the couple. His health and fertility must be unimpeachable, and there should be no family history of genetic diseases. The donor will not be a mirror image of the husband, but an attempt should be made to match physical characteristics. We see no reason to follow Kleegman's procedure of matching the religion of the donor and the couple. Use of RhoGAM makes Rh compatability between the donor and the wife a less crucial issue today, though we still use Rh negative sperm donors for Rh negative women. AID is a private matter between the physician and the couple. Discussions with friends or relatives should be firmly discouraged. Use of friends or relatives as donors raises the potential for emotional problems in the future and should not be allowed. Similarly, requests to mix the husband's sperm with the donor's signifies that the couple may not have made the emotional adjustment to the thought of donor insemination. The husband's semen may also be deleterious to the donor's sperm.

Donor inseminations are useful in azospermia, severe oligospermia, or necrospermia refractory to treatment. They are also useful if the woman has a long history of fetal loss due to Rh sensitization. Here an Rh negative donor would be used. Genetic diseases may on occasion be an indication for donor insemination.

The basal body temperature chart is the most useful guide to the approximate time of ovulation. Initially, an attempt is made to inseminate on the day just before the temperature rise based on reviewing 2 months of charts. Usually one to three inseminations are done each month. Approximately 50% of the successful cases will occur within the first 2 months. If pregnancy has not occurred by that time, a hysterosalpingogram is performed. Approximately 90% of pregnancies that will occur happen within 6 months.

Inseminations can be placed in the uterus, cervix, or vagina. A cervical cap, used by some physicians, does not appear to enhance the success rate. Intrauterine inseminations run the potential risk of infection and of severe pain due to uterine cramping. Certainly, no more than 0.3 cc can be safely instilled into the uterus.

We prefer to inject at the entrance to the cervical canal by means of a polyethylene catheter (Milex Company). The major portion of the semen overflows into the posterior fornix. The overflow collects on the posterior blade of the speculum, and the cervical os is allowed to dip into the pool while the woman rests for 20 minutes with her hips elevated.

Current estimates of the fertility potential of sperm are based on numbers, motility, and morphology as viewed through the light microscope. In the future more sophisticated investigative techniques may uncover other abnormalities. For example, electron microscopic examination of sperm from two infertile males revealed absence of the acrosome, the enzyme-containing caplike structure that covers the anterior portion of the nucleus.

Chromosomal abnormalities can be found in approximately 5 to 7% of males with azospermia or severe oligospermia.[20] Klinefelter's syndrome with an XXY chromosomal complement is one example of an abnormality which can be associated with testicular dysfunction. We do not know whether minor chromosomal abnormalities may handicap sperm which otherwise appear normal in terms of numbers, motility, and morphology.

If the male, on examination of the semen, is thought to have a reasonable potential for fertility, attention is directed to the woman. Failure to ovulate is the major problem in 15% of couples that we see (Chapter 17), while another 20 to 30% will have tubal pathology, and in 5% a cervical factor is associated with the infertility. Tests for all these factors need to be scheduled at specific times in the menstrual cycle.

POSTCOITAL TEST

Estrogen levels peak at the time of ovulation and thus provide maximum stimulation of the cervical glands. This produces an outpouring of clear, watery mucus which may be of sufficient quantity to be noted by the woman. Earlier in the cycle when estrogen output is lower and starting 2 to 3 days after ovulation when progesterone secretion increases, the mucus is thick, viscid, and opaque.

The postcoital test is performed around the time of expected ovulation as determined by previous basal body temperature charts or by the length of prior cycles. Within 8 hours of coitus cervical mucus is removed with a nasal polyp forceps and examined for macroscopic and microscopic characteristics. A 2-hour interval between coitus and examination has been recommended as giving maximum information. Others have suggested that a 16- to 24-hour interval provides a better assessment of sperm longevity. A study by Gibor and associates indicated that there is no drop in the number of sperm at any time during the first 24 hours.[31] There are reports that the number of sperm does decrease after 8 hours, and this is more in keeping with our experience.[32] Therefore, we suggest that the couple have coitus in the morning and that the test be performed early in the afternoon at the latest. It is also suggested that the couple abstain from intercourse for 48 hours prior to the postcoital test.

If the mucus is thick rather than thin, opaque instead of clear, the proximity of the test to ovulation should be determined by the onset of the next period (or by the temperature chart if one is being taken during that cycle). If poor mucus quality is related to inaccurate timing, the test should be repeated in the subsequent cycle. Poor mucus at ovulation time is a physical barrier critically diminishing sperm penetration and requiring alteration to enhance fertility. Buxton and Southam found that 33% of women who had good mucus became pregnant while only 14.5% of women with repeatedly poor mucus achieved a pregnancy.[33] In our clinic, 53.8% with good mucus became pregnant while 37% with poor mucus became pregnant, a statistically significant difference. In all likelihood some of these poor tests are reflections of inaccurate timing. It also points out that poor mucus is not an absolute bar to pregnancy but only indicates a poorer prognosis.

Treatment of poor mucus is best accomplished by giving 0.3 mg of conjugated equine estrogen daily for 8 or 9 days preceding the expected time of ovulation. In a 28-day cycle that would be between days 5 and 13. We see little advantage to continuing the hormone treatment through the luteal phase of the cycle. A theoretical disadvantage of continuous treatment is the evidence that there is an increased risk of vaginal cancer in young girls whose mothers took diethylstilbestrol during the first half of their pregnancy. If estrogen fails to produce a change in the mucus, the dose is increased to 0.625 mg/day. Higher doses may be counterproductive by interfering with ovulation. In the rare cases where 0.625 mg does not change the mucus, it is worth trying one or two cycles on 1.25 or even 2.5 mg. Theoretically, the comparatively high doses of estrogen overstimulate the cervical glands and force out inspissated mucus. Following the cycles on the high dose pills, the dose is dropped back to 0.625 mg daily from day 5 through 13 and the postcoital test is repeated. If there is evidence of chronic cervicitis with thick yellowish mucus, systemic antibiotics are used initially. If this is not successful the cervix is treated with electrocautery or cryosurgery.

Another tactic to overcome the barrier of thick cervical mucus is intrauterine insemination of sperm.[34] This is accomplished using a tuberculin syringe with an attached thin, sterilized polyethylene tube which is threaded through the cervix. Normally after coitus only the sperm enter the uterine cavity and semen remains in the vagina. Intrauterine insemination of even small amounts of semen may stimulate strong uterine contractions and produce an anaphylactic type reaction. For this reason no more than 0.3 cc of semen should be introduced. The intrauterine method allows direct introduction of bacteria into the uterus, and a few cases of tubal infection have been reported following this procedure.

The postcoital test also gives information concerning the male. Absence of sperm requires a review of the couple's coital technique. Repeated cancellations of appointments for the postcoital test may be another clue that there are sexual problems that have not been uncovered by the interview. More important, absence of sperm necessitates a detailed review of the semen specimen.

The necessity of scheduling the postcoital test may produce problems when the couple cannot have sex "on demand." In these cases precise timing must be sacrificed and the woman told to come to the office following unscheduled intercourse.

What constitutes a normal number of sperm in a postcoital test has been a matter of dispute. The estimates range from 1 to over 20/high power field (HPF). More critical than controversy over theoretical normal values is the question of what prognostic value the postcoital test has for the infertile couple. In a study by Buxton and Southam good sperm migration in the postcoital test yielded a pregnancy rate of 48.9%, while with poor sperm migration the conception rate was 31.6%.[33] The poor category included tests in which no sperm, only dead sperm, or rare motile sperm were found. The good classification included those tests in which a few or more motile sperm were found in each HPF. A study from our clinic showed that there was a statistically significant increase in the percentage of pregnancies when there were more than 20 sperm/HPF.[35] There was no statistically significant difference in percentage of pregnancies between groups having 0, 1–5, 6–10, or 11–20 sperm/HPF. It would obscure the issue to call a postcoital test with 21 or more sperm/HPF "normal," suggesting that less than 21 is somehow abnormal. The former gives a better prognosis for pregnancy, but a substantial number of pregnancies occur even when no sperm are found in the postcoital test.

If only immotile sperm are found in the mucus the percentage of pregnancies is significantly lower than when motile sperm are found.

What useful information can be gleaned from the postcoital test? If sperm are found in the mucus it is reasonable assurance that coital technique is adequate. This precludes the need for the woman to flex her thighs following intercourse or to place a pillow under her hips as a means of keeping sperm in the vagina. During normal intercourse sperm rapidly leave the semen pool and enter the cervical mucus. The semen is lost through the vaginal introitus or is broken down by vaginal enzymes. Women should be told that loss of semen is the normal occurrence and not a cause for infertility. If live sperm are found in the cervical mucus the pH is not hostile and the pregnancy rate is higher than if the sperm are all immotile. If there are more than 20 sperm/HPF, the male, in all likelihood, has a sperm count above 20,000,000/cc and the couple has a significantly better chance for pregnancy than if the postcoital test contains less than 20 sperm/HPF. If the mucus is clear and abundant with good spinnbarkheit, the patient has a better chance for pregnancy than if it is thick and sparse. Beyond this basic information little more can be obtained from the postcoital test. There is little advantage in having, for example, 10 sperm/HPF compared to having 1 sperm/HPF.

Intrauterine aspiration of sperm has been advanced as providing a more realistic appraisal of fertility potential.[36] We have not adopted this test in our clinic. Attempts to refine the postcoital test by studying individual fractions from different levels in the cervical canal have not produced convincing evidence of value. Davajan and Kunitake found a greater percentage of motile sperm at the internal os of five women of known fertility compared to five women with unexplained infertility.[37] Evaluation of these data is difficult because the motility of the husband's sperm was not specified. A recent publication by the same group again did not provide data which would warrant making the more laborious fractional postcoital test a routine procedure.[38] They performed fractional tests in 143 infertile couples, of whom 51 had had abnormal routine postcoital tests and 92 normal routine postcoital tests. Of the 92 women who had normal routine tests, 16 had abnormal fractional postcoital tests. All 16 were treated with low dose diethylstilbestrol, and 3 became pregnant. However all 3 had poor spinnbarkheit, a result that should have been apparent also with a routine test. In summary, 143 fractional postcoital tests were performed for a questionable gain of 3 pregnancies. Unless it can be shown more convincingly that the 16 women categorized by the fractional postcoital test are a unique population and can be helped by specific therapy, we see no reason that warrants use of the fractional test.

One of the most difficult problems in infertility is the postcoital test which repeatedly shows only dead sperm despite good mucus. The patient should be cautioned that lubricants such as K-Y Jelly and Surgilube have a spermicidal effect *in vitro* and should not be used by infertile couples. If lubrication is necessary vegetable oil or glycerin can be used without interfering with sperm movement.[39] Re-examination of the husband's semen to check sperm motility is an absolute necessity. Following this, the pH of the cervical mucus is determined at midcycle. If it is below 7, treatment with a precoital alkaline douche (ProCeption, Milex) may be helpful. This must be an extremely rare finding. Thirdly, sperm antibody testing is in order. If none of these factors are abnormal, treatment with ampicillin, 250 mg q.i.d., on the 5th to the 10th day of the cycle may be used as a last desperate try to improve the couple's fertility. This should be continued over three cycles. In rare cases a pregnancy does occur, but it is hard to know whether the ampicillin should be given credit for the success. A more logical approach is the use of intrauterine inseminations.

A postcoital test cannot be considered a substitute for a semen analysis. While 21 or more sperm/HPF is almost always associated with a sperm count above 20 million/cc, the postcoital test gives little information concerning the morphology of sperm in the ejaculate. There are considerably fewer abnormal forms in the cervical mucus compared to the ejaculate. This may represent a filtering effect of the cervical mucus or may indicate that abnormal forms do not have the motility to penetrate the cervical mucus.

TESTS OF TUBAL PATENCY

The convenience of performing a Rubin's test with CO_2 in the office and the avoidance of irradiation have been outweighed by the discomfort of the test and the high percentage of false readings which suggest tubal occlusion. This may result from tubal spasm initiated by the gas.

In our practice hysterosalpingography (HSG) has replaced the Rubin's test except in women who give a history suggestive of dye allergy. The x-ray study is performed 2 to 6 days after cessation of a menstrual flow. If there is a history of pelvic inflammatory disease a sedimentation rate is first obtained and, if elevated, antibiotic therapy is given. The procedure is scheduled for 2 to 3 months in the future. Shortly before, a repeat sedimentation rate is obtained. If masses or tenderness are revealed by the pelvic examination consideration should be given to bypassing the HSG and to evaluating the pelvis by laparoscopy.

HSG should be done under image intensification fluoroscopy and a minimum number of films taken. If one reviews a number of HSG it becomes readily apparent that radiologists have a penchant for ordering repetitive, noninformative films. Too often multiple oblique views are taken to delineate minimal filling defects in the uterus which are of no clinical significance. In our experience the oblique films are of little help even in diagnosing tubal patency. Only three films are usually required—a preliminary before dye is injected, a film showing spill of dye from one or both tubes, and a delayed film to show spread of dye through the peritoneal cavity. It is advantageous if the gynecologist does the actual injection of dye but in most instances this is now done by the radiologist. The dye can be injected using a classic Jarcho cannula with a single tooth tenaculum, or alternatively a suction apparatus can be appended to the cervix and dye injected through a contained cannula. This latter device eliminates the discomfort associated with application of the tenaculum. In either case the cannula should be bubble-free. When Ethiodol, an oil dye, is used there is no need to premedicate the patient or to restrict her to a liquid diet the day of examination. Bowel evacuation by enema is not required. In short, the patient needs no preparation and most certainly does not require an anesthetic.

The dye should be injected slowly so that abnormalities of the uterine cavity are not obscured. Usually no more than 3 to 6 cc of dye are required to fill the uterus and tubes. If the patient complains of cramping, the injection of dye should be stopped for a few minutes and fluoroscopy temporarily discontinued. Spasm is rare with Ethiodol, our preferred medium, but if it does occur slow injection with pauses may be helpful. If the tubes fill but dye droplets do not spill from the ends of the tubes, the uterus should be pushed up in the abdomen by means of the tenaculum or suction cup. This puts the tubes on stretch and may help to release dye from the fimbriated end. The droplets seen coming from the tube are the result of mixing of the oil dye and peritoneal fluid. On occasion, injection of dye into a hydrosalpinx will produce a similar pattern, and the 24-hour film is crucial in differentiating this condition from normal spill.

If dye goes through one tube rapidly and fails to fill the other tube, it usually means that the dye-containing tube presents the path of least resistance. In this situation the nonfilling tube is usually normal. When both tubes were patent on x-ray, the pregnancy rate in our own series was only slightly higher (58%) than when there was unilateral patency (50%).[40] This finding, though, is at variance with an ealier study of Wahby et al. in which only 23% (11 of 48) of women conceived with unilateral patency on Lipiodol hysterosalpingography.[41] With bilateral patency their pregnancy rate was 36%.

While the diagnostic usefulness of hysterosalpingography is unquestioned, its value as a therapeutic procedure in infertility is a subject of some controversy. Whitelaw et al. found no increase in the pregnancy rate following hysterosalpingography.[42] Palmer, though, reported that 75% of patients having a hysterosalpingogram showing tubal patency and whose husbands had normal sperm counts became pregnant within 1 year of the procedure.[43] This was three times the pregnancy rate found by the same author among patients who had not had a hysterosalpingogram. Speculation concerning the precise mode of therapeutic action of the procedure has included the following:

1. It may effect a mechanical lavage of the tubes, dislodging mucus plugs.

2. It may straighten the tubes and thus break down peritoneal adhesions.

3. It may provide a stimulatory effect for the cilia of the tube.

4. It may improve the cervical mucus.

5. The iodine may exert a bacteriostatic effect on the mucous membranes.

If hysterosalpingography does enhance fertility, is the effect seen with both oil- and water-soluble dyes? Gillespie reported a conception rate of 41.3% within 1 year of hysterosalpingography with oil media, while the rate was only 27.3% when water-soluble agents were employed.[44] This is in accord with the experience at the Yale Infertility Clinic.[40] Three groups of infertile patients were compared. One had hysterosalpingograms done with Ethiodol, another had hysterosalpingograms with Salpix, a water dye, and the third had no hysterosalpingograms. Within 1 year of the termination of their infertility workup the group which had Ethiodol hysterosalpingograms had a significantly higher percentage of pregnancies, the great majority of which followed within 7 months of the x-rays. There was no difference between the groups having hysterosalpinography with Salpix and those who did not have x-rays. In addition to its value in enhancing fertility, Ethiodol produces a better film image and a lower incidence of pain on injection compared to water-soluble dyes.

The use of an oil medium has been criticized on grounds that it is only slowly absorbed and may cause granuloma formation. Granulomas probably do not form in normal tubes. It is only the abnormal tube with increased sequestration of dye which is prone to granuloma formation. Granulomas also have been reported following hysterosalpingography with Salpix. An additional fear with oil dye is embolization, a complication which has never occurred in our series. When fluoroscopy is used venous or lymphatic intravasation can be detected immediately and injection of dye halted. In his monograph, Siegler reported nine deaths attributable to HSG.[45] Lipiodol, an oil medium, was used in six of these cases, the last occurring in 1947. Since that time there has been only one fatality, which occurred in 1959 after embolization of a water-soluble dye.

OVULATION

Disorders of ovulation account for approximately 10 to 15% of all infertility problems. These may be anovulation or severe oligo-ovulation. In the latter cases, even though ovulation does occur, its relative infrequency diminishes the woman's chances for pregnancy. If she has periods only every 3 or 4 months, for practical purposes it matters little whether these are ovulatory or anovulatory. She should be treated with clomiphene to increase the frequency of or to initiate ovulation (see Chapter 17), and this can be started immediately, even before other areas have been investigated.

Basal Body Temperature

Women who have menstrual periods at monthly intervals marked by premenstrual symptoms and dysmenorrhea are almost always ovulatory. Indirect confirmatory evidence of ovulation is obtained by use of basal body temperature charts. The temperature can be taken either orally or rectally with a regular thermometer or with special instruments that show a range of only a few degrees and thus are easier to read. It is worth emphasizing that the temperature must be taken immediately upon awakening and before any activity. The woman may be surprised to find that the basal temperatures are substantially lower than the usual 98.6°. Characteristically, prior to ovulation they are in the 97.2°–97.4° range, and after ovulation the basal temperature is over 98°. Days when intercourse takes place should be noted on the chart, and this may give the physician an indication that coital frequency is a problem. Even using temperature charts, no one can pinpoint the exact day of ovulation. A significant increase in temperature is not noted until 2 days after the luteinizing hormone (LH) peak, coinciding with a rise in peripheral levels of progestin to greater than 4 ng/ml.[46] Physical release of the ovum probably occurs on the day prior to the time of the first temperature elevation. This may or may not be marked by a dip in the temperature to the lowest level of the cycle. The temperature rise should be sustained for 10 to 16 days and the reading will then drop at the time of the subsequent menstrual period. If an approximate time of ovulation can be determined by temperature charts, a sensible schedule for coitus is every other day in a period encompassed by 3 to 4 days prior to and including 2 to 3 days after expected ovulation. While this would be ideal, it is unwise to demand rigid adherence to a schedule. This may produce psychologic stress sufficient to inhibit sexual relations. In discussing coital timing the patient will usually want to know the fertilizable life of the sperm and the egg. The information on human gametes is speculative. Cases have been reported when isolated coitus even up to 7 days prior to the rise in basal body temperature has resulted in pregnancy, but this probably represents the limits of biologic variation. Estimates have been made that sperm retain their ability to fertilize for 24 to 48 hours and that the human egg is fertilizable for 12 to 24 hours.

Endometrial Biopsy

This is performed 2 to 3 days prior to the expected period and the histology is read by the criteria outlined by Noyes, Hertig, and Rock.[47] While premenstrual biopsy may present the possibility of interrupting a pregnancy if performed in a conception cycle, the danger is minimal. Buxton and Olson, in their study of biopsies done during the conception cycle, found that only 2 of 26 patients aborted.[48] The alternative of taking the biopsy on the 1st day of menses has three disadvantages: (1) inconvenient time for patient and physician, (2) the tissue is disrupted and often more difficult to interpret, and (3) a slight amount of bleeding may occur at the time of the expected period even if the patient has become pregnant. We have found the Meig's curette (Codman & Shurtleff, Inc.) very suitable for obtaining a small strip of tissue from high on the anterior wall. It is slightly smaller than the usual suction endometrial biopsy instruments.

Inadequate Luteal Phase

Inadequate luteal phase is often an ambiguous diagnosis, and many times it has been invoked as an excuse to warrant the use of clomiphene or other hormones. Moreover, there is considerable confusion surrounding both the diagnosis and treatment of the inadequate luteal phase, and the questions that need answering are:

1. What is an inadequate luteal phase?
2. What means should be used to establish the diagnosis?
3. How frequently is it seen in infertile couples?
4. What is the correct treatment?

The term inadequate luteal phase suggests inadequate production of progesterone by the corpus luteum. The diagnosis is established if the histologic dating of the endometrium is more than 2 days behind the cycle day determined by the onset of the subsequent menstrual flow. There must be more than a 2-day lag in the endometrium, for Tredway et al., using the LH surge to pinpoint ovulation, found that 5 of 11 normally ovulating women had biopsies 2 days out of synchrony with the day of the menstrual cycle.[49] There are obvious difficulties in establishing a diagnosis using the histologic criterion. There can be variations in the interpretations of the same biopsy by different observers. The same endometrium can show varying patterns, and there can be discrepancies between the maturation of the glands and that of the stroma. Despite these drawbacks, biopsy remains the most secure way of diagnosing an inadequate luteal phase.

If the basal temperature chart shows a rise which is sustained for less than 10 days this too can be considered evidence of an inadequate luteal phase. Concern is often expressed when the temperature shows a very slow rise though it remains elevated for the normal length of time. This is of doubtful significance but should be checked by endometrial biopsy.

Serum progesterone levels have been used to confirm the presence of ovulation. Israel et al. found that a single luteal phase serum progesterone of 3 ng/ml or more provided presumptive evidence of ovulation.[50] Abraham et al. suggested that if the sum of three plasma progesterone determinations, taken between 4 and 11 days prior to menses, were equal to 15 ng/ml, ovulation had occurred and there was normal corpus luteum function.[51] However, these levels can be exceeded in cases where the endometrial biopsy shows a lag of 3 days or more.[52] While groups of women with inadequate luteal phase have lower levels of progesterone than do women with normal function, there is an overlap of values.

Many women will have isolated cycles characteristic of the inadequate luteal phase and they do not require treatment. Estimates are that less than 4% of infertile women have repeated cycles with this deficiency, and demonstration of its occurrence in more than one cycle is required before therapy is warranted.[53]

Jones and co-workers at Johns Hopkins have achieved a high conception rate by using progesterone vaginal suppositories (50 mg) daily following the midcycle rise in temperature.[52, 54] The suppositories are not available commercially and must be compounded by a pharmacy. Another tactic is to give injections of human chorionic gonadotropin (HCG) in varying doses 2 to 3 days after the rise in temperature. Either 10,000 international units (IU) can be given at that time as the sole treatment, or smaller doses (2,500–5,000 IU) can be given every 2 to 3 days for four injections. The injection of HCG can delay the onset of menses for up to 7 days. Other treatments include clomiphere and human menopausal gonadotropin. The latter has been used because of evidence that an inadequate luteal phase can result from a deficiency of follicle-stimulating hormone in the proliferative phase of the cycle.[55] Evaluation of any therapy is difficult because a significant number of conceptions occur without treatment. One group of drugs which has been widely used for treatment of the inadequate luteal phase, but which may in fact be deleterious, is the synthetic progestins. Provera, in higher doses than those used in the inadequate luteal phase cases, depresses progesterone levels when given after ovulation.[56]

Endometriosis

While every woman complaining of infertility should be suspected of having endometriosis, the suspicion is heightened if there is progressively severe dysmenorrhea, dyspareunia, or pain on defecation. Beading, nodularity, and tenderness of the uterosacral ligaments are characteristic of endometriosis, as is a uterus in fixed retroversion.

Even if there is a high index of suspicion our policy is to proceed with the routine infertility investigation. If the hysterosalpingogram is normal but pregnancy does not occur within 6 to 7 months after the x-ray, laparoscopy is suggested. This is the same treatment plan that is followed even if there is no suspicion of endometriosis.

It is preferable to establish the diagnosis by laparoscopy before treating the woman with hormones for prolonged periods of time. In addition, significant endometriosis associated with infertility is best treated surgically, with the expectation that conception will occur in approximately 50% of the women.

Hormonal therapy is reserved for two groups of infertile patients. If a few minimal implants are noted in the cul de sac at the time of laparoscopy but the tubes and ovaries are free, then treatment with Ovral, 1 pill a day, is initiated and maintained without interruption for 3 to 4 months. Breakthrough bleeding is managed by increasing the dose of the hormone. There is no report in the literature which proves the efficacy of this therapy, but it seems to be a reasonable approach.

If symptoms recur following conservative surgery for infertility and if pregnancy has not occurred 3 years after the operation, then long term suppression (1 to 2 years) with Ovral can be utilized. If pregnancy has not occurred within 3 years of operation the couple can be told that there is very little chance of conceiving in the future.

When an endometrioma is unexpectedly discovered at surgery in a young woman without other evidence of endometriosis, postoperative use of cyclic combination birth control pills should be prescribed to provide protection against further disease, unless there is a contraindication to their use.

Numerous suggestions have been made concerning the prevention of endometriosis. The most reasonable is avoidance of tubal insufflation, hysterosalpingography, and cervical dilatation during a menstrual flow so that endometrial cells will not be forced out through the tube into the peritoneal cavity.

A logical approach to the prevention of endometriosis would be the use of progestin contraception with its protective effect of decidualization. This should diminish the amount of menstrual debris available for retrograde flow through the fallopian tubes. In all likelihood retrograde flow is the causative factor of pelvic endometriosis.

Preliminary reports suggest that the experimental drug, Danazol, an isoxazol derivative of 17α-ethinyltestosterone, may be useful in the treatment of endometriosis. The drug, which inhibits gonadotropin secretion, is given in doses of 800 mg a day for 3 to 8 months. Side effects include acne, weight gain, irritability, and unilateral tremor of the upper extremity. In a few cases the endometriosis has returned rapidly after discontinuation of the drug.

Mycoplasma

Mycoplasma, a pleuropneumonia-like organism, has been implicated as a possible cause of habitual abortion and salpingitis. Gnarpe and Friberg from

Uppsala, Sweden, reported that infertile couples had a markedly higher prevalence of T mycoplasma in cervical mucus and semen than did a group of fertile women and men. Treatment with doxycycline decreased the numbers of couples with mycoplasma and also was associated with pregnancy in 15 of 52 couples (29%), all of whom had had primary infertility of at least 5 years' duration.[57] However a series of reports from England agreed with these findings in only one respect. They confirmed that treatment with doxycycline could eliminate mycoplasma from the genital tract of the majority of individuals. In this study there was no difference, however, in the frequency of either T strain or mycoplasma hominis between infertile and fertile couples.[58] In a double blind study, treatment with doxycycline for 28 days had no effect on the rate of conception, and the English group suggested that culturing for mycoplasma in the routine investigation of infertility was unrewarding.[59]

We are unaware of any published double blind study from the United States, and our current practice is to culture for mycoplasma only in cases of habitual abortion.

Sperm Allergy

It has been over a decade since Franklin and Dukes sparked interest in the role of sperm-agglutinating antibodies in infertility.[60] Despite the many studies that have appeared in the intervening years, the basic question of whether circulating antibodies in the female interfere with fertility remains unanswered. An attempt will be made here to list the information now available and to hazard some guesses on the role of sperm antibodies in reproduction.

1. There have been four reports of women who developed severe allergic reactions following contact with semen.[61] This is a dramatic illustration of the antigenicity of semen.

2. Approximately 20% of infertile women have sperm-agglutinating antibodies in their serum.[62]

3. In many cases the serum component responsible for the agglutination is not a γ-globulin but rather a β-globulin, possibly attached to a steroid hormone.[63]

4. The only known treatment for sperm-agglutinating antibodies is avoidance of contact between the woman and semen. This necessitates using a condom during intercourse for 3 to 12 months and also avoiding semen exposure through oral-genital or anal contact. The test for agglutinating antibodies is checked every 3 months, and when the reaction disappears or becomes minimal unprotected intercourse is advised around the time of ovulation. Approximately 35% of couples will conceive following this course of action.

5. Some women with sperm-agglutinating antibodies will become pregnant without treatment. This does not necessarily negate the importance of the agglutinating antibodies, because their activity *in vivo* may depend on the vigor of the sperm population that they face. Some sperm are more readily incapacitated by the same antibody than are others.[64] This could also explain the presence of sperm-agglutinating antibodies in women of known fertility.

6. Sperm antibodies can be present despite a postcoital test showing adequate numbers of moving sperm.

7. In infertile women a sperm immobilization test gives a lower percentage of positive tests compared to the agglutination reaction (approximately 5 to 10%), and positive reactions in fertile women are almost nonexistent.[65] The serum component involved appears to be a γ-globulin. Condom therapy does not seem to overcome this antibody.

8. Testing of serum to uncover the reaction may not be the best approach. There are cytotoxic antibodies in the cervical mucus which may not be present in the serum.[66] In addition, there may be tissue-fixed antibodies in the cervical and endometrial tissue which may not be mirrored by circulating antibody.[67] Certainly, it would be advantageous to study cervical mucus and cervical tissue for antibodies not found in the serum. For clinical purposes this is impractical.

9. The evidence for an infertility effect of sperm antibodies in men seems more firmly established than it is in women. Higher titers in males are correlated with diminished chances for conception.[68] Other than clearing genitourinary tract infections, there is no known therapy.

Many workers in the field of infertility feel that sperm-agglutinating antibodies are nonspecific and unrelated to infertility. Some believe that tests for immobilizing antibodies provide the better estimate of immunologic reactions against sperm, while others feel that this test too is meaningless.

It is our impression that there are a few men and women who are infertile on the basis of an immunologic reaction. It is still worthwhile to try to uncover these cases by testing both the male and the female for agglutinating and immobilizing antibodies.

WHEN SHOULD ADOPTION BE ADVISED?

With proper evaluation and therapy, plus some luck, approximately 50% of couples attending an infertility clinic will become pregnant. Of the 50% who do not achieve a pregnancy, the group most in need of counseling are those with unexplained infertility. Despite the absence of pathology, couples with 3 or more years of infertility have a poor prognosis, and the physician should encourage consideration of adoption.

Because of the shortage of adoptable babies, couples are more susceptible now to suggestions of therapy no matter how tenuous their rationale. In the past we have disagreed with some popularly held beliefs and treatments, and we feel that those admonitions are worth repeating.

Women should not be told that they are infertile because they are too nervous. Unless anxiety interferes with ovulation or coital frequency, there is no present evidence that infertility is caused by the usual anxieties besetting a couple attempting to conceive.[69] Despite many anecdotes to the contrary, adoption does not increase a couple's fertility.[70] The treatment of euthyroid infertile women with thyroid has repeatedly been shown to be worthless.[71, 72] A dilatation and curettage (D and C) is not a legitimate part of a routine infertility investigation. It provides minimal information beyond that obtained by endometrial biopsy and is both expensive and potentially hazardous because it subjects the woman to the risk of general anesthesia. There is also no substantial evidence to support the old belief that a woman becomes more fertile following D and C. If a woman has menstrual bleeding that indicates patency of the canal, then dilatation of the cervix for "stenosis" will not improve fertility.

Unfortunately, uterine suspensions are still being performed as a primary treatment for infertility. In a study by Carter et al. it was shown that patients with retroversion of the uterus, unassociated with pelvic adhesions, who were subjected to suspension operations had a lower pregnancy rate than women with retroversion who had no surgery.[73] Uterine suspension is helpful only when it is secondary to operation for other indications such as endometriosis or pelvic adhesions.

The uterus has a tremendous capacity for expansion, given the proper stimulus, and this holds true for every size uterus. Therefore, we do not believe that the so called "infantile" or "hypoplastic" uterus should ever be blamed for infertility. Many young women have been psychologically traumatized because a physician told them that their uterus was too small for pregnancy.

Equally ill advised in the investigation of infertility is the routine ordering of laboratory tests such as skull x-rays, urinary determinations of 17-ketosteroids, and gonadotropins not indicated by clinical judgment. These may be of value in selected cases but certainly not in every case.

The philosophy should not be "try it, it might just work." We have seen too many disillusioned couples who, without any indication, have been given clomiphene, Provera, and low dose estrogen, and then have been treated with husband inseminations. The goals of the practitioner should be to accomplish a thorough investigation, to treat any abnormalities that are uncovered, to educate the couple in the working of the reproductive system, and to give the couple some estimate of their fertility potential. If these goals are achieved by a sympathetic, understanding physician they will satisfy most couples who suffer from infertility.

REFERENCES

1. MacLeod, J, Human Male Infertility, Obstet Gynecol Surv 26:335, 1971.
2. Derrick, FC, and Johnson, J, Reexamination of "Normal" Sperm Count, Urologie 3:99, 1974.
3. Nelson, CMK, and Bunge, RG, Semen Analysis: Evidence for Changing Parameters of Male Fertility Potential, Fertil Steril 25:503, 1974.
4. Amelar, RD, Dubin, L, and Schoenfeld, C, Semen Analysis, Urologie 2:605, 1973.
5. Amelar, RD, Coagulation, Liquefaction, and Viscosity of Human Semen, J Urol 87:187, 1962.
6. MacLeod, J, A Testicular Response during and following Severe Allergic Reaction, Fertil Steril 13:531, 1962.
7. Lemere, F, and Smith, JW, Alcohol Induced Sexual Impotence, Am J Psych 130:212, 1973.
8. Bourne, RB, Kretzchmer, WA, and Esser, JH, Successful Artificial Insemination in a Diabetic with Retrograde Ejaculation, Fer-

til Steril 22:275, 1971.
9. Stewart, BH, and Bergant, JA, Correction of Retrograde Ejaculation by Sympathomimetic Medication: Preliminary Report, Fertil Steril 25:1073, 1974.
10. Stockamp, K, Schreiter, F, and Altwein, JE, α Adrenergic Drugs in Retrograde Ejaculation, Fertil Steril 25:817, 1974.
11. Dubin, L, and Amelar, RD, Etiologic Factors in 1294 Consecutive Cases of Male Infertility, Fertil Steril 22:469, 1971.
12. Charney, CW, Treatment of Male Infertility, in Behrman, SJ, and Kistner, RW, eds., *Progress in Infertility*, Little, Brown, Boston, 1968.
13. Meinhard, E, McRae, CU, and Chisholm, GD, Testicular Biopsy in Evaluation of Male Infertility, Brit Med J 3:577, 1973.
14. Schwarzstein, L, Human Menopausal Gonadotropins in the Treatment of Patients with Oligospermia, Fertil Steril 25:813, 1974.
15. Mellinger, RC, and Thompson, RJ, The Effect of Clomiphene Citrate in Male Infertility, Fertil Steril 17:94, 1966.
16. Foss, GL, Tindall, VR, and Birkett, JP, The

Treatment of Subfertile Men with Clomiphene Citrate, J Reprod Fertil *32:*167, 1973.

17. Sherins, RJ, Clinical Aspects of Treatment of Male Infertility with Gonadotropins: Testicular Response of Some Men Given HCG with and without Pergonal, in Mancini, RE, and Martini, L, eds., *Male Fertility and Sterility*, Academic Press, New York, 1974.

18. Maddock, WO, and Nelson, WO, The Effects of Chorionic Gonadotropin in Adult Men: Increased Estrogen and 17-Ketosteroid Excretion, Gynecomastia, Leydig Cell Stimulation and Seminiferous Tubule Damage. J Clin Endocrinol Metab *12:*985, 1952.

19. Schwarzstein, K, Aparicio, NJ, Turner, D, Calamera, JC, Mancini, R, and Schally, AV, Use of Synthetic Luteinizing Hormone Releasing Hormone in Treatment of Oligo-Spermic Men, Fertil Steril *26:*331, 1975.

20. de Kretser, DM, The Management of the Infertile Male, Clin Obstet Gynaecol *1:*409, 1974.

21. Agger, P, Scrotal and Testicular Temperature: Its Reaction to Sperm Count before and after Operation for Varicocele, Fertil Steril *22:*286, 1971.

22. MacLeod, J, Further Observations on the Role of Varicocele in Human Male Infertility, Fertil Steril *20:*545, 1969.

23. Amelar, RD, and Hotchkiss, RS, The Split Ejaculate, Fertil Steril *16:*46, 1965.

24. Amelar, RD, and Dubin, L, A New Method of Promoting Fertility, Obstet Gynecol *45:*56, 1975.

25. Bunge, RG, Caffeine Stimulation of Human Ejaculated Spermatozoa, Urologie *1:*371, 1973.

26. Schoenfeld, C, Amelar, RD, and Dubin, L, Stimulation of Ejaculated Human Spermatozoa by Caffeine, Fertil Steril *26:*158, 1975.

27. Ericsson, RJ, Langevin, CN, and Nishino, M, Isolation of Fractions Rich in Human Y Sperm, Nature (Lond) *246:*421, 1973.

28. Evans, JM, Douglas, TA, and Renton, JP, An Attempt to Separate Fractions Rich in Human Y Sperm, Nature (Lond) *253:*352, 1975.

29. Ross, A. Robinson, JA, and Evans, HJ, Failure to Confirm Separation of X and Y Bearing Human Sperm Using BSA Gradients, Nature (Lond) *253:*354, 1975.

30. Kleegman, SJ, Therapeutic Donor Insemination, Fertil Steril *5:*7, 1954.

31. Gibor, Y, Garcia, CJ, Cohen, MR, and Scommegna, A, The Cyclical Changes in the Physical Properties of the Cervical Mucus and the Results of the Postcoital Test, Fertil Steril *21:*20, 1970.

32. Danezis, J, Sujan, S, and Sobrero, AJ, Evaluation of the Postcoital Test, Fertil Steril *13:*559, 1962.

33. Buxton, CL, and Southam, AL, *Human Infertility*, Hoeber-Harper, New York, 1958.

34. White, RM, and Glass, RH, Intrauterine Insemination of Husband's Sperm, Obstet Gynecol *47:*119, 1976.

35. Jette, NT, and Glass, RH, Prognostic Value of the Postcoital Test, Fertil Steril *23:*29, 1972.

36. Kleegman, SJ, and Kaufman, SA, *Infertility in Women*, FA Davis, Philadelphia, 1966.

37. Davajan, V, and Kunitake, GM, Fractional in Vivo and in Vitro Examination of Postcoital Cervical Mucus in the Human, Fertil Steril *20:*197, 1969.

38. Moran, J, Davajan, V, and Nakamura, R, Comparison of the Fractional Post Coital Test with the Sims Huhner Post Coital Test, Int J Fertil *19:*93, 1974.

39. Goldenberg, R, and White, R, The Effect of Vaginal Lubricants on Sperm Motility in Vitro, Fertil Steril *26:*872, 1975.

40. Mackey, RA, Glass, RH, Olson, LE, and Vaidya, RA, Pregnancy following Hysterosalpingography with Oil and Water Soluble Dye, Fertil Steril *22:*504, 1971.

41. Wahby, O, Sobrero, AJ, and Epstein, JA, Hysterosalpingography in Relation to Pregnancy and its Outcome in Infertile Women, Fertil Steril *17:*520, 1966.

42. Whitelaw, MJ, Foster, TN, and Graham, WH, Hysterosalpingography and Insufflation, J Reprod Med *4:*56, 1970.

43. Palmer, A, Ethiodol Hysterosalpingography for the Treatment of Infertility, Fertil Steril *11:*311, 1960.

44. Gillespie, HW, The Therapeutic Aspect of Hysterosalpingography, Brit J Radiol *38:*301, 1965.

45. Siegler, AM, *Hysterosalpingography*, Medcom Press, New York, 1974.

46. Moghissi, KS, Syner, FN, and Evans, TN, A Composite Picture of the Menstrual Cycle. Am J Obstet Gynecol *114:*405, 1972.

47. Noyes, RW, Hertig, AT, and Rock, J. Dating the Endometrial Biopsy, Fertil Steril *1:*3, 1950.

48. Buxton, CL, and Olson, LE, Endometrial Biopsy Inadvertently Taken During Conception Cycle, Am J Obstet Gynecol *105:*702, 1969.

49. Tredway, DR, Mishell, DR, Jr, and Moyer, DL, Correlation of Endometrial Dating with Luteinizing Hormone Peak, Am J Obstet Gynecol *117:*1030, 1973.

50. Israel, R., Mishell, DR, Jr, Stone, SC, Thorneycroft, IH, and Moyer, DL, Single Luteal Phase Serum Progesterone Assay as an

Indicator of Ovulation, Am J Obstet Gynecol *112:*1043, 1972.

51. Abraham, GE, Maroulis, GB, and Marshall, JR, Evaluation of Ovulation and Corpus Luteum Function using Measurements of Plasma Progesterone, Obstet Gynecol *44:*522, 1974.

52. Jones, GS, Aksel, S, and Wentz, AC, Serum Progesterone Values in the Luteal Phase Defects, Obstet Gynecol *44:*26, 1974.

53. Murphy, YS, Arronet, GH, and Parekh, MC, Luteal Phase Inadequacy, Obstet Gynecol *36:*758, 1970.

54. Jones, G, Luteal Phase Defects, in Behrman, SJ, and Kistner, RW, eds., *Progress in Infertility*, Little, Brown, Boston, 1975.

55. Strott, CA, Cargille, CM, Ross, GT, and Lipsett, MB, The Short Luteal Phase, J Clin Endocrinol Metab *30:*246, 1970.

56. Johansson, EDB, Depression of the Progesterone Levels in Women Treated with Synthetic Gestagens after Ovulation. Acta Endocrinol *68:*779, 1971.

57. Gnarpe, H, and Friberg, J, T-mycoplasmas as a Possible Cause for Reproductive Failure. Nature (Lond) *242:*120, 1973.

58. de Louvois, J, Blades, M, Harrison, RF, Hurley, R, and Stanley, VC, Frequency of Mycoplasma in Fertile and Infertile Couples, Lancet *1:*1073, 1974.

59. Harrison, RF, de Louvois, J, Blades, M, and Hurley, R, Doxycycline Treatment and Human Infertility, Lancet *1:*605, 1975.

60. Franklin, RR, and Dukes, CD, Further Studies on Sperm Agglutinating Antibody and Unexplained Infertility, JAMA *190:*682, 1964.

61. Halpern, BN, Ky, T, and Robert, B, Clinical and Immunological Study of an Exceptional Case of Reaginic Type Sensitization to Human Seminal Fluid, Immunology, *12:*247, 1967.

62. Glass, RH, and Vaidya, RA, Sperm Agglutinating Antibodies in Infertile Women, Fertil Steril *21:*657, 1970.

63. Boettcher, B, and Kay, DJ, Agglutination of Spermatozoa by Human Sera with Added Steroids, Andrologie *5:*265, 1973.

64. Fjallbränt, B, Cervical Mucus Penetration by Human Spermatozoa Treated with Anti-Spermatozoal Antibodies from Rabbits and Man, Acta Obstet Gynecol Scand *48:*71, 1969.

65. Isojima, S, Li, T, and Ashitaka, Y, Immunologic Analysis of Sperm Immobilizing Factor Found in Sera of Women with Unexplained Sterility, Am J Obstet Gynecol *101:*677, 1968.

66. Parish, WE, Caron-Brown, JA, and Richards, CB, The Detection of Antibodies to Spermatozoa and the Blood Group Antigens in Cervical Mucus, J Reprod Fertil *13:*469, 1967.

67. Schwimmer, WB, Ustay, KA, and Behrman, SJ, Sperm Agglutinating Antibodies and Decreased Fertility in Prostitutes. Obstet Gynecol *30:*192, 1967.

68. Rumke, P, Van Amstel, N, Messer, EN, and Bezemer, PD, Prognosis of Fertility of Men with Sperm Agglutinins in the Serum, Fertil Steril *25:*393, 1974.

69. Noyes, RW, and Chapnick, EM, Literature on Psychology and Infertility: A Critical Analysis, Fertil Steril *15:*543, 1964.

70. Rock, J, Tietze, C, and McLaughlin, HB, Effect of Adoption on Infertility, Fertil Steril *16:*305, 1965.

71. Tyler, ET, The Thyroid Myth in Infertility, Fertil Steril *4:*218, 1953.

72. Buxton, CL, and Herrmann, WL, Effect of Thyroid Therapy on Menstrual Disorders and Sterility, JAMA *155:*1035, 1954.

73. Carter, B, Turner, V, Davis, CD, and Hamblen, ED, Evaluation of Gynecologic Survey in Therapy of Infertility, JAMA *148:*995, 1952.

17

MEDICAL INDUCTION OF OVULATION

CARL GEMZELL, M.D.

Failure to ovulate is a major problem in reproductive disorders. It may be the result of dysfunction at any level of a complex system including higher centers in the brain, the hypothalamic-pituitary-ovarian axis, and the steroid feedback mechanism. It renders the woman infertile, which is the prime reason for attempts at restoration of ovulatory cycles.

Anovulation is the basic deficit in the polycystic ovary syndrome. It is accompanied by amenorrhea, sometimes oligomenorrhea, and, on rare occasions, even apparently regular cycles. It is likely, though, that in most instances, in women with regular cycles anovulation is sporadic. Generally, anovulation is associated with recognizable irregularity of the cycle and it occurs more frequently at menarche and in the premenopausal state.

Anovulation with amenorrhea may be the first and only sign of a pituitary tumor such as a chromophobe adenoma. Pituitary destruction, which may be due to various reasons, such as infarct necrosis at the time of delivery or thrombosis, causes anovulation and amenorrhea. It usually also causes other signs of grave pituitary insufficiency.

In most cases of anovulation, with or without amenorrhea, there are no gross organic lesions of the pituitary or the hypothalamus. Ovulation may cease in connection with the discontinuation of oral contraceptive treatment, severe dieting, or emotional disturbances, but it may also cease without any obvious sign of hypothalamic dysfunction.

A prerequisite for induction of ovulation in women who do not ovulate is the presence of normal ovaries with oocytes and follicles. The lack of oocytes, as in women with primary ovarian failure or with premature menopause, renders treatment impossible (see Chapter 14).

In principle, there are three approaches to ovarian stimulation for induction of ovulation, i.e. two hormonal approaches with human gonadotropin or gonadotropin-releasing hormone (GnRH), and one chemical approach with clomiphene citrate. Human gonadotropins act directly on the ovaries, bypassing the pituitary and the hypothalamus, while clomiphene requires for its action an intact pituitary and hypothalamus.

Gonadotropin-releasing hormone has recently been isolated from the hypothalamus and synthesized.[1] It reaches the anterior pituitary via a portal system and releases both follicle-stimulating hormone (FSH) and luteinizing hormone (LH).

Consequently, it would be an ideal means of stimulating the ovaries in cases of normal pituitary but abnormal hypothalamic function. In women who do not ovulate, GnRH has been shown to increase the release of both FSH and LH from the pituitary, but not enough to stimulate sufficient follicular growth or to induce ovulation of follicles which are primed with human gonadotropins.[2] The reason for this is not clear. It may be that the pituitary of the amenorrheic woman is not adequately adapted to GnRH and following exogenous administration of GnRH it releases insufficient amounts of gonadotropins during too short a time. The amount of GnRH may not have been enough in these trials, and other forms of administration of GnRH may yield better results.

Human gonadotropins seem to be the panacea for induction of ovulation as they only require normal ovaries. It is possible with human gonadotropins to induce ovulation in hypophysectomized women or in women with a pituitary adenoma or necrosis. However, the possibility of complications such as overstimulation leading to cyst formation or multiple pregnancies is a very real danger to the patient and human gonadotropins should only occasionally be used as the first means of induction of ovulation. Clomiphene citrate is relatively safe to use and when administered in daily doses of 50 to 200 mg for 5 days does not give rise to any serious side effects or complications.

CLOMIPHENE

Clomiphene citrate exists as two isomers which have been separated as *cis*- and *trans*-clomiphene. Although preliminary data suggest that *cis*-clomiphene is more potent in terms of inducing ovulation, the two isomers are mixed in the commercial preparation. The mechanism of action of clomiphene is not clear. There is evidence that estradiol uptake by the pituitary and anterior hypothalamus is reduced. It is most likely that the major stimulus for the ovarian response to clomiphene is mediated via the hypothalamus and the pituitary and that the drug acts to release gonadotropins. Evidence is also available that clomiphene has a direct effect on the ovaries. Administered together with human pituitary gonadotropin (HPG), it increases the sensitivity of the ovaries to HPG.

Clomiphene citrate has proven to be an especially useful drug in patients who do not ovulate or who ovulate at intervals greater than 45 days because of a hypothalamic dysfunction. It is essential that estrogen secretion be adequate and that the serum-FSH level be within the normal range. Withdrawal bleeding following Provera can be taken as presumptive evidence of FSH activity. There should be no signs or symptoms of any gross pituitary disease. Women with secondary amenorrhea or oligomenorrhea attributable to deficient stimulation by gonadotropic hormones or to a deranged synthesis of steroid hormones by the ovary often exhibit estrogen production in the normal range. Clomiphene is recommended for these women.[3] Women with amenorrhea following the use of oral contraceptives and women with galactorrhea and amenorrhea belong to this group even if their endogenous estrogen production is low.[4] In all cases of galactorrhea, x-ray tomograms of the sella should be obtained to rule out a pituitary tumor.

Clomiphene therapy is much safer than treatment with human gonadotropins and need not be controlled as strictly. The only absolute contraindication to drug use is the presence of ovarian enlargement. Clomiphene should not be used in women who ovulate regularly. It does not enhance their fertility. Pelvic examination should be performed before and after each course of treatment in order to exclude those who have enlarged ovaries and to rule out a pregnancy before beginning the next course of treatment. If enlarged ovaries are detected clomiphene treatment should be delayed for at least one cycle. In order to obtain information about when and if ovulation takes place the woman should record her basal body temperature. If necessary, determinations of plasma progesterone can be used to reveal an inadequate corpus luteum.

Clomiphene citrate in doses of 50 mg is given for 5 days starting on the fifth day of a cycle or, if the patient is not cycling, on the fifth day after a bleed induced by progesterone or Provera. If after 4 weeks menstruation has not occurred and the patient is not pregnant the dose of clomiphene citrate can be increased to 100 mg/day for 5 days, following a withdrawal bleeding. In subsequent cycles if the temperature remains monophasic the drug dose can be increased to 150 mg and eventually to 200 mg/day. We usually stay at each dose level for two cycles before deciding it has not induced ovulation, and then proceed to the next higher level. At the higher dose visual symptoms may arise such as blurring or scotomata. No permanent eye damage has been reported, but visual problems are sufficient reason to stop the drug. The most troublesome minor side effect is flushing. If there is no response to the 200 mg dose treatment is abandoned and eventually human gonadotropins are initiated. Others have tried to supplement clomiphene with human chorionic gonadotropin but this is usually successful only when there has been a partial response to clomiphene, evidenced by a rise in temperature but failure to sustain the rise for more than 8 or 9 days. If ovulation is induced, however, following any of the doses of clomiphene, therapy is continued at that level for three to six cycles or until conception occurs. If pregnancy does not occur after three ovulatory cycles a postcoital test should be performed to be sure that clomiphene has not interfered with mucus production. If this occurs Premarin, 0.3 mg, or Estinyl, 0.02 mg, can be given from day 5 through day 14 of the cycle. In most series ovulation occurs in 80% of the women and pregnancy in 30 to 40%. Approximately 5% of the conceptions are twins; only rarely are there multiples beyond two.

Women who ovulate with clomiphene but fail to conceive may be candidates for wedge resection of the ovaries. Those who do not respond to clomiphene with biphasic charts can be treated with combinations of clomiphene and human menopausal gonadotropins. There is only limited experience with this combination, which utilizes clomiphene, 100 mg/day for 5 to 7 days, then after skipping a day human menopausal gonadotropin, 2 ampules a day for 4 to 6 days with a drop to 1 ampule for 1 to 2 days, and then an ovulatory injection of human chorionic gonadotropin (10,000 international units (IU)) 48 hours later. The course with the gonadotropins should be monitored by estrogen determinations as described below.

GONADOTROPINS

It is by now well established that in order to induce ovulation in the human, gonadotropins from human sources should be used.[5, 6] They are from two sources: from human pituitaries obtained at autopsy (HPG), or from the urine of postmenopausal women (HMG).[7] Extracts of different potency and ratio between FSH and LH have been used, and almost all preparations give good results. A widely used preparation of HPG contains 25–30 IU (2nd IRP-HMG) of FSH activity and 20–30 IU of LH (2nd IRP-HMG) per mg, with a ratio between FSH and LH of 1:1.

Further purification of this HPG preparation has yielded preparations which based on biological units were clinically less potent, while rather impure preparations with ratios of FSH and LH of 1:6 gave good and consistent results. Consequently, there was little indication that HPG preparations with low LH content were superior to those with high LH contamination. Further purification of the pituitary extract did not seem worthwhile, especially when the purification procedure caused loss of biological activity. However, some preliminary results seem to indicate that in women with the polycystic ovary syndrome, who are sensitive to HPG, preparations with low LH content were preferable to those with high LH contamination.

Extract from postmenopausal urine has been used together with human chorionic gonadotropin (HCG) to stimulate the ovaries and induce ovulation and corpus luteum formation.[8] Two commercial preparations are in common use today. They contain about 75 IU of FSH activity per ampule, with a ratio of FSH to LH of 1:1 (Pergonal) or of 1:2 (Humegon).

There has never been any need to use LH from the human pituitary for induction of ovulation, thanks to the luteinizing effect of HCG, which is readily extracted from pregnancy urine. Human pituitary LH does not prevent overstimulation. If it is used instead of HCG, repeated doses have to be administered, because its biological half-life is shorter than that of HCG.

Several commercial preparations of HCG are available and in general have the same effect on the primed follicle.

Although pituitary and urinary FSH are chemically different, they seem to have the same clinical effect when preparations with equal FSH activity are used. The two preparations administered alternatively to the same women gave similar responses as far as the number of ovulations and pregnancies were concerned and also according to the rise in total urinary estrogen excretion.

SELECTION OF PATIENTS

Pituitary gonadotropic failure is a state which may be seen with an apparently normal pituitary, with a pituitary that is the site of a tumor or necrosis, or with a primary abnormality in the hypothalamic region. A common characteristic of these patients is low levels of serum FSH and LH, although normal levels do not exclude a diagnosis of pituitary insufficiency.[9] Also common in these patients are low serum estrogens indicating inactive ovaries. These patients, who are without any other symptoms of endocrine disorders or congenital malformations, constitute the group which is suitable for treatment with human gonadotropins.

An ideal patient for treatment with human gonadotropins is under 35 with nonfunctioning ovaries, primary or long-lasting secondary amenorrhea, normally developed sex organs, and low gonadotropins. She should be fully investigated, be complaining of infertility, have a normally fertile husband, and show no barriers to conception. Pregnancy should not be contraindicated on medical grounds, and there should be no preferable alternative method.[10]

MONITORING TREATMENT

One of the difficulties in treatment with human gonadotropins is the variation in individual response. There is no fixed dosage schedule for all patients. It has also been apparent that the response of the same patient to the same dose may differ significantly from one cycle to the next. One woman, having aborted seven fetuses after her first treatment, had a single fetus after her second treatment without any change of dosage. There is also a very small range between a dose that will fail to stimulate the follicles at all and one which produces overstimulation. In order to make the best use of the gonadotropins and to avoid complications the treatment should be carefully monitored. The purpose of monitoring gonadotropic therapy is to obtain an ovarian response that compares as much as possible with the ovarian changes that take place during a normal spontaneous ovulation and to avoid overstimulation leading to multiple pregnancies or ovarian cyst formation.

The ovarian changes that take place during a normal ovulatory cycle can be recorded by daily determinations in blood or urine of estrogen and progesterone. The estrogens during the follicular phase reflect the maturation of the follicle, while progesterone is an indicator of the activity of the corpus luteum. By comparing changes in levels of estrogens and progesterone in normal ovulatory cycles with those obtained following stimulation with human gonadotropins it is possible to obtain information about the optimal daily dose of human gonadotropin, the number of days this dose should be administered, when HCG or LH administration should be commenced, if and when ovulation took place, and the hormonal activity of the corpus luteum.

TREATMENT

Daily determination of total urinary estrogens (TE) or plasma estradiol has been used successfully to obtain information about the optimal daily dose of HPG and the number of days this dose should be administered.[11] Increases in plasma progesterone will then confirm that ovulation has taken place and will also provide information on the activity of the corpus luteum.[12]

Following an adequate HPG dose there is usually a latent period of 3 to 4 days without any change in TE. Thereafter TE rises continuously during another 6-day period, with a daily increase of about 50% over the previous day. When a suitable level in urine of TE (80–100 μg/24 hours) or in plasma estradiol (800–1000 pg/ml) is reached, ovulation is induced by the administration of HCG. If the drop in urinary estrogens and the rise in plasma progesterone follow the same pattern as found after a spontaneous ovulation the risk of overstimulation is limited. If, on the other hand, no drop in TE occurs, the rise in plasma progesterone is moderate, and a menstrual bleeding occurs less than 10 days after the HCG administration, ovulation may not have occurred. By 9 days after ovulation the detection of HCG in serum by a special radioimmunoassay can confirm conception.[13]

There are other criteria which can be used to assess ovarian response to HPG. These include gross appearance, sialic acid concentration, arborization pattern and spinnbarkheit of the cervical mucus, and the ability of sperm to penetrate the mucus. However, they are less reliable than the TE excretion and more difficult to evaluate. Some women display a close correlation between ovarian response and the karyopyknotic index, whereas others, mainly because of vaginitis and coitus, fail to do so.

The aim of an HPG treatment of an individual woman is to find the ideal HPG dose that will produce a change in TE and plasma progesterone which approaches as closely as possible the changes found during the normal ovulatory cycle. If this goal is achieved the chances of a normal single conception will be good, and the risk of overstimulation will be negligible. The ideal daily dose of HPG (HMG) might vary from 75 to 750 IU. For the first treatment it is always advisable to start with a low dose of 75 to 150 IU. The following courses could start with the same daily dose as was ideal for the previous one.

HPG and HMG have been administered in many different ways which all more or less give good results. Doses given at intervals of a few days[14, 15] or equal daily doses[6, 10, 16] of human gonadotropins usually provide the same rise in urinary estrogens and the same number of conceptions; but it seems that the divided doses are more difficult to control and, in general, require larger amounts of the hormones.

Ovulation is induced by a rather large dose of HCG which has to be repeated after some days in order to obtain a normal length of the luteal phase. The plasma levels of progesterone should be determined at least three times in order to confirm ovulation.

Human pituitary gonadotropins have been used since 1960 in Uppsala in order to induce ovulation in infertile women. Since 1968 daily estrogen determinations have been done in order to monitor the treatment. During an 8-year period (1960–1967), when 290 patients were treated, the pregnancy rate was 45%, the multiple birth rate was 33%, and the abortion rate was 28% (Table 17.1). Clinical symptoms of overstimulation leading to hospital care occurred in less than 2% of the induced cycles. During a second, 5-year period (1968–1973) when daily estrogen determinations were done, 351 patients were treated. The pregnancy rate was about the same or 41%, but the multiple birth rate had dropped to 17% and the abortion rate to 20% (Table 17.1). Only 0.5% of the treatments ended with symptoms of overstimulation. It was apparent that careful monitoring of treatment with daily estrogen determinations lowered the multiple birth rate by half and probably had some effect on the abortion rate. Most of the multiple pregnancies were twins, and the cases of overstimulation were mild and did not require hospital care. This is crucial because the massively enlarged ovaries, ascites, hemoconcentration, and hypovolemia that accompany hyperstimulation may be life threatening.

The two groups included amenorrheic women with no or low basal estrogen levels, women with primary amenorrhea with pronounced estrogen deficiency, and a few women (7) who were hypophysectomized because of pituitary adenoma. All of these women were very suitable for HPG therapy. It was interesting to note that 84% of the pregnancies occurred after the first two courses with HPG, and an additional 15% became pregnant following the third to the fifth courses. It follows

TABLE 17.1
Use of Human Pituitary Gonadotropins at Uppsala, 1960–1973

	Primary and secondary amenorrhea, 1960–1967	Primary and secondary amenorrhea and "clomiphene failures," 1968–1973	Primary amenorrhea, 1960–1971
	No.	*No.*	*No.*
Patients	290	351	15
Treatment courses	606	759	78
Pregnancies	130	143	21
Singles	63	94	15
Multiple births	31	20	4
Abortions	36	29	2
	%	*%*	*%*
Pregnancy rate	45	41	87
Multiple births rate	33	17	19
Abortion rate	28	20	10

from these results that a woman might be treated three times with HPG, after which the chance of conception is considerably smaller and an alternative treatment might be considered. It also shows that the selection of patients is of great importance.

Among the women who were treated unsuccessfully with HPG some had husbands with signs of impaired fertility, such as low sperm count or increased percentage of abnormal sperm. Some were treated only once or twice, and others showed various reactions, such as poor cervical mucus combined with poor sperm penetration, that might explain their failure to conceive. Also included in this failure group are some women who ovulated after clomiphene therapy but did not conceive. With HPG treatment, only occasionally did they become pregnant.

A total of 15 women with primary amenorrhea were treated during a 10-year period (Table 17.1). They were all highly motivated, and no alternative method was available. All were primed with cyclic estrogen therapy before treatment with HPG. In view of the infantile form of the genital tracts of these patients, it was surprising to find a high rate of conception (87%) together with a low rate of abortions (10%).

In patients with the Stein-Leventhal syndrome, treatment with HPG was not encouraging. Many of these patients were "clomiphene failures," and only a few treated with HPG conceived.

CONCLUSION

Induction of ovulation can be achieved by human gonadotropins or clomiphene citrate. So far gonadotropin-releasing hormone, although highly active in releasing both FSH and LH from the pituitary, has been of little use as a therapeutic agent in the treatment of anovulatory women.

HPG acts directly on the ovaries and thus it has a broader therapeutic use than clomiphene, which requires an intact pituitary and an intact hypothalamus. As HPG treatment is associated with increased risks of complications, clomiphene ought to be used as a first choice. Cost is also a factor, with clomiphene costing between $5 and $20 a cycle while gonadotropins cost between $250 and $500 for one try for pregnancy.

By careful selection of patients and strict control of treatment the best results are achieved. About 84% of the pregnancies following HPG treatment occur during the first two courses of treatment. The best results were obtained in young women with quiescent ovaries who responded in a similar pattern to each treatment.

REFERENCES

1. Schally, AV, Arimura, A, Kastin, AJ, Matsuo, H, Baba, Y, Redding, TW, Nair, RMG, Debeljuk, L, and White, WF, Gonadotropin-Releasing Hormone: One Polypeptide Regulates Secretion of Luteinizing and Follicle-Stimulating Hormones, Science 173:1036, 1971.
2. Nillius, SS, and Wide, LJ, The LH-Releasing Hormone Test in 31 Women with Secondary Amenorrhoea, J Obstet Gynecol Brit Comm 79:874, 1972.
3. Greenblatt, RB, Gambrell, RD, Mahesh, VB, and Scholer, HLF, Clomiphene and its Isomers, in Diczfalusy, E, and Borell, U, eds, Nobel Symposium, Stockholm 15:263, 1970.
4. Shearman, RP, Amenorrhea after Treatment with Oral Contraceptives, Lancet 2:1110, 1966.
5. Gemzell, CA, Diczfalusy, E, and Tillinger, KG, Clinical Effect of Human Pituitary Follicle-Stimulating Hormone (FSH), J Clin Endocrinol Metab 18:1333, 1958.
6. Gemzell, CA, Induction of Ovulation with Human Gonadotropins, Recent Progr Horm Res 21:179, 1965.
7. Donini, P, Puzzoli, D, and Montezemolo, R. Purification of Gonadotrophin from Human Menopausal Urine, Acta Endocrinol 45:321, 1964.
8. Lunenfeld, B, Menzi, A, and Volet, V, Clinical Effects of Human Postmenopausal Gonadotrophin, Acta Endocrinol Suppl 51:587, 1960.
9. Wide, L, Nillius, SJ, Gemzell, CA, and Roos, P, Radioimmunosorbent Assay of Follicle-Stimulating Hormone and Luteinizing Hormone in Serum and Urine from Men and Women, Acta Endocrinol Suppl 174, 1973.
10. Gemzell, CA, Induction of Ovulation with Human Gonadotropins, Proc. 2nd International Congress of Endocrinology, Part II, Excerpta Medica Foundation, 83-2:805, 1965.
11. Brown, JB, MacLeod, SC, MacNaughtan, C, Smith, MA, and Smyth, BJ, A Rapid Method for Estimating Oestrogens in Urine Using a Semi-Automatic Extractor, J Endocrinol 42:5, 1968.
12. Johansson, EDB, and Gemzell, CA, The Relation between Plasma Progesterone and Total Urinary Oestrogens following Induction of Ovulation in Women, Acta Endocrinol 62:89, 1969.
13. Wide, L, and Porath, J, Radioimmunoassay of Proteins with the use of Sephadex-coupled Antibodies, Biochim Biophys Acta 130:257, 1966.
14. Crooke, AC, Butt, WR, and Bertrand, PV, Clinical Trial of Human Gonadotrophins. III. Variation in Sensitivity between Patients and Standardization of Treatment, Acta Endocrinol Suppl 111, 1966.
15. Cox, RI, Cox, TL, and Black, TL, Test for Ovarian Function and Responsiveness Leading to Ovulation Induction, Lancet 2:888, 1966.
16. Gemzell, CA, Induction of Ovulation with Human Gonadotrophins, Int J Gynecol Obstet 8:593, 1970.

INDEX